Palliative Medicine and Hospice Care

Guest Editor

TAMARA S. SHEARER, DVM

VETERINARY CLINICS OF NORTH AMERICA: SMALL ANIMAL PRACTICE

www.vetsmall.theclinics.com

May 2011 • Volume 41 • Number 3

SAUNDERS an imprint of ELSEVIER, Inc.

W.B. SAUNDERS COMPANY
A Division of Elsevier Inc.

1600 John F. Kennedy Blvd. • Suite 1800 • Philadelphia, PA 19103-2899
http://www.vetsmall.theclinics.com

VETERINARY CLINICS OF NORTH AMERICA: SMALL ANIMAL PRACTICE Volume 41, Number 3
May 2011 ISSN 0195-5616, ISBN-13: 978-1-4557-7997-0

Editor: John Vassallo; j.vassallo@elsevier.com

Veterinary Clinics of North America: Small Animal Practice (ISSN 0195-5616) is published bimonthly (For Post Office use only: volume 41 issue 3 of 6) by Elsevier Inc., 360 Park Avenue South, New York, NY 10010-1710. Months of issue are January, March, May, July, September, and November. Business and Editorial Offices: 1600 John F. Kennedy Blvd., Ste. 1800, Philadelphia, PA 19103-2899. Customer Service Office: 3251 Riverport Lane, Maryland Heights, MO 63043. Periodicals postage paid at New York, NY and additional mailing offices. Subscription prices are $262.00 per year (domestic individuals), $427.00 per year (domestic institutions), $128.00 per year (domestic students/residents), $347.00 per year (Canadian individuals), $525.00 per year (Canadian institutions), $385.00 per year (international individuals), $525.00 per year (international institutions), and $186.00 per year (international and Canadian students/residents). To receive student/resident rate, orders must be accompanied by name of affiliated institution, date of term, and the *signature* of program/residency coordinator on institution letterhead. Orders will be billed at individual rate until proof of status is received. Foreign air speed delivery is included in all *Clinics* subscription prices. All prices are subject to change without notice. **POSTMASTER:** Send address changes to *Veterinary Clinics of North America: Small Animal Practice*, Elsevier Health Sciences Division, Subscription Customer Service, 3251 Riverport Lane, Maryland Heights, MO 63043. Customer Service (orders, claims, online, change of address): Elsevier Periodicals Customer Service, Elsevier Health Sciences Division Subscription Customer Service 3251 Riverport Lane Maryland Heights, MO 63043. Tel: 1-800-654-2452 (U.S. and Canada); 314-447-8871 (outside U.S. and Canada). Fax: 314-447-8029. E-mail: journalscustomerservice-usa@elsevier.com (for print support); journalsonlinesupport-usa@elsevier.com (for online support).

Reprints. For copies of 100 or more of articles in this publication, please contact the Commercial Reprints Department, Elsevier Inc., 360 Park Avenue South, New York, NY 10010-1710. Tel.: 212-633-3812; Fax: 212-462-1935; E-mail: reprints@elsevier.com.

Veterinary Clinics of North America: Small Animal Practice is also published in Japanese by Inter Zoo Publishing Co., Ltd., Aoyama Crystal-Bldg 5F, 3-5-12 Kitaaoyama, Minato-ku, Tokyo 107-0061, Japan.

Veterinary Clinics of North America: Small Animal Practice is covered in *Current Contents/Agriculture, Biology and Environmental Sciences, Science Citation Index, ASCA, MEDLINE/PubMed (Index Medicus), Excerpta Medica, and BIOSIS.*

Printed and bound by CPI Group (UK) Ltd, Croydon, CR0 4YY

Transferred to Digital Print 2011

Contributors

GUEST EDITOR

TAMARA S. SHEARER, DVM
Certified Canine Rehabilitation Practitioner; Shearer Pet Health Hospital, Sylva, North Carolina; Founder/Executive Director, Pet Hospice and Education Center, Sunbury, Ohio

AUTHORS

VALARIE HAJEK ADAMS, CVT
Healing Heart Pet Hospice, Appleton, Wisconsin

AZARIA AKASHI, PhD, MCC
Psychologist and Coach, Worthington, Ohio

JOSEPH A. ARAUJO, BSc
Department of Pharmacology, University of Toronto; CanCog Technologies Inc, Toronto, Ontario, Canada

VANDHANA BALASUBRAMANIAN, JD
Solo Practitioner, Chicago, Illinois

THERESA DEPORTER, DVM, MRCVS
Oakland Veterinary Referral Services, Bloomfield Hills, Michigan

ROBIN DOWNING, DVM
Diplomate, American Academy of Pain Management; Certified Canine Rehabilitation Practitioner; Certified Pain Educator; Hospital Director, The Downing Center for Animal Pain Management, LLC, Windsor, Colorado

GARY M. LANDSBERG, DVM, MRCVS
Diplomate, American College of Veterinary Behaviorists; Diplomate, European College of Veterinary Behavioral Medicine (Companion Animal); North Toronto Animal Clinic, Thornhill; Director of Veterinary Affairs, CanCog Technologies Inc, Toronto, Ontario, Canada

KATHRYN D. MAROCCHINO, PhD
Fellow in Thanatology; ABS School of Maritime Policy and Management, Culture and Communication Division, California State University Maritime; The Nikki Hospice Foundation for Pets, "Rosemoor House," Vallejo, California

ANN P. MCCLENAGHAN, BS, CVT
Hearts on the Mend, Willow Grove, Pennsylvania

BERNARD E. ROLLIN, PhD
University Distinguished Professor, Department of Philosophy, Colorado State University, Fort Collins, Colorado

AMIR SHANAN, DVM
International Association for Animal Hospice and Palliative Care, and Compassionate Veterinary Care, Chicago, Illinois

TAMARA S. SHEARER, DVM
Certified Canine Rehabilitation Practitioner; Shearer Pet Health Hospital, Sylva, North Carolina; Founder/Executive Director, Pet Hospice and Education Center, Sunbury, Ohio

ALICE E. VILLALOBOS, DVM, DPNAP
Distinguished Practitioner, National Academies of Practice; Director, Animal Oncology Consultation Service, Woodland Hills; Director, Pawspice Care Clinics at VCA Coast Animal Hospital, Hermosa Beach; Beachside Animal Referral Center, Capistrano Beach, California

Contents

This article outlines the young history of animal hospice by first focusing on the history of human hospice, with special emphasis on the last 200 years. It then examines similarities between the two, showing how human hospice has informed its animal counterpart and defined it as specialized comfort care benefiting terminally ill companion animals in their home setting as well as a unique journey wherein the caregiver understands that quality of death is as important as quality of life. The article includes a bibliography and two specialized reading lists—on human hospice and on the growing field of animal hospice.

There is great flexibility in how palliative medicine and hospice care can be delivered to pet owners. The veterinarian needs to develop a plan based on the professional's individual preferences. Variations in the services that are offered, the location of where the services are delivered, and the composition of the professional team will vary with the veterinarians preferences. Marketing and legal issues must be addressed when considering to offer palliative and hospice care. An organizational worksheet is provided at the end of this article to help with planning.

Starting a palliative or hospice care plan as soon as possible after a pet qualifies allows for better care of the pet and the family. The process is made more efficient by applying the 5-step strategy for comprehensive palliative and hospice care. The veterinarian and staff can immediately begin applying the philosophy of palliative and hospice care by following this protocol and be sure that no area of care is being neglected.

The revised veterinary oath commits the profession to the prevention and relief of animal suffering. There is a professional obligation to properly assess quality of life (QoL) and confront the issues that ruin it, such as undiagnosed suffering. There are no clinical studies in the arena of QoL assessment at the end of life for pets. This author developed a user-friendly QoL scale to help make proper assessments and decisions along the way to the conclusion of a terminal patient's life. This article discusses decision aids and establishes commonsense techniques to assess a pet's QoL.

Robin Downing

When negotiating the challenges of end-of-life care for animal patients with clients, veterinary health care providers must continually engage in ongoing evaluation of the pet's quality of life, as well as assessing the client's quality of life to ensure that the best decisions possible are made. By combining regular physical evaluations, including careful palpation to unmask pain, with open and honest dialog with the client about the pet's day-to-day reality, the partnership of pet owner and veterinary health care team can accept the challenge of anticipating, preventing, finding, and relieving pain in the veterinary palliative care and hospice patient.

Alice E. Villalobos

The "Pawspice" philosophy, which the author introduced at the 2000 American Veterinary Medical Association meeting, focuses on *symptom* management along with a kinder, gentler, or modified approach to *standard* therapy. Many veterinarians have preconceived bias or ingrained beliefs about aging, serious illness, multiple comorbidities, and cancer, which may cause a negative or dismissive approach toward palliative treatment, especially in geriatric pets. Veterinarians and their v-teams must overcome this insensitive attitude about life-limiting disease. This article describes assessment, treatment, and home management of some nonpainful life-limiting diseases, including cancer and age-related decline of vital functions in the Pawspice setting.

Gary M. Landsberg, Theresa DePorter, and Joseph A. Araujo

Physical signs of old age may be obvious, but mental and cognitive changes require more careful observation. Changes in behavior may represent the earliest indications of medical problems, or disorders of the central nervous system, and these may be bidirectional. Cognitive dysfunction syndrome is underdiagnosed and affects a substantial portion of aged companion animals. This article describes potential treatment regimens to address age-related behavioral problems, as well as a framework for investigating differential diagnoses. Early identification of changes in behavior is essential for the adequate treatment and management of medical and behavioral problems, and for monitoring outcomes.

Robin Downing

Veterinary patients in palliative and hospice care have progressive and often degenerative diseases that can cause pain as well as loss of function and decreased quality of life. These patients can often benefit from the application of physical medicine and rehabilitation techniques to maximize comfort and function. Physical medicine and rehabilitation are most effective as adjuncts to pharmacologic pain management. Physical medicine and rehabilitation can decrease the doses of analgesics required to keep these patients comfortable. The blend of physical and pharmacologic medicine allows an optimum balance between maximum comfort and maximum mentation.

Some pet owners may have more difficulty managing a pet's mobility challenges than any other disorder. This problem is especially frustrating because the pet is often otherwise healthy. The decline in mobility is also connected to many disease processes, such as the neuropathies seen in poorly regulated diabetes and the weakness associated with degenerative myelopathy. As death nears, a decline in mobility toward becoming recumbent or moribund is expected. The progression of the mobility disorder will vary according to the disease process. As the pet's mobility declines, the burden of care will increase. This article addresses how to care for pets with mobility changes.

Hygiene, comfort, and safety during pet palliative care and hospice are usually straightforward. The veterinary health care team must coordinate care to ensure that the pet and the family are fully informed and engaged in the process. End-of-life issues, euthanasia, and death are typically not everyday concerns for the pet owner. Pet owners and veterinary patients rely on the veterinary health care team to help create the structure within which the pet will die. The veterinary team can give the family-pet unit the gift of structure and multifaceted comfort. The veterinary profession must take seriously this unique niche of care.

End-of-life care frequently requires owners and veterinarians to make decisions of monumental consequences while feeling they sorely lack essential information. This feeling can be distressing to owners and veterinarians and lead to strains in their relationship. This article illustrates an approach to end-of-life decision making that offers the greatest benefit to the animal, the owner, the veterinarian, the veterinary practice, and, ultimately, the veterinary profession. The article introduces issues and concepts that underlie all companion animal end-of-life decision making — the human-animal bond, quality of life, and veterinarians' nonmedical helping roles — and discusses major end-of-life decisions.

This article discusses tips for veterinarians dealing with terminally ill patients. These tips include veterinarians taking care of themselves physically, mentally, and spiritually and exploring beliefs about pets dying. This article also addresses veterinarians' relationships to pets and owners and their role as facilitator; studying the ethics of end-of-life-treatment; referring owners to other specialists; and taking care of staff.

Euthanasia is a double-edged sword in veterinary medicine. It is a powerful and ultimately the most powerful tool for ending the pain and suffering. Demand for its use for client convenience is morally reprehensible and creates major moral stress for ethically conscious practitioners. But equally reprehensible and stressful to veterinarians is the failure to use it when an animal faces only misery, pain, distress, and suffering. Finding the correct path through this minefield may well be the most important ethical task facing the conscientious veterinarian.

Most veterinary hospice services are provided in the pet owner's home. Recognized standards of care have not yet been established in this emerging field. This article explores the legal implications surrounding the provision of veterinary hospice care in the United States; and provides veterinarians with the legal information necessary to determine whether and how to prepare for offering palliative and hospice care services. The legal issues that may arise in the context of veterinary hospice are largely duplicative of those that arise in the course of other types of small animal veterinary practice.

In providing palliative care and hospice in a veterinary outpatient primary care setting it is important to manage all aspects of the patient's needs as well as the primary disease process, and to understand that veterinary palliative care and hospice do not require a special degree or board certification. They only require compassion for the terminally ill patient and the human family members, a commitment to keeping patients united with their families for as long as they are comfortable, and a willingness to keep a comprehensive perspective on the patient's changing needs as death nears.

This author's experience in oncology proposes "Pawspice," a new concept that offers early supportive care for pets with life-limiting disease, embracing palliative care and standard care. Pawspice offers compassionate and comprehensive symptom relief at diagnosis while addressing life-limiting diseases. The concept of Pawspice is to maintain quality of life with palliative care that improves the patient's debilitating conditions by 30% to 50%, while simultaneously administering standard care via gentle chemotherapy modified for low toxicity. This combination makes Pawspice different than palliative care (pain and symptom relief) or hospice (intense comfort care that precedes imminent death), which prevail in most conventional thinking.

This article is a case report of a veterinarian caring for a golden retriever with nasal cancer. It addresses the 5-step strategy for comprehensive palliative and hospice care protocol, which organizes examinations, consultations, and conversations with clients. The case report presents diagnosis, treatment, and euthanasia.

RELATED INTEREST

Surgical Clinics of North America
April 2011 (Vol. 91, No. 2)
Update on Surgical Palliative Care
Geoffrey P. Dunn, MD, FACS, *Guest Editor*

THE CLINICS ARE NOW AVAILABLE ONLINE!

Access your subscription at:
www.theclinics.com

Preface

The Role of the Veterinarian in Hospice and Palliative Care

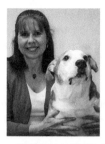

Tamara S. Shearer, DVM, CCRP
Guest Editor

The intent of this issue is to give the veterinary profession the tools to care, not cure, when the burden of treatment has no benefit. The veterinarian's role in providing good palliative and end-of-life care for pets is paramount. Until now, very little information was available on how to apply palliative and hospice care in the veterinary profession even though some veterinarians have been applying the principles of these disciplines for decades. In the past, the knowledge and application of symptom and pain management tools were not as advanced as today. Our ability to relieve suffering and improve quality of life has never been more powerful. These medical advancements give veterinarians more options to treat the symptoms of disease so the profession is able to preserve a longer quality of life in pets struggling with aging, chronic, and terminal illnesses.

Introducing palliative and hospice care as a recognized field of veterinary medicine will help to better serve pets with serious illness. The term *hospice* comes from the Latin word *hospitium*, which means to host. Hospice is defined as a facility or program designed to provide a caring environment for supplying the physical and emotional needs of the terminally ill. The term *palliate* comes from the Latin word *palliare*, which means to cloak or conceal. Palliate refers to alleviating symptoms without curing the underlying medical condition. Palliative care in veterinary medicine addresses the treatment of pain and other symptoms to achieve the best quality of life regardless of disease outcome. It helps families to understand the disease process and to make decisions. Palliative care also helps support the families emotionally. Hospice is a specialized form of palliative care. It focuses on caring for patients that are in the end stages of terminal illness. Hospice care is an extension of palliative care that tends to patients that are nearing death. The foundation of both disciplines relies upon a philosophy of care.

Some interesting studies in human palliative and hospice care support the importance of embracing this type of care for pets. According to the *New England Journal*

Vet Clin Small Anim 41 (2011) xi–xiii
doi:10.1016/j.cvsm.2011.03.018
0195-5616/11/$ – see front matter © 2011 Elsevier Inc. All rights reserved.

of Medicine, human patients that received early palliative care for metastatic lung cancer had better quality of life at the end of life.[1] These patients also experienced an increased survival time. It is reasonable to assume that the same might apply for similar disease processes in pets.

A study of 122 human caretakers showed that a lack of preparedness when a person was dying resulted in a prolonged grieving period of more than 9 months, with major depression. This study demonstrated that caretakers were nine times more likely to be depressed and were more likely to suffer from severe depression for 6-8 months than when loved ones were enrolled in hospice for less than 4 days.[2] Because of the strong bond between some people and their pets, it is reasonable to assume that similar data may apply to the loss of a pet, thus highlighting the need for palliative and hospice care for pet owners.

Requests from pet owners for palliative medicine and hospice care are on the rise. As the human population ages and physicians refer family members into hospice care, exposure to human palliative and hospice care has increased. Those that have had a good experience with loved ones are seeking the same type of end-of-life care for their pets.

It is the veterinarian's role to deliver palliative and hospice care on a case-by-case basis. Not all concepts of palliative and hospice care may apply to every pet owner because of the differences in belief systems of people about pets. The role that culture and religion plays in shaping those views can contribute to the care people seek for their pets.

The degree to which the palliative and hospice care philosophy is followed will vary because of differing viewpoints on dying. While some pet owners choose not to extend supportive care for terminally ill pets (in 2006, according to the AVMA's US Pet Ownership and Demographic Sourcebook, 17.3% of dog owners and 36.3% of cat owners did not use veterinary services), others choose to provide symptom management to keep their pets comfortable as long as possible. Hospice care is most important to families who do not choose or believe in euthanasia because of cultural or religious beliefs. Regardless of pet owner's beliefs, the veterinarian's role is to be there to care, support, guide, and educate. The profession needs to embrace an organized system and philosophy to deliver care to provide the best symptom relief for those pets. This should help prevent the suffering of a pet whose owner hesitates to seek care for fear of being judged about their beliefs about death. The role of the veterinarian should reinforce the commitment to find a solution for the problem and will continue to help no matter what.

With the evolution of palliative and hospice care in the veterinary profession, the veterinarian should consider referral for the specialized care or, better yet, expand the clinic's services to include those services. Organized palliative and hospice care options may minimize the opportunity for substandard care or premature euthanasia because a veterinarian is too busy, is too distracted, or lacks symptom management skills. Palliative and hospice care allows for another alternative instead of performing convenience or premature euthanasia. It helps to insure the pet is comfortable up until the time that the pet dies naturally or until the need for euthanasia is determined with the help of the professional support team and family.

This issue is a collaboration of what we have learned over the years in pain management, symptom management, oncology, rehabilitation, ethics, and behavior. This information is brought together to help pets where there is a decision not to pursue curative treatment, where there is diagnosis of a terminal illness, or if symptoms of a chronic illness are interfering with the routine of the pet. The role the veterinarian plays in palliative and hospice care will continue to evolve with advancements in medicine and the gathering of statistics.

The purpose of this issue is to assist in providing palliative medicine and hospice care to pets in an organized, structured system that applies concepts of human palliative and hospice care where it applies to better serve pets with serious illness. It will provide a guide and resource for veterinary professionals who choose to apply the concept of hospice and palliative care. The potential to influence the standards of care in veterinary medicine has never been greater. Our overall goal should be the improvement of quality of life for the patients that are entrusted to our care and this issue will give the profession the tools to care when the pet cannot be cured.

Tamara S. Shearer, DVM, CCRP
Shearer Pet Health Hospital
1054 Haywood Road
Sylva, NC 28779, USA

E-mail address:
tshearer5@frontier.com

REFERENCES

1. Temel J, Greer JA, Muzikansky A, et al. Early palliative care for patients with metastatic non–small-cell lung cancer. N Engl J Med 2010;363:733–74.
2. Herbert R, Prigerson H, Schultz R, et al. Preparing caregivers for the death of a loved one: a theorectical framework and suggestions for future research. J Palliat Med 2006;9:1164–9.

In the Shadow of a Rainbow: The History of Animal Hospice

Kathryn D. Marocchino, PhD, FT (Fellow in Thanatology)[a,b,*]

KEYWORDS

- Animal hospice • Pet hospice • Veterinary hospice care
- Palliative care • Hospice care • End-of-life care
- Hospice-assisted natural death

Among Native American peoples, there is a haunting and beautiful phrase to describe the often extraordinary moments of interaction between the world of animals and that of humans when both meet, often unexpectedly, in an almost magical form of communion. It is said that when that encounter occurs, and the bond of friendship is strengthened in a unique way, they have walked together "in the shadow of a rainbow." (The saying was widely introduced to the public through the work of Robert Franklin Leslie, whose book *In the Shadow of a Rainbow*, published by W. W. Norton & Company in 1974, recounted the true story of a remarkable friendship between a man and a wolf.) No better description can indeed be applied to the deep relationship established between companion animal and human caregiver during the precious and meaningful time referred to as animal hospice. For although both may have nurtured mutual love and deep respect during a lifetime together, it is the journey they undertake when they enter a hospice experience side by side that defines the personal transformation both undergo. They become one as they walk the path, accepting of each other's weaknesses yet cognizant of their inner strength, and increasingly aware that the journey is about to begin.

It behooves us to better understand what animal hospice is and how it evolved into its present-day form by examining its history in relation to the development of human hospice, from which it derives its basic principles and to which it is closely allied. As the president and founder of the Nikki Hospice Foundation for Pets (the NHFP), the nation's first nonprofit organization devoted to the provision of home hospice care for

No funding support was sought for this work.
The author has nothing to disclose.
[a] ABS School of Maritime Policy and Management, Culture and Communication Division, California State University Maritime, 200 Maritime Academy Drive, Vallejo, CA 94590, USA
[b] The Nikki Hospice Foundation for Pets, 400 New Bedford Drive, "Rosemoor House," Vallejo, CA 94591, USA
* ABS School of Maritime Policy and Management, Culture and Communication Division, California State University Maritime, 200 Maritime Academy Drive, Vallejo, CA 94590.
E-mail address: marocchino@sbcglobal.net

Vet Clin Small Anim 41 (2011) 477–498
doi:10.1016/j.cvsm.2011.03.008
0195-5616/11/$ – see front matter © 2011 Elsevier Inc. All rights reserved.

terminally ill companion animals, it is both a privilege and an honor to offer this article for the reader as an attempt at historically clarifying what may well become one of the fastest-growing and most sought-after specialties in the realm of veterinary medicine.

THE HISTORY OF HUMAN HOSPICE

As a well-conceived concept and a pragmatic sociomedical program, human hospice has brought immeasurable benefits to terminally ill patients and their families on a worldwide scale and has made an enormous contribution to the way we perceive the process of dying. However, hospice originally described a place of charitable refuge where travelers on a difficult journey could find rest and shelter, and appropriately the term comes from the Latin *hospes* (host), *hospitum* (hospitality), and *hospitium* (guest house). One of the older and more famous examples of this type of haven is the Hospice on the Great Saint Bernard Pass, the primary function of which was to offer rest and refreshment to pilgrims and travelers on their way to Rome, Santiago de Compostela, Chartres, or other shrines, where most were hoping for a miraculous cure for their chronic diseases or terminal illnesses. Erected in 962 AD and still maintained by Augustinian monks, it is now more widely know for its St Bernard rescue dogs (introduced during the seventeenth century), although it still functions as a shelter for travelers passing over the Pennine Alps.

However, an even earlier example was the large hospice for pilgrims journeying to Rome erected at Portus at the end of the fourth century by Saint Fabiola, a roman matron profoundly influenced by the ascetic teachings of Saint Jerome and Saint Pammachius, a former Roman senator. Most likely influenced by the hospice of the convent she had resided in while in Bethlehem, Fabiola provided respite for the sick, the weak, and the destitute, thus following in the Christian tradition of giving to the needy and caring for the forsaken.

Hospices that began to cater specifically to the incurably ill began originating in the eleventh century, when the Crusaders allowed those who had no family or who could not afford other accommodation to enter their places of refuge. Religious foundations or Western Christian military orders were typically the providers of hospice care during the Middle Ages, such as the Order of the Knights Hospitaller of St John of Jerusalem in the early fourteenth century, later known as the Knights of Rhodes and subsequently as the Knights of Malta in the sixteenth century, all providing sanctuary for travelers as well as for the sick and dying. Although many of these hospices languished as the orders themselves dispersed or transformed (especially after the Reformation, when many convents, monasteries, abbeys, and priories were closed or became almshouses for the elderly), they were eventually revived in the seventeenth century, when the Company of the Daughters of Charity of Saint Vincent de Paul began establishing itself as a provider of corporal and spiritual works of mercy, specifically to the sick poor.

It was not until the nineteenth century that the true concept of ministering to the dying began to gain momentum. In 1842, Jeanne Garnier formed L'Association des Dames du Calvaire in Lyon, France, and the following year the organization opened a home for the dying. Because of Garnier's remarkable influence (she was the first to use the word hospice to describe a place that cared exclusively for the dying), 6 other establishments began operations between 1874 and 1899, in Paris and New York. These sites were primarily for the poor and destitute who came to hospice as a last resort, and the kind of care provided was more comfort care than pain management. Nonetheless, the palliative care services that currently exist in both cities originated directly from their original foundations.

In 1834, Dublin saw the opening of St Vincent's Hospital under Mary Aikenhead, Superior of the Irish Religious Sisters of Charity. It was the first medical facility in Ireland to be staffed and operated by nuns. Mary died at Harold's Cross in 1858, and the convent where she had spent her final years eventually became Our Lady's Hospice for the Dying in 1879. One of the busiest hospices at the time, it served up to 20,000 people between 1845 and 1945. The Sisters of Charity later opened other facilities in Australia, such as Sacred Heart Hospice for the Dying in Sydney in 1890, followed by others in Melbourne and New South Wales in the 1930s. (Australia's involvement with hospice did not end with these centers, however. The Home for Incurables opened in Adelaide in 1879, and Sydney saw the establishment of the Home of Peace in 1902 and the Anglican House of Peace for the Dying in 1907.) In England, they founded St Joseph's Hospice in 1905, located in Hackney, in the East End of London. (It was here that Dame Cicely Saunders, now considered the founder of the modern hospice movement, worked during the late 1950s and 1960s, when she began developing the most basic principles of the hospice concept as they are known and widely disseminated today.) To the credit of the Order, all of these facilities are still in existence today and operate as modern palliative care units. In the United Kingdom, what is now known as Saint Columba's Hospice opened in London in 1885 as the Friedenheim, followed by the Hostel of God (now Trinity Hospice) in Clapham in 1891, through the efforts of the Sisters of Margaret. By 1905, because of the increasing popularity of the concept, several other hospices had been established in London, and other areas soon followed suit.

Moreover, during the nineteenth century the plight of the terminally ill became more conspicuous in the public eye, primarily because advances in medical science began drawing attention to the importance of caring for the impoverished in improved sanitary conditions. Furthermore, providing good care for the socially disenfranchised satisfied the prevailing societal need to seek justice for the dying poor and simultaneously invoke altruistic values, widely popularized at the time by Christian reform groups and religious zealots who were working assiduously to improve those facilities that were deemed inadequate. Such fervor largely owed its inspiration to publications on the subject that appeared in *Lancet* and the *British Medical Journal*, among the most notable. New facilities such as the Friedenheim in London, which by 1892 represented an enormous improvement over previous institutions, even began focusing on disease-specific patient admissions, such as those with tuberculosis. By the end of the nineteenth century, infirmaries, almshouses, and hospitals had begun the process of medicalizing[1] dying, although they were still a far cry from the radically institutionalized form of dying that is often seen today in many hospital settings, when the patient is not referred to hospice in a timely fashion or not referred at all.[2]

In the United States, where the hospice movement made its greatest strides during the twentieth century, early involvement mirrored what was occurring in the United Kingdom and in Australia. In 1899, the Servants for Relief of Incurable Cancer opened

---

[1] A good case in point, St Luke's Home for the Dying Poor (later known as St Luke's Hospital) opened in London in 1893, founded by Dr Barrett (the first instance of a trained physician spearheading such a facility). Cicely Saunders volunteered here for a time and was inspired by a doctor to attend medical school because she would be more credible as a physician in her quest to aid the terminally ill.

[2] For a compelling treatment of this issue, see *No Place for Dying: Hospitals and the Ideology of Rescue*, by Helen Stanton Chapple, which appeared in print in April 2010 through Left Coast Press. In his review of this excellent book, Brooklyn College's David Balk (Associate Editor for *Death Studies*), comments that "Thanatologists may conclude that a new Cicely Saunders is needed to face down the hospital culture of avoiding death and of sequestering dying from all else human."

St Rose's Hospice in Manhattan and another in New York City proper and then proceeded to establish similar venues in other urban centers such as Philadelphia, Atlanta, St Paul, and Cleveland. Although admirable in their mission to improve care for the dying, who would otherwise have been alone or isolated, these facilities nonetheless were predominantly nurse-based or volunteer-based and not yet integrated into the health care system we are so familiar with. Not until the latter part of the twentieth century did hospice change its direction, sharpen its focus, and dramatically begin its evolution into the type of end-of-life care that now embraces comfort care as well as the palliation of the physical, emotional, spiritual, or social symptoms of the terminally ill, not only in home settings but in hospitals and nursing homes as well.

The modern philosophy of care that constitutes hospice as we know it was largely defined and implemented by Dame Cicely Saunders. Trained as a nurse, Saunders had volunteered extensively in the hospice setting, where she had been advised to become a physician to make a difference in the lives of the terminally ill. While later attending medical school, she volunteered at St Joseph's Hospice in London, eventually taking on a position there after obtaining her degree. In 1967, Saunders opened St Christopher's Hospice in the southern part of London, imbuing her own facility with a medical atmosphere that allowed it to be more academic in nature. Patients admitted to this facility were seeking relief from total pain (defined as physical, psychological, social, and spiritual); the concept of the wayworn traveler seeking repose and a restorative meal had indeed evolved by leaps and bounds. Saunders was adamant about emphasizing pain management and comfort care rather than aggressive treatment or curative care and had a tremendous effect on the way hospice care is provided worldwide today. (Saunders, whose remarkable career as a nurse, social worker, doctor, and writer had earned her the title of Dame by the Queen of the United Kingdom, eventually died in 2005 in the hospice she had founded.)

In Canada, meanwhile, Dr Balfour Mount, a Canadian urological surgeon who had been inspired during his visit to Saunders at St Christopher's Hospice, returned to Royal Victoria Hospital in Montreal and opened one of the first hospice units in the country in 1975. Mount determined that given the prevalence of both the English and French languages in Canada, it would be more appropriate to use the term palliative care (which he coined) instead of hospice. During the next 2 decades, hundreds of palliative care programs were developed throughout Canada, although only a few years ago, official percentages for patients who do have this kind of care available to them still hovered around 5% to 15%, according to statistics gathered by the Canadian Hospice Palliative Care Organization.

In the United States, it was primarily Florence Wald, Dean of the Yale School of Nursing, who introduced Saunders' concept to the medical community and to the public. Inspired by hearing Saunders lecture in the early 1960s, she later invited the British hospice pioneer to serve as a visiting faculty member at Yale and subsequently spent a sabbatical at St Christopher's Hospice. By 1971, she had established Hospice Inc, founded on the same criteria that Saunders had so assiduously laid out.

However, much of the hospice movement was further enhanced by the works and ideas of Swiss psychiatrist Elizabeth Kübler-Ross, who in 1965 began examining societal responses to the needs of the dying, which she found to be grossly inadequate. Her best-selling book, *On Death and Dying*, published in 1969, profoundly influenced the medical profession's response to the terminally ill. Thanks to her work and to that of the other pioneers in this newly emerging field, lack of adequate care for the dying drew immediate attention and helped put into focus the types of care that were available through hospice and palliative care.

Hospice, end-of-life care, or palliative care programs have recently surpassed the 10,000 mark on the international level, with more than 100 countries participating, many of which have already established solid standards for hospice and palliative care. In 1980, the first hospice facility in Africa opened in Harare, Zimbabwe, and many more have flourished since then throughout the continent. According to an international and independent survey of palliative care practices in 2006, jointly commissioned by the National Hospice and Palliative Care Organization (NHPCO) and the United Kingdom's Help the Hospices, 15% of countries around the world offered palliative care services that were integrated into major health care institutions and 35% offered some form of palliative care services, be they limited or localized.

In 1982 Congress approved the Medicare Hospice Benefit, which expanded hospice care availability for the Medicare-eligible population. In 1986, Congress ensured its permanency, making hospice care available to everyone. Now virtually part of the health care scene, hospice care began to increase and improve as various bills were gradually introduced to the Legislature. By 1997, the burgeoning end-of-life movement quietly focused national attention on "quality of life at the end of life" as well as on the need for increased public awareness and improved physician education. But human hospice itself can perhaps best be defined through the words of the NHPCO's philosophy statement, one that has been used prominently by many other agencies and adequately sums up what hospice truly is:

Hospice provides support and care for persons in the last phases of an incurable disease so that they may live as fully and as comfortably as possible. Hospice recognizes that the dying process is a part of the normal process of living and focuses on enhancing the quality of remaining life. Hospice affirms life and neither hastens nor postpones death. Hospice exists in the hope and belief that through appropriate care, and the promotion of a caring community sensitive to their needs that individuals and their families may be free to attain a degree of satisfaction in preparation for death. Hospice recognizes that human growth and development can be a lifelong process. Hospice seeks to preserve and promote the inherent potential for growth within individuals and families during the last phase of life. [...] Physical, social, spiritual, and emotional care are provided by a clinically-directed interdisciplinary team consisting of patients and their families, professionals, and volunteers. [...] The NHPCO defines palliative care as treatment that enhances comfort and improves the quality of an individual's life during the last phase of life. No specific therapy is excluded from consideration. The test of palliative care lies in the agreement between the individual, physician(s), primary caregiver, and the hospice team that the expected outcome is relief from distressing symptoms, the easing of pain, and/or the enhancing of the quality of life. The decision to intervene with active palliative care is based on an ability to meet stated goals rather than affect the underlying disease. An individual's needs must continue to be assessed and all treatment options explored and evaluated in the context of the individual's values and symptoms. The individual's choices and decisions regarding care are paramount and must be followed at all times. (Quoted directly from "Preamble and Philosophy," NHPCO Web site: http://www.nhpco.org.)

Essentially, hospice is a philosophy of caring that respects and values the dignity and worth of each individual, and although it embraces people who are approaching death, it nonetheless cherishes and emphasizes life, by helping patients and their loved ones live each day to the fullest. (For those who wish to read more about human hospice care, one of the best sources is Amazon, whose Web site contains an extensive array of books on the subject, both for professionals and the general public. As of

November 28, 2010, the site (http://www.amazon.com) listed no fewer than 1223 results under the heading "hospice.") And herein can be found its direct link to animal hospice, which so closely resembles its human counterpart, both in principle and in implementation.

THE HISTORY OF ANIMAL HOSPICE

Animal hospice had its beginnings in the late 1980s, when a small group of passionate veterinarians and mental health professionals who thoroughly understood human hospice began formulating the concept of comfort care for terminally ill companion animals, clearly distinguishing it from traditional options that either aggressively treated the patient or led to direct euthanasia with virtually nothing in between. These pioneers—Dr Eric Clough of New Hampshire and his wife Jane (a registered nurse and then director of Optima Health Hospice), Dr Guy Hancock of Florida, Dr James Harris of California, and Bonnie Mader (founder of the nation's first pet loss support hotline at University of California at Davis [UC Davis] in 1989)—began laying the groundwork for the future movement by initially speaking independently about pet hospice in their own practices and later by joining forces and presenting the concept at various conferences.[3]

Throughout those early years, inasmuch as animal hospice (or pet hospice, as it was informally referred to at the time) differed so greatly from what veterinarians were offering their clients at the end of their pets' lives, it was not readily acknowledged, especially because the basic tenet of dying in one's own home was still in a developmental stage in this country in the human field as well. Despite repeated attempts at convincing their colleagues that pet hospice was a viable option, the Cloughs, Hancock, Harris, and Mader soon found that few were ready to follow in their footsteps unless they were familiar with human hospice and with the dying process itself. Nonetheless, their exemplary dedication and perseverance exerted an influence of its own, and they are to be commended for treading what was then uncharted, and at times even hostile, territory.[4]

Clough began introducing animal hospice into his practice, Merrimack Veterinary Associates in New Hampshire, on a gradual basis and by promoting it through a separate brochure that offered it as an ancillary service. Harris helped personal clients who were interested in animal hospice at his clinic in Oakland, California, although numbers were initially small. Mader talked about hospice repeatedly at UC Davis, hoping to enlist the assistance and backing of the School of Veterinary Medicine, but at the time, found little to no support. The transition to hospice within veterinary medicine had not yet come of age.

During the same time, a few pet hospice facilities began forming in various parts of the country as a few enlightened hospice nurses alongside a handful of inspired veterinary technicians familiar with human palliative care began realizing the validity and the potential of the hospice option, some after personal epiphanies convinced them of its viability and others after listening to talks at local and national American Veterinary

---

[3] The first such presentation was entitled "Hospice Concept for Animals" and was delivered jointly by Hancock, Harris, and Mader at the Delta Society's 10th Annual Conference in Portland, Oregon, in October 1991. The same presentation was then given at the Animals and Us 6th International Conference on Human-Animal Interactions in Montreal, Canada, in July 1992.

[4] Clough had already encountered indifference or resistance to the animal hospice idea even as he began to formulate the concept. Some veterinarians who heard him speak at conferences believed the option was unnecessary, irresponsible catering to the client's misguided wishes, or even downright ridiculous (Eric Clough, VMD, Merrimac, New Hampshire, personal communication, 1997).

Medical Association (AVMA) veterinary conferences (where the Cloughs, Harris, and Hancock continued their innovative presentations for several years).[5]

Two such animal sanctuaries were BrightHaven Holistic Retreat and Hospice for Animals in Santa Rosa, California, and Angel's Gate, originally housed in Fort Salonga, New York. BrightHaven (http://www.brighthaven.org/) initially incorporated as a nonprofit organization in 1991 under the acronym CAPT (Cats Are People Too!) but changed its name to BrightHaven in 1993. Founders Gail and Richard Pope mostly euthanized their animals during the first years of BrightHaven's inception but reverted to what they now consider true hospice care in 2004. Angel's Gate (http://www.angelsgate.org/), now in Delhi, New York, is a residential hospice for animals that began operating in 1992, with currently well more than 400 animals in its care. Founder Susan Marino is a registered nurse, licensed veterinary technician, and New York State licensed wildlife rehabilitator and estimates her euthanasia rate at around 5%. In both instances, these pet hospice facilities allow their animal residents to roam freely, and they rely heavily on integrative and alternative forms of therapy as well as on the almost exclusive use of natural raw diets. (Ella Bittel, holistic veterinarian and founder of Spirits in Transition, has said that these 2 nonprofit organizations "may well represent the richest source of animal hospice experience in the United States" (Ella Bittel, Holistic Veterinarian, Buellton, California, personal communication, April 2010).

In 1996, the NHFP (http://www.pethospice.org/) was established and began operations in 1997, formally incorporating as a 501(C)(3) a year later. Named after its founders' beloved silver mackerel tabby, the NHFP became the first nonprofit organization to promote the concept of home hospice care for terminally ill companion animals under the guidance of a veterinary hospice team. Largely a nationwide referral service, it also provides information on hospice products, pet cemeteries, and burial-related products, and offers pet loss support workshops as well as telephone bereavement counseling. As its mission statement implies, the NHFP subscribes to a philosophy (such as that espoused in human hospice programs) that addresses the physical, emotional, and spiritual needs of companion animals and of the people who love them. It consistently advocates the application of a true hospice formulary whenever possible and is heavily involved in education.

In 1997, the Cloughs were invited to become members of the first board of directors, along with Bonnie Mader and Dr Cheryl Scott, a former registered nurse and nurse practitioner who had herself just founded HomeVet Hospice in Davis, California (the first mobile veterinary hospice unit in the state). Not long afterwards, Dr Tina Ellenbogen (a trained pet loss counselor and human hospice volunteer as well as a veterinarian) joined the NHFP as an advisory board member, bringing to the organization the

---

[5] In 1995, Hancock presented "The hospice concept for animals" at the 66th Annual Conference of the Florida Veterinary Medical Association in Tampa, Florida. In 1997, he delivered the talk "Hospice concepts and geriatric animal medicine" at both the North American Veterinary Conference and at the American College of Veterinary Internal Medicine's (ACVIM) 15th Annual Forum, both held in Lake Buena Vista, Florida. The same presentation was repeated in 1998 at the ACVIM's 16th Annual Forum in San Diego, California. Hancock also served as moderator on a panel devoted to "Hospice care for animals" at the AVMA's 136th Annual Convention in New Orleans in 1999. In 2002 and again in 2005, he taught "Hospice concepts for animals," a Technician Masterclass, at the North American Veterinary Conference in Orlando, Florida. In 1998, the Cloughs presented "Helping clients say good-bye: hospice care for pets" at the AVMA Convention in Baltimore, Maryland and directly inspired CVT Ann McClenaghan, who became a spokesperson for animal hospice among veterinary technicians and later presented her own work at the Second International Symposium on Veterinary Hospice Care, held at UC Davis in 2009.

expertise she had gained from her own house-call and consulting practice in Bothel, Washington (http://www.drtinavet.com/), which had begun operating in 1987 but had seen an increase in requests for home hospice care.

In 1998, by personal invitation from Bonnie Mader, the NHFP's board of directors addressed the veterinary public for the first time through individual presentations during the 50th Anniversary Celebration of the School of Veterinary Medicine at UC Davis and the 11th Annual Symposium on Advances in Clinical Veterinary Medicine. The following year, when the Pet Loss Support Hotline at the UC Davis School of Veterinary Medicine marked its tenth anniversary under the aegis of the California Council of Companion Animal Advocates, NHFP board members were invited to return to speak and subsequently participated in an animated panel discussion that clearly showed that challenges lay ahead for the movement. (Much as Clough had encountered years earlier, some panelists were directly questioned as to why veterinarians were allowing their clients to tell them what to do. The same detractors later tried to hinder the Executive Board of the AVMA from approving the *Veterinary Hospice Care Guidelines*, although to no avail.) (The UC Davis Pet Loss Support Hotline ceased operations in June 2009 because of the budget crisis within the overall UC system.)

In 1999, the NHFP's board of directors produced its own *Guidelines for Veterinary Hospice Care*, which were later posted on the organization's Web site. Among other things, the guidelines mention that

> *Sufficient clinical and anecdotal evidence exists to indicate that veterinary hospice care provides great benefits to both pets and clients. Indeed, veterinary hospice care should now be considered an integral part of veterinary medicine and its practice should be regarded as an effective palliative procedure under state veterinary practice acts. It is nonetheless recommended that educational programs be undertaken by veterinarians before they begin offering veterinary hospice care to their clients' pets, and the assurance of education in veterinary hospice care should be central to the ability of the veterinary profession to provide this service.*[6]

More detailed than the AVMA Guidelines published 2 years later, this document was the first of its kind to address the need for a set of working rules to guide veterinarians in applying end-of-life care basics as they pertain to home hospice care for animals. Nonetheless, the guidelines can only go so far in addressing the individual needs of animals in hospice care. As Gail Pope, founder of BrightHaven, has expressed, "Each animal is a different experience, and there cannot [always] be a standard protocol." (Gail Pope, Reiki Master, Santa Rosa, California, personal communication, July 2009).

In 2000, the NHFP's board members once again gave specialized presentations at the Wild West Veterinary Conference, held in Reno, Nevada, thanks to the assistance of Dr Harris, who had been serving on the advisory board of the NHFP since 1998. Also in 2000, Dr Alice Villalobos led a talk about her newly created Pawspice program (http://www.pawspice.com/) during the 137th AVMA Convention in Salt Lake City, Utah, where she introduced her highly publicized Quality of Life Scale, still consistently referred to by veterinarians who suggest it be used by their clients to determine when their pets should be euthanized.

---

[6] For the complete text of the *Guidelines for Veterinary Hospice Care*, see the NHFP 's Web site, at http://www.pethospice.org. The NHFP's records of all client contacts as well as feedback from hospice veterinarians in its database have suggested that since 1996, requests for hospice care have increased from 10% to 30% according to practitioners who offer it as an additional service and often exceed 50% according to those specializing in hospice/geriatric care as one of their primary services.

The following year, the AVMA formally approved the first *Veterinary Hospice Care Guidelines* (later revised in 2007 with no changes). The Guidelines had been created by advisory board members of the NHFP (among others) at the behest of James Harris, who played an instrumental role in their approval as Chair of the Human-Animal Bond Committee. Approval of the Guidelines by the Executive Board of the AVMA took place in April 2001, followed by their publication in the *Journal of the American Veterinary Medical Association* in June of that same year. Although succinct and generic in nature, they nonetheless represent the AVMA's first attempt at producing a document that would cohesively address the main precepts of animal hospice care as the veterinary hospice community envisioned it at that time. Regardless of their brevity and seeming lack of depth, they judiciously adhere to the format of all AVMA Guidelines; they are meant to inform, provide an overview, suggest basic standards, and encourage veterinarians to do their best at providing the utmost in comfort care. They were not meant to be detailed nor to dictate to the veterinary community how hospice should be done, but rather, guide animal health care practitioners in making the right choices vis-à-vis their clients and their animal patients.

In 2003, Dr Tami Shearer, a nationally acclaimed veterinarian, established her Pet Hospice and Education Center in Columbus, Ohio, after years of traveling to her clients' homes to offer the service. The facility, which covered 111.5 m^2 (1200 square feet), was built adjacent to her companion animal hospital, Shearer Pet Hospital. A year later, it incorporated as a 501(C)(3). When she later moved to Sylva, North Carolina, Dr Shearer founded the Shearer Pet Health Hospital (http://www.shearerpethealth.com/) and currently continues to provide animal hospice services to her clients.[7] Dr Shearer is one of the staunchest supporters of the animal hospice movement and has consistently worked on making various treatment modalities, such as low-level laser therapy, available to companion animals in need of pain management. She is the author of 5 books and a winner of the Hartz Veterinarian of the Year award.

During the same year, Colorado State University (CSU), in collaboration with the Argus Institute, launched its Pet Hospice Volunteer Student Outreach Program (http://www.argusinstitute.colostate.edu/), envisioned in 2002 by veterinarians Charles Johnson and Jack Lebel. Originally, the idea had begun to coalesce a few years earlier, thanks to the founders of "Changes: The Support for People and Pets Program" at CSU's Veterinary Teaching Hospital who had connected with the NHFP to discuss potentially beneficial liaisons between their pet loss support program and pet hospice.

In 2006, holistic veterinarian Ella Bittel created Spirits in Transition (http://www.spiritsintransition.org/), a network that offers animal hospice seminars as well as telephone assistance through a help line. As of October 2009, 56% of Dr Bittel's regular clients (out of a cohort of 50) had chosen hospice, and out of all animal hospice patients, 67% died without euthanasia (Ella Bittel, holistic veterinarian, Buellton, California, personal communication, April 2010.) In every instance, caregivers were extremely grateful. As is the case with BrightHaven and Angel's Gate, Spirits in Transition continues its work on the cutting edge of true animal hospice and has made great strides in promoting hospice training for veterinarians alongside public education about quality of life and quality of death. In 2009, Spirits in Transition began offering online classes on animal hospice.

---

[7] A highly versatile and compassionate veterinarian, Shearer's 5-step strategy has been discussed at many conferences as a pet hospice protocol. One of the most valid things she has written about hospicing a companion animal is "The final issue you need to consider is whether your pet is ready to die, not whether you are ready for your pet to die." Honoring the animal's will to live is indeed paramount in animal hospice care.

The same year, the NHFP became the first animal hospice organization to be officially invited to join the National Hospice and Palliative Care Organization (http://www.nhpco.org/) as an associate member. NHFP board members were encouraged to give presentations at future NHPCO conferences, a dialog was initiated between the 2 organizations, and eventually an NHFP advertisement was accepted for inclusion in the Hospice Foundation of America's (HFA) program guide. This annual publication, which actively promotes HFA's Living with Grief educational programs, continues to attract an ever-increasing number of human hospice professionals to animal hospice.

In 2008, the San Francisco Society for the Prevention of Cruelty to Animals (SF/SPCA) inaugurated its Fospice program (http://www.sfspca.org/) as an adjunct service to its long-standing foster program. Currently overseen by Dr Jennifer Scarlett, Director of Shelter Veterinary Services at SF/SPCA and Lead Veterinarian for the Humane Society's Field Services Program, and by Alison Lane, Volunteer Coordinator at SF/SPCA and a graduate of SF/SPCA Dog Academy, Fospice began in the shelter itself when a handful of volunteers started to take special needs and terminally ill animals into their homes to care for them through a hospice approach while they were in foster care. The program has now extended to the community at large and has been increasing over the past 2 years.

The first of its kind ever implemented in a shelter setting, it is commendable not only as an innovative model for other facilities but also for its capacity to provide abandoned animals at the end of their lives with the opportunity to enjoy the safety of a home environment and human companionship, simultaneously providing medical support and a safety net for people interested in caring for older or physically/mentally challenged pets, many of which are eventually adopted by their Fospice providers. However, candidates for Fospice must have a nonpainful life-limiting condition that can be managed in a home setting, and for the duration of their home stay, they are regularly examined by SF/SPCA veterinarians, who decide on the "right time" for euthanasia.[8]

Virtually at the same time, A Chance for Bliss Animal Sanctuary (http://www.achanceforbliss.com/), located in Penryn, California, formally incorporated as a 501(C)(3). Its mission statement declared it to be committed to the care and welfare of animals, particularly dogs and horses, with a special emphasis on senior and special needs pets. All animals that find their way to the sanctuary become permanent residents "benefiting from the comfort and security of having a loving, caring forever home" and the organization continually promotes "the inherent worth of all beings, regardless of age, condition, or any other factor." (Quoted directly from the A Chance for Bliss Web site, at http://www.achanceforbliss.com.) Providing these residents with hospice care is the natural segue of this philosophy.

In March 2008, in what became a historic moment for the animal hospice movement, the NHFP, in conjunction with the Assisi International Animal Institute (http://www.assisianimals.org/), organized the First International Symposium on Veterinary

---

[8] To the great credit of the overseers of this remarkable program, recent discussions with the NHFP's advisory board members, and a personalized training session in acupressure and energy work by Tom Wilson, PhD, has led Fospice coordinators to develop an interest in alternative and integrative therapies for their foster animals and to gradually consider the feasibility of hospice-assisted natural death for some of their charges instead of reporting a 100% euthanasia rate. In 2009, Dr Scarlett and Allison Lane were invited to give a presentation on their Fospice program at the Second International Symposium on Veterinary Hospice Care, held at the UC Davis School of Veterinary Medicine. For more on hospice-assisted natural death, see footnote 9.

Hospice Care, held at UC Davis and hosted by the UC Davis School of Veterinary Medicine. This groundbreaking event brought together professionals from a wide-ranging variety of fields: from veterinarians, veterinary technicians, and students to mental health and hospice professionals, nurses and hospice volunteers, shelter personnel and animal welfare groups, animal chaplains and pet loss counselors, psychologists and social workers, funeral directors and death educators, business managers of veterinary practices and small clinics, and even lay people interested in promoting the concept to a wider audience in their respective geographic areas.

The conference was enormously successful and inspired many attendees to begin their own animal hospice programs and/or further explore a new field they knew little about. Although the groundwork for the event had begun 10 years earlier, it was obvious that the symposium would not have been so successful had it taken place sooner. Despite the audience's readiness to accept the concept and the enthusiasm that prevailed throughout, panel discussions at the end of each presentation indicated again, as in the past, that new challenges awaited. In essence, not only was the need to define animal hospice in a more cogent way clearly voiced, but it soon became apparent that 2 divergent groups were forming (those who interpreted animal hospice as ending in a hospice-assisted natural death[9] with euthanasia as a last resort and those who saw it as palliative care preceding inevitable euthanasia). It was decided that these issues would be further explored in the next symposium, which is being planned for late summer 2011.

During the same year, Valarie Hajek Adams, a Certified Veterinary Technician (CVT) in Appleton, Wisconsin, opened Healing Heart Pet Hospice as a nonprofit program under the auspices of the Healing Heart Foundation, an organization that sponsors programs honoring the spirit of the human-animal bond. Supported by 2 veterinarians as well as Adams and another CVT, the organization is devoted to providing care for end-of-life pets in their own homes. Although operations have been largely confined to Northeast Wisconsin, interest has already been sparked in other areas of the state, and the program is expected to grow quickly.

In 2009, the NHFP and the Assisi International Animal Institute organized the Second International Symposium on Veterinary Hospice Care, hosted once again by the UC Davis School of Veterinary Medicine. Because the conference focused on expanding many of the topics that had been previously presented, it attracted an even more diverse audience and subsequently included a greater number of talks by holistic veterinarians.

Also that same year, Dr Amir Shanan (founder of Compassionate Veterinary Care in Chicago, Illinois [http://www.compassionatevet.com/] and a long-time animal hospice provider) created the International Association for Animal Hospice and Palliative Care (IAAHPC), the nonprofit status of which is currently pending. Inspired by the first symposium in 2008, Shanan's objective was ultimately to make the IAAHPC (http://www.iaahpc.org/) an umbrella organization for various approaches to end-of-life care for animals, and accordingly he agreed to begin laying the groundwork for a new set of standards for animal hospice care that would improve on what was currently available.

Also in 2009, For Paws Hospice in Pinellas County, Ozona, Florida (http://www.forpawshospice.org/) received its nonprofit status. Founded by former banking

---

[9] Often the term natural death by itself carries with it a negative connotation in that many veterinarians and caregivers alike think that the animal is left to die as in the wild, to its own devices and with no palliation. In order to differentiate between this naturalistic type of dying and true hospice care, the NHFP has been advocating the consistent use of the term hospice-assisted natural death, akin to what we see in human hospice, where death is neither hastened nor postponed.

executive Nancy Weikle after her own experiences with human hospice, the organization now boasts the presence of professionals from the nursing, chiropractic, and veterinary fields on its staff. The mission of For Paws Hospice is to provide support to families who are in need of pet care assistance as well as pet hospice care, and offers referrals to animal service providers and to financial aid and care programs that support local rescue organizations.

In 2010, Synergy Animal Hospice (http://www.synergyanimalhospice.org/) began operating as a 501(C)(3) in Bend, Oregon. Founded by Sharen Meyers, a licensed clinical social worker at Partners in Care Hospice who had given a vibrant presentation on the unequivocal relationship between human and animal hospice at the Second International Symposium on Veterinary Hospice Care, Synergy (by its own definition) is dedicated to extending hospice care to the families of Central Oregon whose animals are experiencing a life-limiting disease process, including grief support for anyone coping with an anticipated or current loss of a cherished animal companion.

That same year, advisory board members of the NHFP met with representatives from the board of directors of the National Hospice and Palliative Care Organization in Washington, DC during the NHPCO's 25th Management and Leadership Conference. The NHFP formally proposed a collaboration to help the animal hospice movement gain momentum and to adhere to true hospice fundamentals and, by the same token, complement the care provided by human hospice so as to include companion animals alongside other family members.

The 2 groups primarily discussed how the NHPCO can embrace animal hospice alongside human hospice, validating both as part of 1 intrinsic and mutually beneficial whole; how the NHFP can best assist other animal hospice organizations in becoming members of the NHPCO, in either a provider capacity or an associate capacity; how the NHFP can implement workshops to show NHPCO human hospice members how developing an animal hospice program adjacent to their own human hospice program can benefit both people and animals; how both partners can jointly create groundbreaking avenues that can lead to insurance coverage for animal hospice and liability insurance for cadres of volunteers who are eager to serve hospice animals and their families; and how both need to find common ground that fosters a greater understanding of hospice, both for human and animal family members, among the public at large and among important constituents, which can deeply affect the future of hospice in this country at all levels.

Also in 2010, the NHFP, BrightHaven, Angel's Gate, Spirits in Transition, Synergy Animal Hospice, and A Chance for Bliss Animal Sanctuary formed the GRACE Consortium (Gratitude and Respect for Animals and their Care at the End of Life), which will apply for nonprofit status. The working mission statement of the organization is as follows: "Promoting awareness of animal hospice in its true sense of fostering respect for animals as sentient beings, developing and sharing a solid base of resources, creating and providing a nationwide support system for animal hospice, and building a community of empowerment that recognizes the time of grace that precedes death and embraces the spirit."

Ideally, the organization will ask other like-minded animal hospice sanctuaries, facilities, clinic-based or university-based programs, private practices, or referral services for home care to join as affiliate members if they can subscribe to the GRACE philosophy and show an interest in promoting its basic objectives. At the time of its inception, GRACE was well on its way to becoming the first animal hospice consortium of its kind in the country.

The history of animal hospice does not end here. Since the NHFP officially launched the veterinary hospice movement in the late 1990s in a public way, interest in the concept has grown tremendously. The organization (which now serves as an important resource for animal hospice care in the home setting) has received thousands of inquiries from across the nation as well as from abroad, mainly from veterinary universities, private practitioners, human hospice providers, and lay people within the community interested in establishing animal hospice programs of their own. The NHFP continues to provide assistance and encouragement to anyone seeking information, largely through published and online materials, telephone consultations, training seminars, and on-site workshops.

As the movement has progressed, many other animal welfare nonprofit organizations, animal sanctuaries, human hospice facilities with adjacent pet hospice units, and private veterinary practices or clinics have followed suit across the nation, emerging in virtually every state and adding themselves on a quasi monthly basis to the growing number of adherents to this cause. Since the NHFP began tracking these entities in 1998 (an often difficult task unless direct contact is established, a third party reveals its existence, or an animal hospice provider's Web site becomes readily accessible during an Internet search) it has found that several of them are increasingly making efforts at preserving the NHFP's original intent of true hospice (advocating hospice-assisted natural death with euthanasia as a last resort), especially when these agencies have been founded by human hospice nurses or volunteers, mental health professionals, and/or veterinarians with backgrounds in human hospice. Of course, this is not always the case.[10]

Although an exhaustive list of facilities or programs offering animal hospice care and/or information, referrals, and resources is difficult to provide here, a handful of the most prominent ones on a nationwide basis is listed later (with their respective Web sites when applicable) in an attempt to give the reader an idea of how prevalent this concept is becoming and how well prepared these providers present themselves to be in terms of compassion, hospice expertise, and a desire to serve both their animal patients and their human caregivers. Among these organizations are both nonprofits and for-profit organizations, with a further distinction between facilities that take in candidates on a permanent basis and those that attempt to place some of them in temporary well-screened foster homes or put them up for adoption (the animal's health permitting or if it is simply suffering from geriatric issues easily dealt with through minor palliation). Moreover, many of these organizations offer pet loss support services as well.

- Angel's Paws (http://www.angelspaws.com/)
- Animal Hospice Compassionate Crossings (http://www.animalhospice.org/)
- Bittersweet Animal Hospice and Grief Recovery Services (Tel. 707-965-9304)
- Blessing the Bridge (http://www.blessingthebridge.com/)

---

[10] As the coordinators of the CSU Pet Hospice Program have been quick to point out in an excellent article, published in the *Journal of Veterinary Medical Education* in 2008, "With any novel program, it has taken time to achieve 'buy in' within the community. Hospice care for pets is a relatively new concept nationally and veterinarians may not consider offering hospice care for their patients. Some veterinarians may not be aware of the concept of hospice for companion animals or the existence of a regional program. *Others may be resistant to offering Pet Hospice to their clients because of a misunderstanding of the hospice philosophy. Sometimes the term 'hospice' is associated with palliative care in which euthanasia is not an option* [author's italics]. The goal of the Pet Hospice program is to support pet owners and their families as they transition from a terminal diagnosis to the death of their pet. The decision to euthanize is solely that of the client and Pet Hospice volunteers support the decision they make in conjunction with their veterinarian." Clearly, hospice-assisted natural death is often not considered an acceptable option by more traditional practitioners because they are assuming euthanasia is being completely disregarded; on the contrary, this alternative sees euthanasia as a last resort, but one that is always available if truly needed when all other forms of palliation have failed, and there is both intense pain and suffering.

- Buttercup's Pet Hospice (http://www.buttercupspethospice.com/)
- Caring for Creatures Animal Sanctuary (http://www.caringforcreatures.com/)
- Kindred Spirits Animal Sanctuary (http://www.kindredspiritsnm.org/)
- Old Dog Haven (http://www.olddoghaven.org/)
- Pawsitive Memories (http://www.pawsitive-memories.com/)
- Peaceful Passings Inc (http://www.peacefulpassings.org/)
- The Clyde Fund (http://www.theclydefund.org/).

Furthermore, as more and more veterinarians add themselves to the NHFP's online database (several dozen more will be added within the next few months), it has become apparent that animal hospice is gradually but decisively becoming another important service that veterinary providers are more willing to offer now as they see a growing need (and hear more insistent requests) on the part of their clientele. In the interest of tracking this information, and to make it ever more accessible to the public at large, the author respectfully requests that readers who become aware of such practices, facilities, or programs contact the NHFP so these resources can be verified and ultimately included in our system.[11]

SUMMARY

What the animal hospice movement needs to chart its own course, hold true to its directives, and realize itself as a unique end-of-life care program that has tremendous potential to heal the souls of its participants is a meeting of the minds between professionals in the human hospice field and within the veterinary community. Only then will a reasonable discourse initiate that allows both parties to rationally commit to the conceptualization of what is best in both worlds for the sake of the companion animal and its family. When veterinarians come to appreciate the enormous value of learning about human hospice principles as a top priority in their quest to grasp the most important facets of hospice care, and when hospice professionals bridge the gap by embracing animal hospice programs and facilities in their midst, we will have come a long way.

I am reminded here of Guy Hancock's words, written to me just before the First International Symposium on Veterinary Hospice Care, where they were shared with the participants:

The importance of the psychosocial and spiritual components of hospice care must be emphasized. My fear is that vets will only focus on the medical and nursing parts. The perspective I've developed serving on the board of the human hospice is that the nursing/medical aspects serve as a base to enable the other two parts, which are actually more important. One of the principles of human hospice care is to keep the patient in charge. Human hospice was founded because nurses and others saw the problems caused by having the medical establishment in charge of decisions rather than the patient. Dedication to serving the needs and wants of the client/patient is a key aspect of hospice care. The veterinary community has an opportunity to avoid repeating the mistakes the medical profession made that made human hospice emerge as alternative care rather than mainstream care. Human hospice has now become nearly mainstream, but it has taken forty years. (Guy Hancock, DVM, St Petersburg, Florida, personal communication, December 2007)

---

[11] The author can be contacted at the corporate headquarters of the NHFP either by email at info@ pethospice.org or by calling (707) 557-8595. Such referrals will be gratefully acknowledged as the nationwide collaborative efforts they are toward helping the NHFP establish a uniform tracking system for animal hospice providers, regardless of their category or their philosophy.

By the same token, Eric Clough's *Thoughts About Hospice Care for Pets, Once Removed*, which he and his wife Jane asked me to share at that first symposium, ring just as true:

> We believe that a new approach is necessary. [...] Those of us who have witnessed the impact of hospice care and kind death at home need to work to make the image of hospice care more acceptable, more appealing. We need to focus on what we can do, what hospice can do to provide care at the end of life. [...] We need to have the courage to say what we can offer that will make a difference at the end of life: to give pet owners the tools to provide their pets with comfort, safety, shelter so that the time they have together is meaningful and memorable. As professionals, as volunteers and as pet owners, we need to truly believe that it is an honor to have the opportunity to care for the pets who have loved us unconditionally, to bear witness and to provide safe passage at the end of life. (Eric Clough, VMS, Kennebunk, Maine, personal communication, January 2008)

Over the past fifteen years, I have often been asked what message I personally would like to send to the mainstream veterinary community in the United States about embracing pet hospice, and although in the past I have spoken on this issue in a more concise fashion, I would like to answer that question here in a more expansive way because it sums up all that animal hospice represents for the NHFP. It is the philosophy we have come to live by (Brief portions of these comments were originally published in the online article, "Vet involvement key to success of pet-hospice movement," by Ranny Green, Features Writer for the Seattle Kennel Club, August 31, 2010. [http://www.seattlekennelclub.org/success-of-growing-pet-hospice-movementcontingent-on-greater-veterinary-involvement/]).

Since 1998, when it first incorporated as a 501(C)(3), the NHFP, the nation's first nonprofit organization devoted to the provision of home end-of-life care for terminally ill companion animals, has been promoting the concept of animal hospice to the veterinary community and to the public at large. Its message is clear, powerful and unequivocal: hospice as we know it for our fellow humans can be effortlessly applied to our animal companions once the stakeholders involved in its implementation (ideally, the veterinary hospice team) understand its basic tenets, believe in its value, and agree to assist the animal patient in a manner that is both consistent with hospice code and respectful of the animal's will to live. The NHFP is proud to announce that, as an associate member of the National Hospice and Palliative Care Organization, its recent partnership with this human hospice group has initiated a new dialog between human and animal hospice that will likely see these 2 branches merge under 1 umbrella.

But what does animal hospice really mean? Animal hospice means providing the best comfort and palliative care possible for a terminally ill animal so that its caregivers can make use of every modality available to achieve proper pain management (if needed) and strive for a level of comfort that allows the animal to live the remainder of its life as comfortably as possible. Animal hospice does not categorically mean palliative care preceding euthanasia nor does it mean postponing death to assuage the emotions of the caregiver. Animal hospice does not mean allowing the animal to die a natural death with no intervention, but rather, it seeks to allow a hospice-assisted natural death wherein euthanasia is always available for extreme cases but is also seen only as a last resort.

Animal hospice means understanding the significance of quality, meaningful time between the animal and the caregiver and respecting the depth of the human-animal bond as well as comprehending the extraordinary importance of the strong spiritual, psychosocial, and emotional needs of both animal and caregiver and meeting those needs accordingly. Animal hospice means working with both the animal and its family as a single unit and appreciating that they are part of the same equation as well as being willing to learn a new and master the principles of true hospice alongside one's own veterinary training.

Animal hospice means honoring the animal's will to live and understanding that it transitions in its own time and at its own pace, with death being neither hastened nor postponed. Animal hospice means embracing the animal's final journey as a moment of transcendence and growth and recognizing that, ultimately, our animals want us to be there when they depart. Animal hospice means doing the utmost to assist caregivers as they companion their animals by supporting them, explaining the alternatives available to them, preparing them for the challenges they are facing, and assuring them that they are not alone. Animal hospice means being willing to fully understand the stages of the dying process, recognizing its importance as the final stage of living, and making a commitment to both animal and caregiver to be with them along each step of the journey.

Animal hospice means understanding the distinction between pain and suffering, appreciating the existential discomfort associated with the process of dying, but seeing them in their proper perspective. Animal hospice means informing the caregiver of the costs associated with the hospice experience and working closely with the family when expenses are an issue, never losing sight of the psychological and physical well-being of the animal (and by extension, its human family) but meeting the needs and wishes of both so they complement one another.

Animal hospice means seeing through the veil and viewing death not as an enemy to be feared but as a doorway to other states of being. Animal hospice means accepting that we have done our best with what we have been given during a specific moment in time but never feeling regret. Animal hospice means being willing to give death a chance, without allowing fear, apprehension, or our own discomfort to guide our decisions but rather, accepting death as a moment of grace and coming to realize that we are still learning, every step of the way. Animal hospice means allowing our animals to teach us what they know about death: far more than we can ever hope to know.

Animal hospice means acknowledging that every case is unique and may belie what traditional veterinary medicine has taught us and that we must be prepared for whatever comes, taking each day one at a time. Animal hospice means being humble enough to concede that when the disease has won, it is time to consider comforting end-of-life care instead of aggressive treatment that often leads nowhere. Animal hospice means respecting the right of the caregiver to choose a hospice-assisted natural death for an animal without being made to feel guilty. Animal hospice means believing in the strength of compassion, the power of love between humans and their animals, and in the endlessness of all life. Animal hospice means "I will be there for you when the time comes, and I will dance with you until the end of the song."[12]

BIBLIOGRAPHY

Canadian Hospice Palliative Care Association. Fact sheet: hospice palliative care in Canada. 2004. Available at: http://www.chpca.net/uploads/files/english/resource_doc_library/Factsheet-HospicePalliativeCareinCanada-2004-09-08.pdf. Accessed March 4, 2011.

Chapple H. No place for dying: hospitals and the ideology of rescue. Walnut Creek (CA): Left Coast Press; 2010.

---

[12] See Tom Wilson, PhD, "Dancing until the end of the song: reflections on animal hospice," presented at the Second International Symposium on Veterinary Hospice Care (SISVHC), held at UC Davis in September 2009, for more information on this theme. The presentation was published in the *Proceedings of the SISVHC* in December 2009.

Clark D. Cicely Saunders: founder of the hospice movement: selected letters 1959-1999. New York: Oxford University Press; 2005.

Clark D. Cradled to the grave? Preconditions for the hospice movement in the UK, 1948–67. Mortality 1999;4(3):225–47.

Clark D. Hospice in historical perspective. In: Kastenbaum R, editor. Macmillan encyclopedia of death and dying. New York: Macmillan; 2003.

Clark D. Palliative care history: a ritual process. Eur J Palliat Care 2000;7(2):50–5.

Clark D. Total pain: the work of Cicely Saunders and the hospice movement. APS Bulletin 2000;10(4). Available at: http://www.ampainsoc.org/pub/bulletin/index.htm.

Clark D, Seymour J. Reflections on palliative care. Buckingham (UK): Open University Press Ltd; 1999.

Connor S. Hospice and palliative care: the essential guide. 2nd edition. New York: Routledge; 2009.

Connor S. Hospice: practice, pitfalls, and promise. Washington DC: Taylor & Francis; 1997.

Feldberg GD, Ladd-Taylor M, Li A. Women, health and nation: Canada and the United States since 1945. Montréal: McGill-Queen's University Press; 2003.

Forman WB, Kopchak Sheehan D, Kitzes JA. Hospice and palliative care: concepts and practice. 2nd edition. Sudbury (MA): Jones & Bartlett Publishers; 2003.

Foster Z, Corless IB. Origins: an American perspective. Hosp J 1999;14(3–4):9–13.

Hallenbeck J. Palliative care perspectives. New York: Oxford University Press; 2003.

Humphreys C. "Waiting for the last summons": the establishment of the first hospices in England 1878–1914. Mortality 2001;6(2):146–66.

James N, Field D. The routinisation of hospice. Soc Sci Med 1992;34(12):1363–75.

Kiernan SP. Last rights: rescuing the end of life from the medical system. Waterville (ME): Macmillan; 2007.

Lewenson SB, Herrman EK. Capturing nursing history: a guide to historical methods in research. New York: Springer Publication; 2007.

Lewis MJ. Medicine and care of the dying: a modern history. New York: Oxford University Press; 2007.

Poor B, Poirrier GP. End of life nursing care. Toronto: Jones and Bartlett; 2001.

Robbins J. Caring for the dying patient and the family. London: Harper & Row; 1983.

Saunders C. "And from sudden death." Frontier 1961:1–3.

Saunders C. Care of patients suffering from terminal illness at St Joseph's Hospice, Hackney, London. Nursing Mirror 1964;14:vii–vix.

Saunders C. Drug treatment in the terminal stages of cancer. Curr Med Drugs 1960; 1(1):16–28.

Siebold C. The hospice movement. New York: Twayne Publishers; 1992.

Spratt JS, Hawley RL, Hoye RE. Home health care: principles and practices. Delray Beach (FL): GR/St. Lucie Press; 1996.

The Nikki Hospice Foundation for Pets Archives. Marocchino K. A brief history of animal hospice. Research Annals; 2010.

Wright M, Wood J, Lynch T, et al. Mapping levels of palliative care development: a global view. J Pain Symptom Manage 2008;35(5):469–85.

FURTHER READINGS

Further (Selected) Reading on Human Hospice

Aoun H. On being a doctor: from the eye of the storm, with the eyes of a physician. Ann Intern Med 1991;116:335–8.

Aries P. The hour of our death. New York: Oxford University Press; 1991.

Barley N. Grave matters: a lively history of death around the world. New York: Henry Holt; 1997.

Baxter DJ. The least of these my brethren: a doctor's story of hope and miracles on an inner-city AIDS ward. New York: Crown; 1997.

Bernardin J. The gift of peace. Chicago: Loyola Press; 1997.

Bernat JL, Gert B, Mogielnicki RP. Patient refusal of hydration and nutrition: an alternative to physician-assisted suicide or voluntary active euthanasia. Arch Intern Med 1993;153:2723–8.

Brookes T. Signs of life: a memoir of dying and discovery. New York: Random House; 1997.

Byock I. Dying well: the prospect for growth at the end of life. New York: Riverhead Books; 1997.

Cassell CK. The patient-physician covenant: an affirmation of Asklepios. Ann Intern Med 1996;124:604–6.

Cassell EJ. The nature of suffering and the goals of medicine. New York: Oxford University Press; 1991.

Cassell EJ. Recognizing suffering. Hastings Cent Rep 1991;21:24–31.

Council on Ethical and Judicial Affairs, American Medical Association. Decisions near the end of life. JAMA 1992;276:2229–33.

Council on Scientific Affairs, American Medical Association. Good care of the dying patient. JAMA 1996;275:474–8.

Cowart DS. Confronting death in one's own way. Pain Forum 1995;4:179–81.

Cummins RO. Matters of life and death: conversations among patients, families, and their physicians. J Gen Intern Med 1992;7:563–5.

de Hennezel M. Intimate death: how the dying teach us how to live. New York: Knopf; 1997.

Field MJ, Cassel CK, editors. Approaching death: improving care at the end of life. Washington, DC: National Academy Press; 1997.

Garfield CA. Psychosocial care of the dying patient. New York: McGraw-Hill; 1978.

Godkin MA, Krant JJ, Doster JJ. The impact of hospice care on families. Int J Psychiatry Med 1983;13:153–65.

Grey A. The spiritual component of palliative care. Palliat Med 1994;8:215–21.

Harmon L. Fragments on the deathwatch. Boston: Beacon Press; 1998.

Hastings Center. Guidelines on the termination of life-sustaining treatment and the care of the dying. Briarcliff Manor (NY): The Hastings Center; 1987.

Jaffe C, Ehrich CH. All kinds of love: experiencing hospice. Amityville (NY): Baywood Publishing; 1997.

Kamm FM. The doctrine of double effect: reflections on theoretical and practical issues. J Med Philos 1991;16:571–85.

Kübler-Ross E. On death and dying. New York: Macmillan; 1969.

Kübler-Ross E. The wheel of life: a memoir of living and dying. New York: Scribner; 1997.

Levine S. Who dies? An investigation of conscious living and conscious dying. New York: Doubleday; 1982.

Lo B. Improving care near the end of life: why is it so hard? JAMA 1995;274:1634–6.

Lynn J. An 88-year-old woman facing the end of life. JAMA 1997;277:1633–40.

Marquis DB. Four versions of the double effect. J Med Philos 1991;19:515–44.

McCue JD. The naturalness of dying. JAMA 1995;273:1039–43.

McKann RW, Hall WJ, Groth-Juncker A. Comfort care for terminally ill patients: the appropriate use of nutrition and hydration. JAMA 1994;272:1263–6.

Mermann AC. Spiritual aspects of death and dying. Yale J Biol Med 1992;65:137–42.

Miyaji N. The power of compassion: truth-telling among American doctors in the care of dying patients. Soc Sci Med 1993;36:249–64.

Morrison RS, Meier DE. Managed care at the end of life. Trends Health Care Law Ethics 1995;10:91–6.

Nuland SB. How we die: reflections on life's final chapter. New York: Knopf; 1994.

President's Commission for the Study of Ethical Problems in Medicine and Biomedical and Behavioral Research. Deciding to forego life-sustaining treatment: a report on the ethical, medical and legal issues in treatment decisions. Washington, DC: US Government Printing Office; 1983.

Quill TE. A midwife through the dying process: stories of healing and hard choices at the end of life. Baltimore (MD): Johns Hopkins University Press; 1997.

Quill TE, Cassel CK. Nonabandonment: a central obligation for physicians. Ann Intern Med 1995;122:368–74.

Seale CF. What happens in hospices: a review of research evidence. Soc Sci Med 1989;28:551–9.

Sharp J. Living our dying: a way to the sacred in everyday life. New York: Hyperion; 1996.

Solomon MZ, O'Donnell L, Jennings B, et al. Decisions near the end of life: professional views on life-sustaining treatments. Am J Public Health 1993;83:14–23.

Sullivan RJ Jr. Accepting death without artificial nutrition or hydration. J Gen Intern Med 1993;8:220–4.

SUPPORT Principal Investigators. A controlled trial to improve care for seriously ill hospitalized patients: the study to understand prognoses and preferences for outcomes and risks of treatment (SUPPORT). JAMA 1995;274:1591–8.

The Hospice Foundation of America. In: Doka KJ, Davidson J, editors. Living with grief: when illness is prolonged. Washington, DC: Taylor & Francis; 1997.

Webb M. The good death: the new American search to reshape the end of life. New York: Bantam; 1997.

Further Reading on Animal Hospice[13]

2nd Chance for Pets. Until it's time for me to go: pet hospice care. The Companion. A Quarterly Newsletter 2005.

AAHA Senior Care Guidelines Task Force. AAHA senior care guidelines for dogs and cats. J Am Anim Hosp Assoc 2005;41(2):81–91.

AAHA/AAFP Pain Management Guidelines Task Force Members. AAHA/AAFP pain management guidelines for dogs and cats. J Am Anim Hosp Assoc 2007;43: 235–48.

American Animal Hospital Association. Hospice care–ending life with compassion (online article). 2010. Available at: http://www.healthypet.com. Accessed October 19, 2010.

American Veterinary Medical Association. Guidelines for veterinary hospice care (revised in 2007, March) [booklet]. AVMA; 2001.

---

[13] The titles listed here represent works written by veterinarians or other professionals, caregivers who have personally hospiced their companion animals, or writers commissioned by specialized animal welfare publications, although a select few have also appeared in animal journals or science magazines. For copies of articles geared more toward the general public (that have appeared in pet periodicals or newspapers), please contact the Nikki Hospice Foundation for Pets. CD-ROMs of the entire Proceedings from both the First and Second International Symposia on Veterinary Hospice Care can also be obtained directly from the NHFP. Readers are encouraged to contact the author if they come across other titles not listed here that they believe should be included.

Birk D. Hospice care for animal companions. Animal News (The Newsletter of Alliance for Animals, Inc) 2006;24(1).

Bishop G, Long CC, Carlsten KS, et al. The Colorado State University Pet Hospice Program: end-of-life care for pets and their families. J Vet Med Educ 2008; 35(4):525–31.

Bittel E. Leaving this life, in rhythm with nature. Holistic Horse, Integrative Therapies for Horse and Rider; 2007. Issue 51.

Bittel E. Hospice for horses–taking time to say farewell. Equine Wellness 2009;4(4).

Bittel E. Embracing death's journey with our animals. Alternatives Magazine, Resources for Cultural Creativity; 2007. Issue 42.

Bittel E. Veterinary hospice care post conference reflections. J Am Holistic Vet Med Assoc 2008;27(2).

Bowen E. Building the bond: Dr. Eric Clough modeled his pet hospice program after human hospice care. Vet Econ 1997.

Bradley P. More than a pet: a holistic guide to animal hospice, compassionate pet death and euthanasia. Conway (AR): Enlightened Marketing; 2009.

Carmack BJ. Loss and grief: dimensions in veterinary hospice care. The Latham Letter; 2009;30(2).

Congalton D. Pet hospice offers alternative to euthanasia. Veterinary Product Staff; 1999.

Congalton D. Veterinarians urged to explore hospice option. Veterinary Product News July 1999.

De Louise D, Lane M. Pet hospice: caring until the end. ASPCA Animal Watch; 2001.

Downing R. Pets living with cancer: a pet owner's resource. Lakewood (CO): AAHA Press; 2000.

Ginsburg L. Creature comforts–Fido's best friend in the end. Natural Solutions Magazine; 2006.

Hancock G, Yates J. Client services for geriatric pets. Number 1. In: Goldston RT, editor, Veterinary clinics of North America, small animal practice, vol. 19. Philadelphia: WB Saunders; 1989.

Hancock G. What is hospice or end-of-life care? [online article]. The American Association of Human-Animal Bond Veterinarians. 2002. Available at. http://www.aahabv.org. Accessed November 15, 2010.

Hancock G. Client services for geriatric pets. In: Hoskins J, editor. Geriatrics of the dog and cat. 2nd edition. Philadelphia: WB Saunders; 2003.

Hancock G. The human animal bond. In: Sirois M, editor. Principles and practice of veterinary technology. 2nd edition. St Louis (MO): Mosby; 2004.

Hancock G. Client services for geriatric pets. In: Sirois M, editor. Principles and practices of veterinary technology. 2nd edition. Philadelphia: WB Saunders; 1995.

Harty E. Pet hospice care–making the best of a hopeless situation. 2000. Available at: http://www.vetcentric.com/magazine. Accessed November 25, 2000.

Israel S. The long goodbye: losing a pet. Positive Thinking; 2007.

Israel S. Go gently into that good night–hospice care for animals. Animal Wellness 2005;7(4).

Kehoe L. Making peace with death. The Whole Dog Journal 2002.

Lagoni L, Morehead D, Butler C. The Bond-Centered Practice: The Future of Veterinary Care. Proceedings of the 1999 ACVIM Forum. Chicago: American College of Veterinary Internal Medicine; 1999.

Mader B. House calls, hospice and comfort rooms: the rewards of providing for clients' needs, Proceedings of the 50th Anniversary Celebration of the School of Veterinary Medicine at UC Davis and the 11th Annual Symposium on Advances in Clinical Veterinary Medicine. Davis (CA): University of California at Davis School of Veterinary Medicine; 1998.

Marocchino K. Honoring life by respecting death: the work of The Nikki Hospice Foundation for Pets, Proceedings of the 50th Anniversary Celebration of the School of Veterinary Medicine at UC Davis and the 11th Annual Symposium on Advances in Clinical Veterinary Medicine. Davis (CA): University of California at Davis School of Veterinary Medicine; 1998.

Marocchino K. The Nikki Hospice Foundation for Pets: its mission and goals. Veterinary Syllabus of the Wild West Veterinary Conference, Reno, NE, October, and the PAWS Conference Proceedings of the First Summit on the healing power of the human-animal bond: lessons learned from the AIDS epidemic. San Francisco (CA): Wild West Veterinary Conference and PAWS (Pets Are Wonderful Support) Conference; 2000.

Marocchino K. The Nikki hospice foundation for pets: a humane option for companion animals. A Publication of the Benicia Vallejo Humane Society. Four Paws Press 1999;2(3).

Marocchino K. Bringing hospice home. Vet Econ 1998.

Mathews K. Nonsteroidal anti-inflammatory analgesics in pain management in dogs and cats. Can Vet J 1996;37:539–45.

Medina J. A matter of choice: hospice care provides a humane option for companion animals. Canine Practice 1999;24(5).

Monti DJ. Pawspice an option for pets facing the end. JAVMA News. October 1, 2000.

Mott M. Growing trend: hospice for pets. LiveScience; 2007.

Nagy K. Pet hospice care. WebVet; 2008.

New Jersey Veterinary Technicians and Assistants, Inc. The Nikki hospice foundation for pets. NJVTSA Newsletter 2008.

Nolen RS. Protecting pet hospice. JAVMA News. December 15, 2007.

Ogilvie GK. Hospice and bond centered practice. Proceedings of the 1999 ACVIM Forum. Chicago: American College of Veterinary Internal Medicine; 1999.

Osborne M. Pet hospice movement gaining momentum. J Am Vet Med Assoc 2009; 234(8):998–9.

Reynolds R. Blessing the bridge–what animals have to teach us about death. Novato (CA): New World Library; 2001.

Rezendes A. More veterinarians offer hospice care for pets. J Am Vet Med Assoc 2006;229(4):484–5.

Rodier L. Moving from cure to care: veterinary hospice care considerations for your canine companion. The Whole Dog Journal 2010.

San Filippo M. Veterinarian to discuss growing field of pet hospice at AVMA Convention. JAVMA News. July 26, 2010.

Scott C. Home hospice for pets: an option for the terminally ill animal companion. Proceedings of the 50th Anniversary Celebration of the School of Veterinary Medicine at UC Davis and the 11th Annual Symposium on Advances in Clinical Veterinary Medicine. Davis (CA): University of California at Davis School of Veterinary Medicine (in-house publication); 1998.

Shearer T. Final decisions and coping with loss (Part 7). In: The essential book for dogs over five. Columbus (OH): Ohio Distinctive Publishing; 2002.

Shearer T. Hospice and palliative care. In: Gaynor JS, Muir WW, editors. Handbook of veterinary pain management. 2nd edition. St Louis (MO): Mosby Elsevier; 2008.

Shearer T. Developing a pet hospice care center. The Latham Letter 2009;30(1).

Smith A. A new option: mobile veterinary hospice care. The Latham Letter 2009; 30(1).

Stepherson L. Pet hospice care at home: loving your pet through the end. 2010. Available at: http://www.Amazon.com. Accessed December 6, 2010.

The Latham Foundation. Veterinary hospice care. The Latham Letter 2008;29(4).

The Nikki Hospice Foundation for Pets and Assisi International Animal Institute. Proceedings of the First International Symposium on Veterinary Hospice Care. Davis (CA): The NHFP and AIAI; March 28–30, 2008.

The Nikki Hospice Foundation for Pets and Assisi International Animal Institute. Proceedings of the Second International Symposium on Veterinary Hospice Care. Davis (CA): The NHFP and AIAI; September 5–7, 2009.

Tremayne J. Focusing on the end. Veterinary Practice News July 2008.

Villalobos A. Conceptualized end of life care: 'Pawspice' program for pets, Proceedings of the AVMA Conference. Salt Lake City (UT). Summer: American Veterinary Medical Association; 2000.

Villalobos A. Pawspice. In: Withrow SJ, Vail DM, editors. Withrow & MacEwen's small animal clinical oncology. 4th edition. Philadelphia: Elsevier Saunders; 2007.

Villalobos A. Hospice: a way to care for terminal pets. North American Veterinary Conference Clinician's Brief. NAVC; 2009.

Villalobos A. Feline pawspice. In: August J, editor, Consultations in Feline Internal Medicine, vol. 6. Philadelphia: Saunders Elsevier; 2010.

Villalobos A. Bonding with patients, veterinarians. Veterinary Practice News July 2010.

Villalobos A. Reflections on the International Symposium on Veterinary Hospice Care. Veterinary Practice News. April 28, 2008.

Villalobos A. Pet hospice nurses the bond. Oncology Outlook in Veterinary Practice News. September 1999.

Wohlfarth J. A gentle departure: hospice care for pets [special issue]. Pet Life 1998.

Delivery Systems of Veterinary Hospice and Palliative Care

Tamara S. Shearer, DVM, CCRP[a,b,]*

KEYWORDS

• Pet hospice • Palliative • Death • Dying • House call

Because palliative medicine and hospice care refer to a philosophy of care, there is great flexibility in how it can be delivered to pet owners. The veterinarian needs to develop a plan based on the professional's individual preferences. The delivery system of hospice and palliative care is dependent on 3 areas that need defining. First, the services that will be offered to the pet owner must be defined. Once the services have been defined, the facility and location of the services will become evident. Third, the professional team that will deliver care needs to be organized. Marketing and legal issues must be addressed when considering to offer palliative and hospice care. An organizational worksheet is provided at the end of this article to help with planning.

When starting hospice and palliative care services, one of the first steps is to define what services will be provided and what services will be referred. This helps dictate the type of facility that will be needed to carry out the services. The choice of services can be divided into offering full-service health care or offering consultation care. Services such as advanced diagnostics or palliative surgery require a fully equipped practice. If a veterinarian wants to offer more integrative care, which might include rehabilitation or overnight accommodations for pet owners, extra space will be required to meet that need in the form of a therapy area and upgraded comfort rooms. The veterinarian should also consider an area for providing daycare services for debilitated patients that need care while their owners work. Other choices might include using a referral system to get the pet additional help for acupuncture, chiropractic, rehabilitation, and a pain management.

Veterinarians should not be discouraged if they choose not to financially invest in a full-service hospital because most palliative medicine and hospice care can take place through consultations or a house call service. Most states require a house call or consulting veterinarian to have a base hospital where a pet can be referred in

---

The author has nothing to disclose.
[a] Shearer Pet Health Hospital, 1054 Haywood Road, Sylva, NC 28779, USA
[b] Pet Hospice and Education Center, 16111 State Route, 37 Sunbury, OH 43074, USA
* Shearer Pet Health Hospital, 1054 Haywood Road, Sylva, NC 28779.
E-mail address: tshearer5@frontier.com

Vet Clin Small Anim 41 (2011) 499–505
doi:10.1016/j.cvsm.2011.03.001
0195-5616/11/$ – see front matter © 2011 Elsevier Inc. All rights reserved.
vetsmall.theclinics.com

case of an emergency. If a pet is referred for a house call or to a consulting veterinarian for hospice care, it is recommended the pet be transferred back to the referring veterinarian if hospitalization or diagnostics are needed to maintain the relationship between the primary caregiver, pet, and pet owner. No matter what type of practice, it is encouraged to have the hospice or palliative care veterinarian use the pet's referring practitioner as one would use an attending physician in human hospice. This approach keeps the communication open between the referring veterinarians and promotes more referrals.

There are advantages and disadvantages with any method of delivering palliative medicine and hospice care. One advantage of choosing a full-service hospital to deliver care is that it allows the patient to have more treatment options. It also provides a well-organized area to care for pets. It usually allows for better accessibility to support staff during hours of operation. For example, if a pet develops acute diarrhea and is in need of intravenous fluids as part of its supportive care, it is likely that the patient could receive the care immediately and under staff supervision in a fully equipped hospital. Diagnostics such as radiographs or blood tests would also be immediately available. If another palliative care patient was in need of help, there would be staff to accommodate that pet's needs at the same time. The disadvantages include difficulty ensuring a peaceful environment when performing other general wellness health care in the same place. Despite the best efforts to maintain a peaceful environment, it is not possible 100 percent of the time because of the unpredictability of animal behavior. It only takes 1 vocal pet to tip the environmental tone of being quiet and peaceful to being noisy and chaotic. Arrival of a trauma case can also change the ambience of the environment. Care must be taken with a full-service hospital's higher operational expenses because an improper budget may affect profitability, and that can add to the disadvantages when trying to provide palliative medicine and hospice care.

One advantage of using consultation services or house call services to deliver care is the ease of creating a peaceful environment. Typically, a consultation service or house call practice can only see 1 pet at a time, so it minimizes the disruptions found at a general practice. There is a lower overhead because the expenses of a larger hospital are not applicable. For example, there is lower or no mortgage payment, fewer staff, and less equipment associated with a house call practice. When using a small consultation office or a house call service, a veterinarian can often achieve the same outcome with a patient as one working out of a large facility. Disadvantages include having fewer treatment options available or having to refer a patient if the health status changes. Veterinarians are limited to seeing 1 patient at a time, therefore they can only help 1 pet at a time and not multiple pets that might require care. A limited number of patients translates into less income generated but, with care, may be profitable, if a careful budget is followed, because of the low overhead.

Once the services are defined then one can try to modify, renovate, or provide a space that allows nursing care to be carried out in the best possible manner. It is recommended to reserve a special place in the hospital to provide the proper physical environment to deliver palliative care or hospice consultations. The facility should promote peacefulness to enhance a relationship-centered environment, which is important in providing palliative medicine and hospice care. Whether a veterinarian is building a new facility or renovating an existing hospital, consideration for the same criteria should exist. If the existing hospital does not have an appropriate area, or has limited space to deliver palliative medicine and hospice care, then perhaps a large storage room might be converted into a consultation area. Space may also exist at the end of a wide hallway that could be converted into a small consultation room. An examination room face-lift can provide space by removing the examination table and existing seating and replacing it with a low-sided love seat or couch. The lighting should be changed from fluorescent to a warmer light. Medical educational posters should be removed and replaced with framed art.

If there is no room suitable for comfortable consultations, veterinarians should consider leasing a small office space near the existing hospital. When considering an off-site facility, take into account zoning laws and whether or not the landlord is pet friendly. Sometimes an office can double as a small classroom where support groups could meet. The addition of a separate clinic wing or office space within walking distance of the existing clinic would be ideal. When building a new facility, providing the proper environment is paramount for the comfort of the pet and the pet owner. The practice owner should choose whether overnight comfort rooms for the pet owner should be part of the design. If a specialized area is not available to provide hospice or palliative care, it is still better to offer the service but care should be taken to make sure the pet is comfortable in the chosen environment.

Environmental enrichment is a process in which the surroundings are manipulated to minimize stress and promote relaxation. Maybe more important than where the services are provided is making sure they are delivered in a proper atmosphere. Part of modifying the facility's environment includes providing nonslip flooring, which is a necessity when caring for debilitated pets to prevent them from falling. Rubberized, cushioned flooring is best; however, many brands require specialized cleaning procedures. If the budget does not allow for permanent nonslip flooring, then more affordable floor runners can be used. If using linkable, rubberized floor tiles like the ones used in children's play areas, care must be taken to prevent urine from leaking between and under the tiles. Garage floor rubber mats are affordable and waterproof, and are available in various sizes to cover the entire floor surface of a room.

Another requirement for enriching the environment includes making sure the area is kept at a comfortable temperature for the pets, and balancing that temperature so it is comfortable for pet owners too. In addition to adjusting the environmental temperature, the hospital should provide additional warmth in the form of blankets, in case a pet is chilled. A fan can provide extra cooling for a pet or pet owner if they become too warm. A fan can also make a pet with a mild breathing difficulty feel more comfortable by blowing the air toward the pet's face.

The environment should be quiet with a minimum of noise distractions. Care should be taken during a consultation or hospice stay to minimize any interruptions when the staff are working with the pet and pet owner. In a busy practice, soft music can buffer background noise. If a room is in use, a code system can be used to alert other staff about the seriousness of the visit. An example of a code system may include putting a colored flag on the door handle.

Ideally, seating should be available for all of the family members, which is difficult in many settings because of restricted space. However, it is more important to have ample area for a large dog to stretch out on the floor or have a low-sided bed or couch where the pet is comfortable. Pillows can provide comfort for family members who prefer to be on the floor with the pets.

Pheromone diffusers for both feline and canine patients may minimize stress in the hospital or office. These pheromones are identical to the ones produced by the cat or dog while nursing newborns. Research has shown that these pheromones reduce stress.[1] Soft, quiet music may also provide comfort. Care should be taken to make sure that the music is not played so loud that it interferes with communication. Studies show that classical music may have a more relaxing effect compared with other forms of auditory stimulation. A music choice called *Through a Dog's Ear* has proved to minimize stress and was created by Joshua Leeds, a psychoacoustic expert who has used animal bioacoustics technology to develop the soundtrack. This music minimizes anxiety and may lower heart rate.[2]

Additional features that compliment a hospice and palliative care facility for pets include applying feng shui concepts to create a healing and relaxing environment. Feng shui is an ancient Chinese art of improving different aspects of life by enhancing the environment according to the traditions of harmony and energy flow.[3] For example, using the color tones of green enhances growth, energy, vitality, and hope, whereas yellow and earth tones promote health, grounding, and connection. Placement of furniture, water features, and plants can change the energy of the environment according to feng shui. There are many resources on the subject from books to consultants to provide advice about this concept to enhance the environment of a facility.

If a specialized area is not available to provide palliative or hospice care, and enhancement of the environment is not possible, it is still better to offer the services than not to have them available. Because palliative and hospice care are based on a philosophy, the person or team delivering the service is the most important aspect when helping a pet.

The professional team that delivers the palliative and hospice care needs to be put together after the services have been defined and the facility has been developed. Some veterinarians and staff may have a natural ability or calling to care for chronically or terminally ill patients. However, not all veterinarians and staff are suited to providing palliative medicine and hospice care, just as not all veterinarians enjoy working up a complicated dermatology case.

There is a set of personality traits possessed by an individual that may contribute to providing better hospice and palliative care. These traits include the ability to be a good listener and to be tolerant and empathetic. Being patient also helps in coping with all aspects of care because, even when following a protocol to guide pet owners through hospice and palliative care, it is common for the families to have a lot of questions. It is important to let pet owners take their time in decision making to ensure a better emotional outcome once the pet dies, as long as it does not interfere with the pet's quality of life. The ability to show and share a compassionate attitude helps to support the family. Good leadership and communication skills help guide families with decision making and allow for better coordination of a care plan. Also, the ability to maintain good composure and remain calm despite one's own feelings is an asset. When developing a palliative and hospice care plan, the capability to be creative and detail oriented makes for a more effective protocol.

Bell, a 9-year-old greyhound, is an example of how the traits of creativity and patience of her caretakers helped her regain her mobility while in palliative and hospice care. Bell had a rear limb amputation after a diagnosis of osteosarcoma. She had long-term postoperative complications that interfered with her ability to walk. Once her complications were managed, she was at a place in her recovery where rehabilitation could begin. However, by this time she was profoundly weak and had lost the will to get up. To motivate Bell, one staff member brought out our very tolerant office cat to spark an instinctual desire to chase or hunt. Bell became more animated and tried with all her might to chase the cat, who did not care that Bell was barking. This stimulation accelerated her rehabilitation through motivation. She was able to meet the goal of walking again. Without this creative incentive, Bell's recovery would have been slower.

The veterinary hospital owner or administrator should choose what type of palliative and hospice care team works best for a practice. The veterinarian or highly trained veterinary technician needs to be the team leader for palliative or hospice care.

Many veterinarians and staff perform the duties of many professions. With experience, some veterinarians and veterinary technicians have become proficient in delivering the care provided by social workers, psychologists, and spiritual leaders. For some, this may be a dangerous practice that may lead to compassion fatigue.[4] Because a veterinarian cannot be available 24 hours a day, 7 days a week, using an interdisciplinary team to deliver palliative and hospice care makes good sense.

In a human hospice, an interdisciplinary team is always called on to carry out the care of the human patient.[5] The team works to initiate treatment while also coordinating drugs, supplies, and equipment to support the care of the patient. They teach family members how to care for their loved one. They also provide spiritual and emotional support. There are some similarities between the human palliative and hospice teams and a veterinary team (eg, **Table 1**).

In human palliative and hospice care, the attending physician may refer patients into hospice care or visit with the patients. The attending physician works with a support team of hospice physicians, hospice nurses, and other professionals to initiate treatment plans and change treatment plans as a patient declines. In the veterinary profession, the pet's general practitioner may be the palliative care or hospice care provider or may be the referring veterinarian. Human hospice nurses are skilled in recognizing pain and symptoms that compromise the quality of life of the patients they treat. They work to keep patients comfortable by managing medications and working with the families. They are in charge of obtaining medical equipment and supplies. They provide hands-on care for the patients and report changes in the patient's health to the physician. In the veterinary profession, this role would be assumed by registered veterinary technicians or specially trained veterinary assistants. Highly skilled veterinary technicians are capable of heading the palliative and hospice care programs in a hospital.

Social workers help provide emotional support and may help with planning both the future and the financial components of care. At the time of writing this article, there are few social workers employed in small animal general practices. Larger institutions have known for years that social workers help to complement the medical components of care. If a practice does not employ a social worker, arrangements can be made with local social workers who have an interest in animal welfare to help these families.

Volunteers or home health aides help families with tasks that include personal hygiene of the loved one. They may also provide help through cleaning and shopping for the families. Veterinary assistants, kennel staff, and volunteers may fill this role for pet owners.

Spiritual support in human hospice is often performed by a chaplain who may work alone or with the family's minister. As with the social worker, arrangements can be

Table 1	
Similarities between the human and the veterinary palliative and hospice team	
Human Care Team	**Veterinary Hospice Team**
Doctor/attending physician	Veterinarian
Hospice nurses	Veterinary technicians and assistants
Social worker	Social worker
Volunteers	Volunteers
Chaplain or spiritual counselor	Chaplain or spiritual counselor
Bereavement counselor	Bereavement counselor

made with the family's spiritual leader or outside clergy. Individuals must have an interest in animal welfare to help support these families. It is important to find clergy who are nondenominational.

Bereavement counselors are specially trained professionals in grief counseling. Human hospice recognizes that some family members may need additional support after the loss of a loved one. Some larger communities already have grief counselors and pet loss support facilitators who serve this role. In general, bereavement counseling is poorly developed in the veterinary profession. Most follow-up with families who have pets that have died is short in duration and may only consist of a sympathy card. Much can be done to develop a better way to care for families that have lost pets by applying the same principles used to help people.

Large practices may find it rewarding to have a complete hospice support staff, such as a social worker or even a clergy member, to support the pet owner in a similar way as a human hospice. Some small practices may find the cost of employing these professionals prohibitive. If a veterinarian cannot financially afford to employ all members of an interdisciplinary team, then they can refer the pet owner to these professionals outside the scope of their practice.

Another advantage of using an interdisciplinary team is that members of a hospice and palliative care team will have different views about the pet and the family because some of those members might have a different perspective of a pet's situation. It is important to listen carefully to all information by all team members when designing or changing a plan to provide the family with the best care.

Marketing palliative and hospice care services might include contacting emergency and referral hospitals and local veterinary clinics about the added service to the community. It is recommended that part of the palliative care team meet with area emergency and specialty clinics to let them know the services that they can provide so they know that palliative and hospice care is available. It is also important to let general practitioners in the area know that these services are now available in the community. Some busy veterinary practices may choose to refer some of their patients to a hospice care specialist because of the additional time commitment required to provide good end-of-life care. Free media exposure through the Internet, newspaper, radio, and television may be solicited through a press release describing the benefits of palliative and hospice care for pets, and will let pet owners know that there is a palliative and hospice care service available.

Unlike the human medical profession, the veterinary profession lacks the financial support of subsidized care in the form of Medicare, Medicaid, health maintenance organizations, and widespread insurance plans. In human medicine, even the cost of bereavement counseling is covered by Medicare. Most pet insurance companies honor claims to care for the health needs of pets but, at this time, only a minority of pet owners purchase insurance for their pets.[6] Palliative and hospice care fees should be based on the time invested by the veterinarian and staff in caring for the pet. There are regional economy variations, so a veterinary consultant may help define what is fair. If a family cannot afford care but seeks help for their pet, a clinic may choose to subsidize care through donations of time, money, or supplies.

When developing a hospice program, the practice owner should inquire with the American Veterinary Medical Association about additional liability issues associated with hospice care because of the need to see patients outside the office setting. Complete details on the legal aspects of providing palliative and hospice care are discussed by Amir Shanan elsewhere in this issue.

Because hospice and palliative care are based largely on a philosophy, it is important to apply those concepts so the actual location of the delivery of care can vary.

A professional wanting to practice this philosophy should not be restricted by physical constraints and inability to afford a facility. Wherever the patient is seen, efforts need to be made to use a team approach for better care of the pet and family. The veterinarian and staff can immediately begin applying the philosophy of palliative and hospice care after the delivery system is in place by following the strategy described in the article by Tamara S. Shearer elsewhere in this issue.

Checklist for palliative and hospice care services
- List veterinary medical services provided
- Choose the following:
  - New facility, modify a facility, offer house calls or consultations
- Facility modification through environmental enhancement
- Organize hospice team
  - Veterinarian
  - Veterinary technician
  - Assistants
  - Volunteers
  - Social worker
  - Clergy
  - Bereavement counselor
- Define fees
- Marketing strategy
- Review liability insurance and consider legal aspects.

REFERENCES

1. Kim YM, Lee JK, Abdel A, et al. Efficacy of dog appeasing pheromone (DAP) for ameliorating separation-related behavioral signs in hospitalized dogs. Can Vet J 2010;4:380–4.
2. Wells DL, Graham L, Hepper PG. The influence of auditory stimulation on the behavior of dogs housed in a rescue shelter. Anim Welfare 2002;11:385–93.
3. Alexander S. Feng shui. In: Alexander S, editor. 10 minute feng shui, easy tips for every room. Gloucester (MA): Fair Winds Press; 2002. p. 2–11.
4. Cohen SP. Compassion fatigue and the veterinary health team. Vet Clin North Am Small Anim Pract 2007;37:123–4.
5. Wittenberg-Lyles E, Parker D, Demeris G, et al. Interdisciplinary collaboration in hospice team meetings. J Interprof Care 2010;3:264–73.
6. Burns K. Pet health insurance gains ground in North America. Schaumburg (IL): JAVMA News; 2007.

Pet Hospice and Palliative Care Protocols

Tamara S. Shearer, DVM, CCRP[a,b,*]

KEYWORDS

• Pet hospice • Palliative • Death • Dying • Euthanasia
• Protocol

Until 10 years ago, there was no standard protocol to help guide veterinarians through the care of a chronically or terminally ill pet until the 5-step strategy for comprehensive palliative and hospice care was developed.[1] Following this 5-step protocol allows the veterinarian and staff to feel confident that no process of care has been neglected. It is designed to promote care on a case-by-case basis.

Many circumstances warrant a recommendation of entering a pet into palliative or hospice care. A decision not to pursue curative treatment or a diagnosis of a terminal illness qualifies for this type of specialized care. When symptoms of a chronic illness interfere with the routine of the pet, then a patient and the family can benefit from a palliative and hospice care program. These care services can also be used if a pet has a disease in which curative treatment has failed or if a pet requires long-term intensive care. Progressive illnesses and traumas that have health complications associated with them also meet the criteria. A thorough examination of the pet and discussion with the pet owner help determine if the pet should enter into palliative or hospice care (**Box 1**).

If a diagnosis fits these criteria, entering into a palliative or hospice care plan as soon as possible after a diagnosis is the best way to have a meaningful effect on a patient's end-of-life care. If possible, the program should start even before the symptoms of disease develop.[2] The 5-step strategy for comprehensive palliative and hospice care helps provide the protocol to start palliative or hospice care (**Box 2**).

EVALUATION OF THE PET OWNER'S NEEDS, BELIEFS, AND GOALS FOR THE PET

When starting hospice and palliative care the most critical of the 5 steps is evaluation of the pet owner's needs, beliefs, and goals for the pet. Honoring and respecting the

The author has nothing to disclose.
[a] Shearer Pet Health Hospital, 1054 Haywood Road, Sylva, NC 28779, USA
[b] Pet Hospice and Education Center, 16111 State Route, 37 Sunbury, OH 43074, USA
* Shearer Pet Health Hospital, 1054 Haywood Road, Sylva, NC 28779.
E-mail address: tshearer5@frontier.com

Vet Clin Small Anim 41 (2011) 507–518
doi:10.1016/j.cvsm.2011.03.002
0195-5616/11/$ – see front matter © 2011 Elsevier Inc. All rights reserved.

Box 1
Circumstances that warrant palliative or hospice care

A decision not to pursue curative treatment

A diagnosis of a terminal illness

Symptoms of a chronic illness interfere with the routine of the pet

Curative treatment has failed

A pet requires long-term intensive care

A pet has a progressive illness or trauma with associated health complications

---

pet owner's psychosocial concerns enhance the trust the pet owner has in the team and make for a better client-patient-doctor relationship. Ideally, the veterinarian, the primary care support staff member, and a social worker should be present for this part of the protocol.

Investigation of the pet owner's needs through asking open-ended questions helps to understand and define the needs of the pet and pet owner. Open-ended questions are those that require more than a "Yes" or "No" answer. These needs and goals should be shared with the entire hospice team and should be respected throughout the care.

An important part of this discussion should include additional information about the pet's relationship to the pet owner. An overview of the pet owner's support system of family and friends is helpful. The staff should obtain contact information for these important people for future reference.

The owner's needs, beliefs, and goals are shaped by past experiences, both negative and positive. For example, a pet owner whose previous animal died prematurely as a result of a surgical intervention to improve quality of life may avoid surgery with another pet. However, if a previous pet had a procedure that improved quality of life, like a pet having pericardial effusion removed from surrounding the heart, the pet owner might be more likely to opt for palliative procedures of that magnitude in the future. Pet owners also have different physical, psychological, social, and spiritual needs depending on the disease. Past experiences and quality-of-life challenges associated with cancer among human family members may affect the choice of care if a pet develops neoplasia.

Information about the pet's activities of daily living help to shape a tailored plan for that family. See the article on mobility challenges by Tamara S. Shearer elsewhere in this issue for a complete set of questions to evaluate the pet's activities. A determination of other activities that the pet engages in is important because the long-term plan should try to preserve these activities for as long as possible.

Preferences for testing to track the disease trajectory should be determined in this step. The pet owner may need an explanation or examples on how this decision might

---

Box 2
Five-step strategy for comprehensive palliative and hospice care

1. Evaluation of the pet owner's needs, beliefs, and goals for the pet

2. Education about the disease process

3. Development of a personalized plan for the pet and pet owner

4. Application of palliative or hospice care techniques

5. Emotional support during the care process and after the death of the pet

---

affect the comfort of the pet. For example, in chronic kidney disease, maintaining a proper phosphorus balance may improve the comfort of the pet by avoiding the effects of secondary hyperparathyroidism. Also, anemia secondary to lack of erythropoietin production by the kidneys can be identified and managed. These parameters can be monitored through simple blood tests. It may help to define an answer by asking about past experiences with the pet's acceptance of medical care. For example, how does the pet behave for blood tests?

Preferences regarding hospitalization versus outpatient or home care should be discussed in advance and are also shaped by past experiences. Pet owners should be asked to describe how the pet acts when it is at a veterinary hospital or away from home in a boarding kennel. Exceptions may sometimes occur that disrupt the original preferences. Even although a pet owner may choose to have the pet cared for at home, there may be a medical crisis that may require a short stay in a hospital environment and the pet owner may change their mind. One example is if a pet develops severe diarrhea and a course of intravenous fluids is indicated to stabilize the patient.

The veterinarian or staff member should discuss whether the pet owner would like additional professional help outside the palliative or hospice care team to advise on supportive care. Examples of outside professionals include veterinary internists, oncologists, pain management specialists, rehabilitation practitioners, certified acupuncturists, alternative medicine specialists, and pet nutritionists.

Financial concerns of the family should be addressed but should not alter the sharing of treatment options for the pet. It is common for pet owners with little means to find the resources to get the best care for their pets. Any financial constraints should be respected when developing a personalized plan. In step 3 (development of a personalized plan), the appropriate way to respectfully discuss financial limitations without leaving out important care options is outlined.

There is benefit in finding out in advance details surrounding preferences near the end of life. By the end of this step, the veterinarian should have a good understanding of the family's beliefs about death and dying. How the pet dies and where the pet dies should be discussed. The pet owners should be asked about their beliefs in euthanasia, natural death, and the use of proportionate palliative sedation as an option for their pet if symptom management fails to keep their pet comfortable. Proportionate palliative sedation is a technique used in human hospice care to provide relief of symptoms that are not manageable.[3] This method of symptom relief is not meant to hasten death or to end life but to relieve symptoms. This technique can be applied in veterinary medicine if a pet owner does not believe in euthanasia or the family needs more time before saying goodbye.

It is also important to know in advance if the pet owner wants to be with their pet at the time of death. The pet owner should be prepared in advance for the choices available when making final arrangements so they have time to pick the best option for the family.

When there is conflict between family members' beliefs, the veterinarian and care team must sometimes take a leadership role to help resolve disputes concerning the pet's care. The team must take into account the psychosocial concerns discussed in the initial visit, yet advocate on the pet's behalf. Good communication and education about a disease is helpful. The veterinarian should reinforce the commitment to find a solution for the problem and continue to help no matter what. Referring back to the psychosocial beliefs or revisiting the initial discussion is also helpful when there is conflict (**Box 3**). A pet owner's goals and priorities may vary and transform as the disease progresses. Their perspective may also change once they are educated about the disease process.

Box 3
Psychosocial concern assessment

Past medical experiences

    Past positive medical experiences

    Past negative medical experiences

    Details from the past that need to be avoided

Preferences for testing to track illness trajectory

    Tracking the illness through testing for increased chance of improving quality of life

    Tolerance of pet for blood being drawn and comfort level around veterinary staff and hospitals

Preferences regarding hospitalization versus outpatient or home care

    Pet's behavior when it is at a veterinary hospital or away from home in a boarding kennel

Preferences regarding outside professional help for specialty care

    Interest in rehabilitation services or medical specialist like an oncologist, cardiologist, neurologist, or internist

    Alternative medicine specialist

    Acupuncturist

Role of financial concerns in health care choices

Belief regarding death and euthanasia

    Preferences on where a pet dies

    Pet owner's desire to be present

    Choice of how to handle the remains

EDUCATION ABOUT THE DISEASE PROCESS

Education about the disease process is best performed by the veterinarian and technical support staff. A good understanding of the disease process enables the pet owner to make informed decisions about their pet's care. A veterinarian should be able to share the stages of the disease process with the pet owner plus discuss what to expect when the pet is dying. The details of the information shared should be based on the pet owners' need to know. The discussion should include information about the disease and its trajectory, information about nutritional support for chronically or terminally ill pets, symptom management options, and enlightenment on death and dying (**Box 4**).

Box 4
Education about the disease process

1. Discussion about illness trajectories and the specific disease

2. Discussion about nutritional support

3. Discussion about recognition and symptom management

4. Discussion about death and dying

Illness Trajectories and Specific Disease Information

A discussion of the pet's disorder by categorizing the disease trajectory helps with the planning of the care and the understanding of the dying process associated with different illnesses. An illness trajectory is a generalized pattern that a group of diseases follow, which may affect how a veterinarian and family deal with a chronic or terminal illness. In human medicine there are 4 illness trajectories that we can apply in veterinary medicine to help explain changes throughout the course of a disease and the events surrounding death.[3]

The first trajectory is when there is a short period of decline before death. In this type of illness a pet maintains most of its health until later in the course of disease, when there is a predictable decline. This timeline of decline can vary over a course of weeks or months. An example is certain types of neoplasia.

The second trajectory is when there is a chronic illness often followed by sudden death after the pet is no longer capable of compensating for its illness. In this disease pattern, the burden of care increases with time as the symptoms become more numerous and intense. At times, the disease may wax and wane or even stabilize, but the pet never reclaims its health and slowly declines. Examples of this second trajectory include chronic kidney disease, liver failure, and congestive heart failure.

The third trajectory is when there is progressive deterioration of a condition. A pet with these diseases has a prolonged trajectory and requires increasing care over time. Secondary complications like decubital ulcers and urinary tract infections are common with these types of illnesses. Examples of a trajectory 3 illness are degenerative myelopathy and cognitive dysfunction.

The forth trajectory is when there is a sudden, severe neurologic or circulatory injury or insult. Trauma, intervertebral disc herniation, and saddle thrombus are included in this trajectory, as is an ischemic event in the brain. This type of insult results in extreme impairment that affects the pet's mobility and ability to function without extraordinary care.

A study in the *Journal of Pain and Symptom Management* reported that people in the last month of their life with end-stage kidney disease have symptom burdens equal to or greater than that of people with cancer. The symptoms most reported include lack of energy, itching, drowsiness, dyspnea, poor concentration, pain, poor appetite, swelling, dry mouth, constipation, and nausea.[4] Sharing information obtained from human hospice studies may help a pet owner understand how the pet might feel as the disease progresses and prepare them for more aggressive symptom management.

If a definitive diagnosis is not known, information can still be shared about common side effects of chronic and terminal illnesses. The most reported side effects of human disease processes include pain, dyspnea, nausea or vomiting, constipation, reflux, anorexia, pruritus, urine retention, fatigue, and neurologic symptoms.[5] The pet owner should be prepared to manage some of these symptoms despite the diagnosis. Because pets lack the ability to communicate some of their symptoms and the magnitude, it is better to anticipate and overtreat these symptoms as long as there are no side effects.

Nutritional Support

Part of the education process should address the nutritional components associated with the pet's illness. Information regarding nutritional support is important because there are many misconceptions about support options and the loss of appetite at the end of life. The veterinarian should explain the risks and benefits of the various options. Pets that have a good appetite may be fed a prescription diet or home-cooked meals formulated for the specific disease process, but if a pet is not interested in food, a variety of creative options can be considered, such as offering favorite foods and hand feeding. Supplementing or relying on feeding tubes, such as esophagos-tomy, nasogastric, and percutaneous endoscopic gastrostomy tubes may be consid-ered for certain disease processes when the pet is hungry but not capable of eating, such as if the pet has an oral tumor or a swallowing disorder. Assisted feeding may also be helpful to support a pet that has a prolonged disease trajectory but otherwise good quality of life. Force feeding by putting food in a pet's mouth should not be rec-ommended and should be discouraged in a palliative or hospice care plan when the pet refuses food, is nauseous, is vomiting, cannot swallow, or is nearing death. The inability or refusal to swallow is a sign that death is near; if that is the case, the pet no longer requires nutrition. Food may create more problems such as aspiration pneu-monia, digestive upset, and the worsening of azotemia. Aggressive intravenous fluid therapy at end of life may create side effects such as pulmonary edema from volume overload, but subcutaneous fluids may help electrolyte disorders and general malaise if a pet is expected to live for several more days.[3]

Symptom Recognition and Management

Pet owners should be educated on how to recognize disease symptoms that can inter-fere with quality of life and what help is available to alleviate the symptoms. In human medicine some debilitated patients cannot communicate their need for pain and symptom relief. This characteristic is also true of the animal population. When in doubt about a pet's comfort, it is better to overtreat for symptoms than to undertreat the symptoms to ensure everything is being done to enhance quality of life. It is important for the pet owners to report health changes so the team can promptly tend to any side effects to prevent suffering. The pet owner should be taught how to recognize pain, nausea, dehydration, constipation, dyspnea, melena, anemia, urinary tract infections, and urinary obstructions.

Information should be shared on how the administration of additional fluids to control dehydration can prevent constipation. Pet owners need to know that there are combinations of drugs and physical rehabilitation techniques like transcutaneous electrical nerve stimulation (TENS) and laser therapy to manage pain and that there are oral and injectable medications to relieve nausea. See the articles on pain manage-ment and symptom management elsewhere in this issue for detailed information on pain and symptom relief.

It is important to discuss in advance what to do when symptom management is not working and there is a dramatic decline in quality of life. The use of proportionate palliative sedation and integrating proven alternative options like acupuncture, massage, and some herbal therapies into the care plan is especially important when symptom management is failing. A drug combination of opioids, midazolam, and phe-nobarbitol called proportionate palliative sedation is sometimes used in human medi-cine to relieve symptoms.[3] This method of symptom relief is not intended to hasten death or to end life but to relieve symptoms. Because of the body's weakened state, many drug combinations may have a double effect. For example, if an opioid is used to reduce the anxiety associated with dyspnea and used to control pain, it may also cause respiratory depression in a weak patient and increase the risk of death. The veterinarian should use combination sedatives, anesthetics, opioids, and antianxio-lytics with care in a weak patient.

These techniques can be applied in veterinary medicine if a pet owner does not believe in euthanasia or the family needs more time before saying goodbye when choosing euthanasia to prevent suffering when other forms of support cannot manage disease symptoms. Instead of abandoning the care when the pet may need it most, veterinarians can use these tools to bridge a disconnect that exists between feeling helpless when symptoms cannot be managed.

Death and Dying

Education and the preparation for the death and dying process should start at the beginning of entering into a palliative or hospice care plan. This is the first step in the preparation for bereavement.[3] After a diagnosis there is much individual variation when discussing life expectancy with pet owners. Even in human medicine, a prediction of the time remaining before death after a diagnosis is made does not always correlate with the estimates of doctors. Statistical averages can serve only as a general guideline and do not tell us exactly how long a particular patient has to live, so good skills of observation can be helpful. A description of the dying process, whether by natural disease progression or by a euthanasia intervention, should be shared with the pet owner based on the specific disease trajectory before the death of the pet. The amount of detail of events should be adjusted according to the pet owner's need to know.

The symptoms of the disease and dying process may vary depending on the illness and the metabolic condition of the pet. For example, a pet owner should be warned that in disease trajectory 2 there may be moments of temporary improvement that may cause confusing moments even during the active dying phase. There are specific signs of approaching death that may indicate that death is becoming nearer. Just like not all symptoms of a disease in an individual are the same, not all signs of death are the same. As a palliative care patient graduates into hospice care, a pet owner should be aware of how to recognize if a pet is actively dying. Most commonly, during the dying process a pet eats less and sleeps more to the point that there is no appetite and there is somnolence. The pet is usually not mobile and there is extreme weakness. The pet owner may notice irregular and shallow respirations, and low blood pressure causes cold extremities. There may be increased respiratory noise in some patients. Eyes are often unable to close while resting, and the pet blinks less, if at all.

There are some disease processes in which the pet experiences the symptoms associated with its disease process before death, as with metastatic lung disease or heart disease, in which a phase of profound respiratory distress can be experienced by the pet. Seizures secondary to electrolyte imbalances and azotemia can also be witnessed and can hasten death. The pet owner needs to know about these potential consequences of the pet's disease process.

If the pet owner has indicated that euthanasia is an option when a pet's quality of life is poor or if they can no longer care for the pet, then education about euthanasia should be discussed. A review of the process, what the pet experiences, and what the pet owner sees is paramount in the education of the euthanasia process. The details should be tailored to the pet owners' need to know and the veterinarian's protocol for euthanasia. The explanation should include what drugs are used, how they are administered, and how long they take to work. Next, explain what reflexes might be witnessed by the pet owner, including a description of breathing changes, occasional vocalization, urination, and defecation. It should also be mentioned that the eyes remain open and that involuntary nerve or muscle twitching plus gurgles from the bowels are normal.

Support staff should seek continuing education that focuses on the needs of chronically and terminally ill pets plus attend pain and symptom management seminars to be better prepared to educate pet owners. The veterinarian should delegate some of the educational process to the support staff so they can begin work on designing a medical plan to help care for the patient.

DEVELOPMENT OF A PERSONALIZED PLAN FOR THE PET AND PET OWNER

The development of a personalized plan for the pet and pet owner should take into consideration the psychosocial beliefs of the family and their desires for the pet. These parameters should have been discussed in detail in step 1. Being respectful of these beliefs, the veterinarian's prime responsibilities are to preserve quality of life by preventing side effects of disease and setting up a plan that works for the pet and family (**Box 5**). This plan includes organization of a care team that meets the emotional needs of the pet owner too. Before sharing the plan with the pet owner, it is paramount that the plan and the prognosis be coordinated with the entire team to avoid the family's receiving mixed messages about the care. Because each team member may have a different perspective to share, there may be differing views on the pet's care, which should be taken into consideration when developing a plan.

It is important to take into consideration the challenge to correctly balance care with side effects of the treatment when creating a plan (see **Box 5**). The care plan is also dependent on how much the pet owner can contribute, because that dictates how much outside support is needed.

Twenty-four-hour Care

The first step for peace of mind for the pet owner is to make sure the pet owner knows how to get help at any time of day that an owner or the animal is in a crisis. This situation is where the team approach plays an important role in sharing care responsibilities so the entire burden does not fall on 1 individual, who in the past was usually the veterinarian. After hours, a contact person should be available for the pet owner, and the support team should also refer to that person. The palliative or hospice care team should incorporate a pet-loss support hotline and emergency clinic contact information for the pet owner for additional after-hours care.

There is value in having written instructions in case of a crisis from the hospice veterinarian to the emergency clinician that outlines the preferred treatment of the patient. For example, if Fluffy is in a hospice care plan the following letter can accompany her to the emergency clinic:

Dear Emergency Staff,
    Through consultation with our hospice team, Mrs Doe chooses to treat the side effects of Fluffy's disease and opts not to have diagnostic procedures performed. We hope that this simplifies your role and that you can focus on symptom management. We respect your judgment and appreciate your insight if drastic changes occur in the pet's health. As part of the hospice team, we would like

---

Box 5
Care plan development

1. Arrangements for 24-hour care

2. Treatment option choices

3. Set up home care environment

4. Preparation for death

to be part of the decision-making support system, even if it is after hours, for Mrs Doe and Fluffy if she needs additional help.

Sincerely,
Palliative and Hospice Care Team

The Importance of Treatment Options

The treatment options need to match the beliefs and needs of the pet owner and to be in the best interest of the pet. When designing a plan it is important to treat all processes that interfere with quality of life. For example, a veterinarian should treat a painful otitis, even in a dying pet, to prevent additional discomfort from the infection or inflammation in the ear.

The doctor should always give all of the supportive treatment options despite any financial constraints. It is important for the veterinarian to educate the pet owner about all options for care in case the owner chooses to invest more in the pet's care. This statement acknowledges that the team was listening to the pet owner about financial constraints but allows for the complete discussion of treatment options: "I know that you shared with me concerns that you had limited resources when it came to Fido's care. In case that changes, or in case you come across someone who is having similar problems, I want you to be informed about all of the choices available."

When designing a plan, special care must be taken to lessen the side effects of polypharmacy therapy. It is important to obtain a complete list of medications that a pet has been prescribed to avoid drug interactions such as serotonin syndrome or reactions between a nonsteroidal antiinflammatory and corticosteroids. Appropriate drug therapy must take into consideration side effects and drug interactions.

For pets that are difficult to medicate, oral medicines can be compounded into a more palatable medication. Also, many medicines can be given as a subcutaneous injection that the pet owner can be taught to administer.

Alternative care choices should be offered if the pet owner is open to the additional aids in keeping their pet's stay comfortable. These services should be provided by veterinarians who have an understanding of palliative and hospice care philosophy.

Setting up Environment at Home

The personalized plan should include helping the pet owner to set up an area in their home to care for their pet if off-site care is not an option. If the pet is still mobile, it is important to provide flooring with good traction to minimize the risk of falls. This objective can be accomplished by laying down rugs with rubber backing or using floor runners that do not slip and slide. The rubber backing serves a double purpose because it is waterproof and protects the underlying floor if a pet is urinary incontinent. Pet owners should block off stairways to prevent falls for pets that are unstable. Furniture should be moved to prevent a pet from falling into sharp edges or getting stuck between objects. For pets that are allowed on furniture, human beds could be lowered and/or steps or ramps provided. Mobility-impaired pets often cannot use steps and ramps because their steep inclines make them difficult to navigate. For more details on how to help a mobility-impaired pet, see the article elsewhere in this issue.

A social location should be selected so the pet can be part of the interactions among normal family activities, especially if that is what the pet is used to. Some families move their own sleeping area to another area of the house if the pet can no longer climb stairs to sleep in the bedroom. Other pet owners put pet carriers in the bed with them to keep an incontinent or mobility-impaired pet close at night. Pet carriers are also helpful for pets that wander at night. No matter where the pet sleeps, bedding that is soft and easy to clean should be recommended. It is helpful to have at least 2 sets of bedding in case it gets soiled. Stay-dry beds and mattress covers help with hygiene.

All locations where the pet may reside should have access to water so they do not have to go to another location. This strategy minimizes the risk of dehydration. Access to food should also be made easily available. It is important for some pets with disabilities to be fed with elevated feeders or even hand fed if their mobility problem interferes with normal eating posture. Access to a litter box should be made easier by moving it close to the cat, lowering the sides, and increasing the size of the box. Some cats learn to use a hygiene pad sprinkled with kitty litter instead of a litter box.

Based on the pet's needs, thermal comfort should be adjusted for the individual. Some short-coated lean pets prefer warmth whereas other pets that are overweight or the thick-coated northern breeds like cool temperatures. If an outdoor pet cannot be brought inside, care must be given to protect it from temperature extremes that contribute to fly-strike in the warmer months and frostbite or freezing when it is cold.

The environment during the last hours of life should be made as peaceful as possible for the pet and the family by dimming the lights and playing soft music, as discussed elsewhere in this issue. The pet owner may consider letting the pet choose its favorite spot. Some pets have a favorite spot in the yard or woods. Other options may be added to enhance a relaxing environment according to the family's preferences.

Preparation for Death

When designing a palliative or hospice care plan, the veterinarian must respect the pet owner's choice when it comes to euthanasia or natural death. The details surrounding the death of the pet should already have been discussed in the previous protocol steps. The palliative and hospice care team must advocate on behalf of the pet if there is a failure in care provided by the family or hospice support staff and the pet is clearly suffering. The veterinarian and hospice team must provide solutions to prevent suffering. As discussed earlier, the use of proportionate palliative sedation is a technique often using a combination of pain blockers, sedatives, and antianxiety drugs to provide relief of symptoms that are not manageable. Some alternative methods to relieve pain like massage, acupuncture, therapy lasers, and TENS may also help to manage symptoms before death. More details on pain and symptom management can be found elsewhere in this issue.

APPLICATION OF PALLIATIVE OR HOSPICE CARE TECHNIQUES

The fourth step includes applying and teaching the hospice or palliative care techniques that have been outlined in the personalized plan. Technical support staff should review the techniques required to care for the ill pet with the pet owner. It is recommended that the pet owner have written instructions and be shown the technique and then they should demonstrate the technique (**Box 6**). For example, a pet owner should be shown how to give subcutaneous fluids by the support staff. The pet owner should then demonstrate the technique in front of the staff member. Written instructions should be distributed for clarification and review.

All medications should be reviewed and the pet owner should understand the use and the frequency of each drug. Information about how to recognize a side effect of the drug should be reviewed (**Box 7**).

If any technique is awkward or uncomfortable for the pet owner, the task must be practiced or delegated to another individual to minimize stress and maintain a good relationship between pet and owner. If a pet owner is having difficulty medicating a pet, consider having the medication administered in a different form or made into

---

Box 6
Technique teaching tips

1. Provide technique demonstration

2. Provide written information describing the technique

3. Have the client repeat the technique in front of staff

4. If needed, provide compounded medications for ease of administration

5. Provide a list of medication side effects

---

a different flavor. If a pet does not take oral medications, many tolerate subcutaneous injections, and this technique can be taught to most pet owners.

Depending on the care plan and the pet's disease, the veterinary staff should show how to express a bladder to help a pet urinate. They should teach how to use assistive devices to aid in mobility. They need to demonstrate how to apply ophthalmic medications such as eye lubricants. There are efficient ways that technical staff can share to maintain hygiene in debilitated patients that keep the pet comfortable and make home care easier. See the article elsewhere in this issue for more care tips. There should always be a technical support team member for the pet owner to contact if, and when, problems develop in performing any technique.

EMOTIONAL SUPPORT DURING THE CARE PROCESS AND AFTER DEATH

Emotional support during the care process and after the death of the pet is one of the most important steps in palliative and hospice care. Even although this step is listed as fifth, it is important that it begins the moment a pet is diagnosed with a chronic or terminal disease.

In addition to the veterinary staff, social workers, psychologists, and bereavement counselors help provide emotional support during the care process. They can help families with planning the future and financial components of care. If a practice does not employ a social worker, arrangements can be made with local social workers who have an interest in animal welfare to help the family. For spiritual support, a pet owner may choose to work with a minister of their choice. If the team uses outside spiritual support, it is important for that professional to respect the cultural traditions and spiritual beliefs of the pet owner.

After the death of a pet, bereavement counseling should last as long as necessary. In a human hospice the bereavement follow-up may last for more than 1 year. An initial assessment by the hospice team helps determine the duration of care that may be

---

Box 7
Medication side effect list for clients

1. A rapid decline in condition, especially after starting a new medication

2. Restlessness, excitability, salivation, licking of lips, or trembling after administration of a medication

3. Lack of appetite or vomiting after giving medication

4. Change in bowel movement consistency, frequency, or color

5. Development of skin irritation or itching

6. Development of depression or disorientation after administration of a medication

---

needed. The veterinary staff should be able to recommend more services to help pet owners grieve the loss of a pet, especially if the pet owner is depressed or has special needs. Many larger communities have pet-loss support groups that help with the bereavement process. If grief becomes complicated, then referral to a licensed professional should be considered.

Veterinarians and staff should also recognize and be able to help surviving pets that are suffering with behavioral changes secondary to the death of a companion animal. If a pet is having difficulty, a pet owner could spend time with that pet by walking, grooming, or playing, being careful not to create separation anxiety. Background noise like a television or radio may be provided when the pet is left alone. If a pet's appetite declines sometimes sitting with the pet at mealtime helps. Also, in some situations, adoption or fostering a new pet may be helpful, but only if the pet experiencing the loss is social.

SUMMARY

Starting a palliative or hospice care plan as soon as possible after a pet qualifies allows for better care of the pet and the family. The process is made more efficient by applying the 5-step strategy for comprehensive palliative and hospice care. The veterinarian and staff can immediately begin applying the philosophy of palliative and hospice care by following this protocol and be sure that no area of care is being neglected.

REFERENCES

1. Shearer T. Hospice and palliative care. In: Gaynor J, Muir W, editors. Handbook of veterinary pain management. St Louis (MO): Mosby; 2010.
2. Temel J, Greer JA, Muzikansky A, et al. Early palliative care for patients with metastatic non-small-cell lung cancer. N Engl J Med 2010;363:733–42.
3. Quill T, Holloway R, Shah M, et al. Primer of palliative care. 5th edition. Glenview (IL): American Academy of Hospice and Palliative Care; 2010. p. 160.
4. Murtagh F, Addington-Hall J, Edmonds P, et al. Symptoms in the month before death for stage 5 chronic kidney disease patients managed without dialysis. J Pain Symptom Manage 2010;40:342–52.
5. von Gunten CF. Interventions to manage symptoms at the end of life. J Palliat Med 2005;8:88–94.

RECOMMENDED READINGS

Levine D, Millis D. Rehabilitation of the geriatric patient. In: Bochstahler B, Levine D, Millis D, editors. Essential facts of physiotherapy in dogs and cats. Babenhausen (Germany); 2004. p. 272–6.
Gaynor J, Muir W, editors. Handbook of veterinary pain management. St Louis (MO): Mosby; 2010.
Manning A. Physical rehabilitation for the critically injured veterinary patient. In: Millis D, Levine D, Taylor R, editors. Canine rehabilitation and physical therapy. Philadelphia: Saunders; 2004. p. 404–10.
Taylor R, Millis D, Levine D, et al. Physical rehabilitation for geriatric and arthritic patients. In: Millis D, Levine D, Taylor R, editors. Canine rehabilitation and physical therapy. Philadelphia: Saunders; 2004. p. 411–25.
Shearer T. The essential book for dogs over five. Columbus (OH): Ohio Distinctive Publishing; 2002.
Villalobos A. Canine and feline geriatric oncology: honoring the human-animal bond. Ames (IA): Blackwell Publishing; 2006.

Quality-of-life Assessment Techniques for Veterinarians

Alice E. Villalobos, DVM, DPNAP[a,b,c,*]

KEYWORDS

- Quality-of-life scale • Quality-of-life assessment
- End-of-life care • Pawspice care • Pet hospice
- Palliative care • Terminal disease

Society has embraced the human-animal bond with love and respect, requesting veterinarians to provide more quality-of-life (QoL) measures for pets at the end of life. The revised veterinary oath commits the profession to the prevention and relief of animal suffering. There is a professional obligation to properly assess QoL and confront the issues that ruin it, such as undiagnosed suffering. The need is particularly acute when families are caring for aging, ailing, or terminally ill pets, especially pets with advanced or recurrent cancer. It is time for the profession to systemically embrace palliative care, pet hospice, and/or Pawspice care. Pawspice starts at the diagnosis of a life-limiting disease. It focuses on symptom mitigation, kinder, gentler standard care, and transitions to hospice when needed. There are no clinical studies in the arena of QoL assessment at the end of life for pets. Therefore, the information presented here is based on the experience of like-minded colleagues worldwide and this author's forty-plus years of experience caring for thousands of oncology patients and escorting the incurable to the end of life. Out of necessity, this author developed a user-friendly QoL scale to help everyone involved make proper assessments and decisions along the way to the inevitable conclusion of a terminal patient's life. The QoL scale guides highly bonded pet owners, who might be in denial, to consider issues that are difficult to face. Pet owners must ask themselves if they are truly able to provide enough care to maintain their ailing pet properly. This article discusses decision aids and establishes commonsense techniques to assess a pet's QoL by using the HHHHHMM (hurt, hunger, hydration, hygiene, happiness,

[a] Pawspice at VCA Coast Animal Hospital, Hermosa Beach, CA 90254, USA
[b] Pawspice at Beachside Animal Referral Center, Capistrano Beach, CA 92627, USA
[c] Animal Oncology Consultation Service at Animal Emergency and Care Center, Woodland Hills, CA 91364, USA
* Pawspice at VCA Coast Animal Hospital, Hermosa Beach, CA 90254.
E-mail address: pawspice@msn.com

Vet Clin Small Anim 41 (2011) 519–529
doi:10.1016/j.cvsm.2011.03.013
0195-5616/11/$ – see front matter © 2011 Elsevier Inc. All rights reserved.

vetsmall.theclinics.com

mobility and more good days than bad days[1]) QoL scale (**Table 1**). The acronym prompts easy recall for the veterinary team (V-team) during discussions with clients.

THE HHHHHHMM QoL SCALE

How do veterinarians know when a chronic, comorbid condition starts to ruin a pet's QoL? Most older pets have 1 or more comorbid conditions such as painful osteoarthritis (OA), obesity, or organ disease. When a life-limiting disease or cancer and its related treatment exert added burdens on a compromised pet, how will the effect on QoL be determined? Who is capable of monitoring that pet? How are they making their decisions? At what point should caregivers abandon further curative therapy? What obligation does the V-team have to provide palliative care or preserve their clients' hope for a beloved pet's well-being? Veterinarians are frequently asked, "When is the right time to euthanize my beloved pet? How will I know?" These questions can be emotionally draining and difficult to answer without assessment guidance

Table 1 The HHHHHMM QoL scale. Pet caregivers can use this scale to evaluate the success of their Pawspice program. Patients are scored on a scale of 1 to 10	
Score	Criterion
H: 0–10	Hurt: adequate pain control, including breathing ability, is first and foremost on the scale. Is the pet's pain successfully managed? Is oxygen necessary?
H: 0–10	Hunger: is the pet eating enough? Does hand feeding help? Does the patient require a feeding tube?
H: 0–10	Hydration: is the patient dehydrated? For patients not drinking enough water, use subcutaneous fluids once or twice daily to supplement fluid intake
H: 0–10	Hygiene: the patient should be kept brushed and cleaned, particularly after elimination, avoid pressure sores and keep all wounds clean
H: 0–10	Happiness: does the pet express joy and interest? Is it responsive to things around it (eg, family, toys)? Is the pet depressed, lonely, anxious, bored, or afraid? Can the pet's bed be near the kitchen and moved near family activities so as not to be isolated?
M: 0–10	Mobility: can the patient get up without assistance? Does the pet need human or mechanical help, such as a cart? Does it want to go for a walk? Is it having seizures or stumbling? Some caregivers believe euthanasia is preferable to amputation, but an animal with limited mobility may still be alert and responsive and can have a good QoL as long as the family is committed to quality care
M: 0–10	More good days than bad: when bad days outnumber good days, QoL might be too compromised. When a healthy human-animal bond is no longer possible, the caregiver must be made aware that the end is near. The decision needs to be made if the pet is suffering. If death comes peacefully and painlessly, that is OK
Total	A total >35 points is an acceptable QoL for pets to maintain a good Pawspice

Adapted from Villalobos A, Kaplan L. Canine and feline geriatric oncology: honoring the human-animal bond. Ames (IA): Blackwell Publishing; 2007. Table 10.1, p. 304. Original article, Villalobos A. QoL scale helps make final call, VPN, 09/2004; with permission.

and decision aids. Today's clients browse and use decision aids from the Internet while their attending doctor might be unaware.[2]

Based on their species, animals have certain needs and desires that should be recognized and respected by their caretakers. The Five Freedoms of Animal Welfare developed in the United Kingdom are: (1) freedom from hunger and thirst, (2) Freedom from discomfort, (3) freedom from pain, injury, or disease, (4) freedom to express normal behavior, (5) freedom from fear and distress (fawc.org.uk/freedoms.htm). The Five Freedoms list was developed for farm animals, but it is applicable for all pets. If pet owners, with their hospice V-teams, are able to maintain these basic desires with a satisfactory level of comfort, then there is justification in preserving the life of a beloved ill pet during the steady decline toward death. How can pet care-givers confidently determine what is satisfactory?

The HHHHHMM QoL scale (see **Table 1**) provides useful guidelines for caregivers to help sustain a positive and rewarding relationship that nurtures the human-animal bond at the end of life. This simple-to-use tool recruits the entire V-team to discuss criteria in the examination room. It provides a framework to assess various aspects of home care and the well-being of failing patients. The straightforward QoL scale, with its objective scoring, automatically helps family members face reality without guilt feelings or confusion. It asks people to quantify their observations as they struggle through the difficult decision-making process of whether to maintain their pet in decline or to elect the gift of euthanasia.

The V-team can use the QoL scale to provide specific guidance for family members to correct deficient criteria by at least 30% to 60%. These improvements can create a remarkable rejuvenation in a failing pet's well-being. V-team staff might say some-thing like, "Our goal is to educate you and help you maintain the best QoL possible for Bella's comfort with no hurt, hunger, or hydration problems and good hygiene and happiness. We'll help you with mobility issues. We want Bella to have more good days than bad days." The V-team can teach clients to assess and control pain and provide good nutritional and hydration support. When discussing hygiene, staff can demonstrate wound care techniques; teach clients to prevent decubital ulcers by using egg crate mattresses, soft bedding, and body rotation; and teach clients to prevent self-soiling with strategic elevation, absorbent towels, diapers, and so forth.

When family members use the QoL scale to assess the basic criteria, they may realize that they need to improve certain aspects of their home care to properly main-tain their pet's comfort. A well-managed end-of-life care program allows more quality time for tender, private moments and sweet conversation to be shared between family members and their beloved pet.

MONITORING AND CORRECTING PATIENT CRITERIA WITH THE QoL SCALE

The most important QoL factors to educate pet owners to competently monitor are recognizing pain, including proper respiration; maintaining adequate nutrition and hydration; and detection of sepsis, depression, and frustration. The V-team must ask themselves these questions: if this pet owner was properly trained to monitor vital func-tions, temperature, administer subcutaneous fluids, and give prescribed medications and sufficient nutrition, can this pet have QoL and live longer at home? Is it in the pet's best interest to be at home with familiar, consistent routine and surroundings[3]? Should the pet remain in the hospital? Hospitalized pets are susceptible to the same hospitalism syndrome (failure to thrive) that infants and geriatric people acquire when hospitalized. Hospitalism occurs because infants and geriatric patients were only handled when wet, being fed, or medicated. Efforts to avoid hospitalism for end-of-life pets are justified. These efforts include offering the hospice option for pets in subacute and acute terminal crises. Dogs with hemoabdomen from ruptured splenic or hepatic hemangiosarcoma are often reluctantly euthanized in the either/or model after triage at emergency clinics. If surgery is declined because of the poor prognosis or financial constraints, there should be a third option. Upset pet owners feel rushed, and pushed to euthanize their pet in the either/or model. If the family wants more time, patients can and should be released, with a signed consent form, to go home with steroids, visceral pain medication, and a belly wrap for the home hospice vigil and home euthanasia. Occasionally, red blood cells are resorbed and some dogs might rally for a week or 2 and provide their families with a more extended farewell.

No Hurt: Pain Assessment Techniques

To prevent suffering, it needs to be recognized. Pain assessment aids and questionnaires for use by pet owners may yield variable results because of owner ignorance, inexperience, and bias. The V-team should assess for all types of pain during the examination while asking questions and educating pet owners to empower them to detect their pet's pain. The desperate pain of respiratory distress or pulmonary embolism is the top priority, outweighing all other criteria. Respiratory distress must be relieved or there is no QoL for the pet and no humane justification to continue the hospice.

When pet owners feel that their pets are having trouble breathing or might be in pain, the V-team should acknowledge the pet owners for knowing their pets intimately. Patients who have cancer often feel their pain more resoundingly at night. Cancer pain has multiple pathways and involves stimulation of nociceptors, tissue damage, inflammation, peripheral and central sensitization, and wind-up pain making superficial attempts at pain management insufficient. Alleviation of cancer pain requires multimodality therapy tailored to the patient's condition and organ function. It should be provided preemptively to observe whether the patient feels and sleeps better with therapy.

Several pain scales for V-team assessment of acute and chronic pain in dogs and cats are available from Colorado State University (CSU), North Carolina State University, University of Montreal, Europe, and other places. Education on the multiple pathways and plasticity of chronic pain in various diseases and using available assessment techniques will increase V-team awareness and detection of previously undiagnosed and undertreated pain in ill, aging, and terminal pets.[4] Detection of pain in cats is more difficult. For instance, physical examination may not detect feline OA pain.[5] The key is to ask specific questions about subtle mobility and behavior changes.[6]

A unique description of OA-related lesions in cats using magnetic resonance imaging found that structure does not dictate pain and functional evaluations using gait analysis and accelerometry.[7]

Pain may respond to 1 or a combination of pharmaceuticals, nutraceuticals, physical (rehabilitation) therapy, and complementary medicine techniques such as acupuncture, chiropractic, low-level laser therapy, and low-level sonic vertical vibration therapy. Pain management is an extensive topic with recent board certification via the International Veterinary Association of Pain Management (IVAPM). Pain management is discussed to greater detail in many other resources[8,9] and elsewhere in this issue in the articles by Downing.

No Hunger: Dealing with Anorexia and Poor Nutrition

Monitoring the patient's weight is essential. Malnutrition, weight loss, and cachexia develop quickly in anorectic animals if pet owners are not educated regarding minimum caloric intake or resting energy requirement (RER). Appetite stimulants such as mirtazipine at one-eighth of a tablet per cat once a day or at the end of the day, or ciproheptidine at 1/4 to 1/2 of a tablet twice a day per cat along with coaxing, hand feeding, or gentle force-feeding with wholesome, flavorful foods might restore and maintain adequate nutrition intake. If the pet drops 10% of body weight or more and is not consuming its RER for 3 to 5 days, then feeding tube placement must be considered as the next best option to prevent decline from starvation. Enteral feeding maintains gut health. Cats suffer from anorexia readily and often do well with esophageal feeding tubes. The technique has been modified several times since it was first described.[10] Some doctors and pet owners eschew the idea of feeding tubes for end-of-life care; however, the patient needs adequate nutrition if the hospice is to continue. Use blended or liquid recovery diets to help maintain proper nutritional and caloric intake.

Nutritional support and immunonutrition may be the only therapies that pet owners may allow for their end-of-life pet. Old age, illness, stress, and fatigue lower the immune status of animals. This result is characterized by a reduced ability to present antigen to T lymphocytes. Aging and obesity are associated with low-level chronic inflammation. These comorbid conditions create a less-efficient or altered immune response, placing the patient at risk for infections, diabetes, autoimmune diseases, and neoplasia. Providing good nutrition and modulating nutraceuticals for ill, geriatric, and ambulatory end-of-life patients can actively and positively influence their innate immune system receptors located in the gut, which is the largest immune organ in the body. Many pet owners are pleased with the QoL benefits that high-quality, targeted immunonutrition brings to their aging and ill pets.[11]

Every effort should be made to control nausea and vomiting that may be contributing to the pet's anorexia. Maropitant (Cerenia) acts centrally as an antiemetic and antinausea agent. Recently, maropitant has been documented to provide a significant visceral analgesia effect, providing added comfort for palliative and hospice patients.[12] Reglan, Anzimet, and Zofran are widely used and excellent antiemetics. Famotidine and sucralfate may also help provide gastrointestinal comfort care.

No Hydration Problems

Educate clients about adequate fluid intake per kilogram (22 mL/kg/d). Educate clients to assess for hydration by the pinch method. Teach subcutaneous (SQ) fluid techniques as a way to supplement the fluid intake of ailing pets. This saves the client money and keeps the pet healthier. Giving SQ fluids can make a huge difference in QoL.

Good Hygiene

Some pets, especially cats with oral cancer, have difficulty keeping clean. They are demoralized. The odor and hypersalivation associated with necrotic, oral tumors can be offensive and cause social rejection by family members. Use antibiotics to control odor. Dampen a sponge with diluted lemon juice and hydrogen peroxide. Gently stroke the face, paws, and legs of the patient (mother tongue). This technique helps clean the fur and soothe the unkempt cat. Dogs enjoy facial grooming and massage as well.

If the patient has an open, weeping, necrotic nonmalignant, chronic wound, it may need bacterial culture, debridement, and partial closure to promote healing. Teach owners the modern principles of wound care. Gentle cleaning with saline rinses or sprays, wound surfactants to lift away bacteria without tissue damage, and moist bandages to promote healing are helpful.[13] Malignant wounds are difficult to care for. Some respond to palliative radiation therapy. Some need intense pain control because of haunting allodyna. Many pets need protective bandages or body suits to avoid self-mutilation. This topic is discussed in the article by Adams and McClenahan elsewhere in this issue.

Happiness: The Serum Fun Factors

QoL includes psychosocial well-being, which might be contentment enriched with fun. Happiness generates physiologic and mental well-being and longer survival times.[14] This author likes to call the effect of happiness the serum fun factors. It is important to instruct pet owners to create frequent moments of enjoyment for their pets. Many end-of-life pets cheer up and look forward to these uplifting events. The Pawspice model follows pediatric cancer care, which strives to entertain children with enjoyable programs. End-of-life pets need to derive some pleasure from being alive and some enjoyment (being petted and talked to) for a part of their day and to have fun if at all possible.[15] Ask these questions: does the pet express joy and show interest in the family? Is the pet responsive to caressing and the environment? Is the pet depressed, lonely, anxious, bored, or afraid? Is the pet isolated? Can the pet's bed be moved closer to family activities?

Mobility: A Variable Criterion

The necessity for mobility seems to be dependent on the weight and species of the patient. Cats and small lap dogs can and do enjoy life with much less need for handling their own mobility than large and giant breed dogs. The QoL scale score for mobility is acceptable from 0 to 10. The answer to the mobility question has viable and variable scenarios. "She would be impossible to pick up and carry around. For the same reason (her size) her ability to control her urine and stool output is important." This statement was made by Dr Robin Downing regarding Murphy, her Great Dane, who survived osteosarcoma for 3 years and became the CSU Limb Sparing Mascot.

Utilitarian pet owners may be rigid in their mobility requirements for their dog(s). Some pet owners are regretfully willing to euthanize their pet rather than elect amputation of a limb. Some pet owners might unwittingly allow their dog to bear a painful limb for months before electing the gift of euthanasia. Some pet owners and cultures (eg, Sweden) have the honest, but teleologic, feeling that amputation is mutilation. They believe that amputation is not fair to the animal.[16]

Nursing care of immobile large dogs is demanding and may be physically impossible for many pet owners to deal with. Can the dog be lifted up and taken outdoors for daily eliminations? Will a harness, a sling, or cart help? Can the cat be helped into the litter box to eliminate with assistance? Is there a feline QoL scale[17]? Is medication helping? Is there a schedule with family members willing to change the position and rotate the pet every 2 hours? Atelectasis and decubital ulcers must be avoided. Is the bedding material soft enough? Can an egg crate mattress be used and set up properly to avoid decubital ulcers? Is there a role for a pet mobility cart or an Evans standing cart (jorvet.com)? These items can greatly facilitate keeping pets with limited mobility and allows them to experience joy and well-being. For more in-depth information, read the article by Dr Tamara S. Shearer elsewhere in this issue.

More Good Days than Bad Days

If a terminal pet experiences more than 3 to 5 bad days in a row, QoL is too compromised to continue the hospice and the HHHHHMM QoL score drops to less than 35. When a healthy, 2-way interactive human-animal bond is no longer possible, it is time let go. All family members who make the effort to work with the QoL scale will become self-aware that the end is near. The final decision needs to be made if the pet suffers breakthrough pain despite adjusted multimodal analgesics. The veterinary oath clearly binds the V-team to prevent suffering. When death draws near, pets can be given heavy sedation to relax them before receiving the gift of a bond-centered euthanasia at home, at their local pet hospital, or at an emergency clinic.

Do Not Let a Pet Suffer to Death

Because of cultural, religious, or personal beliefs, a few pet owners and a small contingent of veterinarians and counselors prefer natural death to assisted death. When a pet owner has this bias, it is difficult and disheartening for the V-team to compromise their personal ethics to justify caring for an emaciated, dehydrated, depressed, terminal patient that must endure further deterioration, pointless pain, and suffering until liberated by death. When a veterinarian or pet hospice counselor has this bias, it affects how they think and how they influence their client's decision making for their terminal pet when the bad days persist without any good days. The attending doctor or counselor may be sincerely attempting to respect the owner's wishes while caring for the patient. However, they may be totally unaware of how they are manipulating their clients into withholding the mercy of euthanasia for the pet, if or when it is needed. This situation is another version of the either/or scenarios mentioned earlier that withhold hospice as a third option from family members for incurable pets and pets in acute and subacute crisis. By withholding options in the either/or model, the attending doctors are practicing the strongest form of coercion.[18]

It is fortunate if a pet is able to die at home in a painless and peaceful state. This outcome is ideal and acceptable, and is most predictable when using veterinary supervision that includes proper pain control and home euthanasia services. Not all terminal animals receive professional help or are able to pass away peacefully and naturally at home. Some dying pets suffer greatly and go into terrible respiratory distress and thrash about and become agonal before death. This outcome is not natural. In the wild, debilitated animals naturally become prey. Sick animals in the wild do not survive long enough in decline to endure the angst of suffering to death. Witnessing a house pet's traumatic death can be a horrible experience for loving family members who did not want their beloved pet to suffer this pointless indignity without having the option of humane euthanasia. Family members feel guilty and are haunted for years with these harsh memories. The right thing to do for pet owners who prefer a natural death is to provide adequate pain medication, instruct them to use the QoL scale, and have a backup plan in case their pet goes into a distressful crisis and needs professional help to change worlds. Caregivers should know where to go 24/7 for immediate assistance for the gift of euthanasia to avoid a beloved pet's futile and unnecessary suffering to death.

EMOTIONAL SUBJECTIVE-OBJECTIVE-ASSESS PLAN FOR ASSESSMENT OF CLIENTS

An essential part of pet hospice and Pawspice includes emotional support of family members. Most pet owners who seek end-of-life care have strong attachment to their pets. When that attachment is threatened by disease or cancer, distress is a natural consequence.[19] The V-team should expect that end-of-life pet owners are dealing with emotional issues such as anxiety, anticipatory grief, worry, fear, and feelings of being inadequate to meet the demands of their sick pet's care.[20] To complicate matters more, the recession has financially humbled millions of families who worry about being unable to afford the cost of care for their beloved pets.

Because most members of the V-team are not trained in psychology, it is helpful to use assessment tools. In 2000, Laurel Lagoni and Carolyn Butler, who directed the Argus Center at CSU, adapted the subjective-objective-assess plan (SOAP) for medical charts, as a format to assess the emotional status of clients. They proposed questions for the V-team to assess client emotions. This set of questions became the Emotional SOAP (E-SOAP) (**Table 2**). Although CSU uses the Calgary-Cambridge Guide to the Medical Interview for instruction (skillscascade.com/handouts/Calgary-cambridgeframework.pdf), Lagoni and Butler are happy to contribute their E-SOAP assessment tool for the hospice V-team.

Every member of the hospice V-team should recognize, acknowledge, and respect their clients' human-animal bond. The V-team needs to understand that the human

Table 2
Emotional SOAP

Medical Variable		Emotional Variables
How do you think this animal is doing? Physical appearance Body language and demeanor Interactions with the owner What is the reason for this visit? What does your intuition tell you about this patient?	**S | S** **Subjective** *What do you feel/notice/suspect?*	How do you think this owner is doing? Physical appearance Body language and demeanor Interactions with the pet What might the owner need from you? What does your intuition tell you about this owner?
What does the owner tell you about this animal and the presenting problem? What is the important medical history? What do you find on physical examination?	**O | O** **Objective** *What are the facts?*	What does the owner tell you about his/her feelings and relationship with this pet? What is the important emotional history? What do you find on the Family-Pet Relationship Information Form?
What past experiences and knowledge can you draw on for this case? What diagnosis can you rule in based on your collected information?	**A | A** **Assessment** *What can you conclude from an overall synthesis of the data?*	What past experiences and knowledge can you draw on for this case? What emotional needs and support-based services can you rule in as potentially applicable to this case?
What options can you recommend and offer for treatment? What is the time frame for treatment? What is the cost of treatment? What is the treatment follow-up?	**P | P** **Plan** *What treatment and support options are available to owners?*	What options/resources (supportive people, finances, time) are available to this owner? What is the time frame for support? What is the cost of the recommended support services? What is the support follow-up?

Courtesy of Laurel Lagoni and Carolyn Butler, Fort Collins, CO.

emotions they witness are a normal part of every recheck and follow-up in end-of-life care. It is also important to realize that emotions can be obvious, well-hidden, and, occasionally, out of control. It is best to consciously begin the E-SOAP when entering the examination room. Asking questions with kindness and sincerity may reveal the hidden emotions and attachment that are the basic drivers of the end-of-life program.

S: subjective. Be aware of how you feel about or sense your client's emotional state. What do you notice about the client's appearance? What do you suspect this client may need? The subjective questions to ask yourself include How do I think this pet owner is doing? What might this person need from me or the V-team? What does my intuition tell me about this pet owner? What do I notice about my client's physical appearance, their body language and demeanor, and interactions with their pet? Know that some people mask fear and nervousness by asking numerous questions or they ask the same question rephrased. Others may act out or be submissive or react with inappropriate laughter. If you suspect this behavior, it is important to ask questions such as, How are you doing with all this stress?

O: objective. Questions must be asked to establish the facts. What does the owner tell you? What is the important emotional history? How does this pet fit into the pet owner's life? What is their human-animal relationship like? Does the pet sleep on the bed? Are there other pets in the household? Does the pet owner have a family? Is the pet like a child to this person?

A: assess. Gathering the subjective and objective information in the E-SOAP helps to evaluate whether there is emotional discord or trauma in the situation. The information will help the attending doctor and staff to determine whether the family or the primary caretaker's attitude is accepting of their pet's pending death.

P: plan. Developing an appropriate plan may not be easy. The either/or plan would be to either offer support yourself or to refer the client for counseling. This author firmly believes that all members of hospice V-teams should be willing and able to provide on-the-spot emotional support for their clients. Emotional support is readily accomplished by offering clients sincere acknowledgment and validation of the special bond that they share with their beloved pet. Say something like: "We know that you and Bella share a very special bond. It's natural for you to feel heartbroken. We understand your pain." In addition, the V-team should, at least superficially, address the client's basic emotional concerns. Many pet owners ruin good days of their pet's life by suffering with anticipatory grief. Point this out. Say something like: "Try to focus on the good days because Bella is very much alive and still with you right now!" When clients remain depressed or upset and are unable to derive any comfort from the V-team's efforts, then refer them for professional counseling. Be prepared to give some immediate grief assistance and hand the client a pet loss workbook or a grief pamphlet. Keep this necessary information handy for clients when professional grief counseling is indicated, especially if they are overly depressed or suicidal. Present this information with concern and compassion for their grief.[20]

Laurie Kaplan, MSC, who organized and edited the manuscript for this author's client-friendly veterinary textbook, *Canine and Feline Geriatric Oncology: Honoring the Human-Animal Bond,*[1] is a pet loss therapist, family counselor, and author. Laurie's pet loss workbook, *So Easy to Love, So Hard to Lose,* is an excellent grief processing tool for pet owners who need and want help dealing with their intense grief. Laurie's instructional book, *Help Your Dog Fight Cancer,* has helped thousands of pet owners manage the day-in and day-out home care of sick dogs. Her books are available on line at helpyourdogfightcancer.com. *Pets Living with Cancer: A Pet Owner's Guide,* by Dr Robin Downing (published by AAHA Press) and *Speaking for Spot* by Dr Nancy Kay, ACVIM, are also helpful resources for clients.

The E-SOAP is a handy assessment tool (see **Table 2**) The first 2 steps (subjective and objective) provide the assessment technique for helping the V-team gather intuitive and objective information about the pet owners' emotional QoL. The third and fourth steps (assess and plan) provide the V-team with the authority and support to assess and make a plan of action to provide clients who are caring for terminal pets with the emotional support that they deserve. In this author's experience, few pet owners seek professional help for themselves. They make excuses or say they cannot afford to spend more money. For this reason, effective and spontaneous communication skills are important and should be required for every member of the hospice V-team. Each person who provides care for end-of-life pets should be able to, at the very least, offer kind and compassionate words of comfort to clients with a hand on the shoulder or an appropriate hug. Grief-stricken clients desperately need empathy and comfort, when they need it, which is generally on the spot.

USE A FRAMEWORK FOR ETHICAL DECISION MAKING

One can access the Framework for Ethical Decision Making by Mike McDonald at www.ethics.ubc.ca by clicking *Documents* then *Framework for Ethical Decision Making*. The agenda urges all involved parties, including attending doctors, specialists, hospital staff, and the family, to reach consensus and comfort with their decisions, especially in their final decisions. If there is reluctance or disagreement, the attending doctor needs to work harder to provide the family with more options. Adapting this framework for animals, the V-team must prioritize the pet's best interests and QoL. Embracing a compassionate and professional attitude, all V-teams should offer palliative or hospice care for incurable patients. The more hopeful clients with ambulatory pets might prefer Pawspice care, which combines gentler versions of standard care, immunonutrition, and palliative care, and which transitions into hospice when needed.[21] There is no perfect choice, but the course taken should be reasonably acceptable to those involved in the circumstances (McDonald M. An ethical decision making framework [unpublished document], University of British Columbia Center for Applied Ethics, 2002, http://www.ethics.ubc.ca).

SUMMARY

V-teams and pet owners have an ethical obligation to maintain QoL for terminal pets. This obligation can be fulfilled by using QoL assessment techniques. The HHHHHMM QoL scale is a user-friendly tool that directs caregivers to assess and score their pet on essential criteria: monthly, weekly, daily, or hourly on an as-needed basis. The V-team can educate the family to conscientiously monitor and improve their pet's QoL score if suboptimal to an acceptable status. The hospice V-team can also assess the emotional QoL of pet owners using the E-SOAP technique and support the emotional needs of family members. The V-team can validate the human-animal bond. Using the Framework for Ethical Decision Making can help clients feel justified with keeping their feeble pets in hospice and out of the mindless machinery of medicine that coerces so many human patients and their families into electing overtreatment at the end of life.[22] "Primum non nocere. First, do no harm." Hippocrates.

REFERENCES

1. Villalobos A, Kaplan L. Canine and feline geriatric oncology: honoring the human-animal bond. Hoboken (NY): Blackwell Publishing (Wiley-Blackwell); 2007.

2. Brace C, Schmocker S, Huang H. Physicians' awareness and attitudes toward decision aids for patients with cancer. J Clin Oncol 2010;28:2286–92.
3. Stella JL, Lord LK, Buffington CA. Sickness behaviors in response to unusual external events in healthy cats and cats with feline interstitial cystitis. J Am Vet Med Assoc 2011;238(1):67–73.
4. Lascelles BD. Supportive care for the cancer patient. In: Withrow SJ, Vail DM, editors. Small animal clinical oncology. 4th edition. St Louis (MO): Saunders Elsevier; 2007. p. 291–346. Chapter 16.
5. Klinck MP, Frank D, Rialland P, et al. Psychometric validation of pain and quality of life questionnaires in osteoarthritic cats. ACVB/ABSAB Veterinary Behavior Symposium. Atlanta (GA), July 30, 2010.
6. Klinck MP, Frank D, Guillot M, et al. Owner-observed behavior changes in the home as tools in the diagnosis and therapeutic monitoring of feline osteoarthritis. University of Montreal, with permission, pending validation and publication. Montreal, Canada, 2010.
7. Guillot M. Evaluation of osteoarthritis-associated pain in cats: novel information from a pilot study. University of Montreal, with permission, pending validation and publication. Montreal, Canada, 2010.
8. Gaynor JS, Muir WW. Handbook of veterinary pain management. St Louis (MO): Mosby Elsevier; 2008.
9. Jones K, Villalobos A, Ellenbogan T, et al. IVAPM guidelines: pain management for end of life care. Nashville (TN): IVAPM Web site; 2011.
10. Rawlings CA. Percutaneous placement of a midcervical esophagostomy tube: new technique and representative cases. J Am Anim Hosp Assoc 1993;29. 526–30.
11. Twedt D. Chronic vomiting: a practical clinical approach, SVMA syllabus. Denver (CO): SVMA; 2011.
12. Satyaraj E. Immunonutrition, Nestle Purina Nutrition Forum: changing paradigms in nutrition. St Louis (MO): Nestle Purina; 2008.
13. Hendrickson DA. Advanced wound care, SVMA syllabus. Denver (CO): SVMA; 2011.
14. McMillan FD. Emotional maltreatment in animals. In: McMillan FD, editor. Mental health and well-being in animals. Ames (IA): Blackwell Publishing; 2005. p. 167–79. Chapter 12.
15. Rollin BE. Animal happiness, a philosophical view. In: McMillan FD, editor. Mental health and well being in animals. Ames (IA): Blackwell Publishing; 2005. p. 235–42.
16. Rollin BE. Oncology and ethics. AVMA Proceedings. 2004.
17. Villalobos A. Feline Pawspice. In: August JR, editor. Feline internal medicine, vol. 6. St Louis (MO): Saunders Elsevier; 2009. p. 811–24. Chapter 68.
18. Yeates JW, Main DC. The ethics of influencing clients. Views: Commentary. J Am Vet Med Assoc 2010;237(3):263–7.
19. Voith VL. Attachment of people to companion animals. Vet Clin North Am Small Anim Pract 1985;15(2):289–95.
20. Choen SP, Fudin CE, editors. Animal illness and human emotion. Prob Vet Med 1991;3(1):1–37.
21. Villalobos AE. "Pawspice" an end of life care program for terminal patients. In: Withrow JS, Vail DM, editors. Withrow & MacEwen's small animal clinical oncology. 4th edition. St Louis (MO): Saunders/Elsevier; 2007. p. 327–33.
22. Temel JS. Early palliative care for patients with metastatic non–small-cell lung cancer. N Engl J Med 2010;363(8):733–42.

Pain Management for Veterinary Palliative Care and Hospice Patients

Robin Downing, DVM, CCRP, CPE

KEYWORDS

• Palliative care • Maladaptive pain • Windup • End-of-life

Our obligation as veterinary health care providers is to advocate on behalf of beings that cannot advocate for themselves. Dr Lloyd E. Davis wrote in 1983[1] that "[o]ne of the psychological curiosities of therapeutic decision making is the withholding of analgesic drugs, because the clinician is not absolutely certain that the animal is experiencing pain. Yet the same individual will administer antibiotics without documenting the presence of a bacterial infection. Pain and suffering constitute the only situation in which I believe that, if in doubt, one should go ahead and treat."

Palliative care in the health care arena means to treat the symptoms of a disease without the intention of curing it. In the context of end-of-life care, palliative strategies are designed to alleviate any symptoms of disease that compromise the comfort of the patient, whether or not the disease is a life-limiting condition that results in death. Palliative care maximizes quality of life in those animal patients who are approaching their death.[2] Applying the principles and practices of palliative care and hospice to pets is a relatively new phenomenon. And because pain is a major factor in diminished quality of life, pain management plays a critical role in applying palliative care and hospice principles to pets.

Appropriate pain management at the end of life and in the face of life-limiting disease is a function of striking a balance between risks and benefits. For instance, a palliative care or hospice patient might benefit from nonsteroidal antiinflammatory drugs (NSAIDs) despite safety concerns. It may be that the benefit of taking the NSAID in terms of pain relief and reduction of inflammation is worth the potential risk to kidney and liver function in order to maximize quality of life. Another aspect of achieving balance during palliative care occurs during the use of narcotics for pain as we do our best to achieve adequate pain control without creating a state of sedation or somnambulance.

The author has nothing to disclose.

The Downing Center for Animal Pain Management, LLC, 415 Main Street, Windsor, CO 80550, USA

E-mail address: drrobin@downingcenter.com

Vet Clin Small Anim 41 (2011) 531–550

doi:10.1016/j.cvsm.2011.03.010

The World Health Organization defines palliative care as "active total care of patients whose disease is not responsive to curative treatment. Control of pain...is paramount. The goal of palliative care is achievement of the best quality of life for patients and their families...Palliative care provides relief from pain and other distressing symptoms." (extracted from *Cancer Pain Relief and Palliative Care*. Technical Report Series 804. Geneva, Switzerland: World Health Organization; 1990).

One step that must be taken as a pet enters palliative care and hospice is the articulation of goals of care; crafting the goals of care may involve developing a formal document, or it may require only a simple outline. These goals vary from family to family, but it is reasonable to expect some commonality. Examples of goals of care that may be applied to the veterinary patient include the following: longer life, relief of symptoms, improved mobility, improved appetite, and good patient hygiene.[3] Regardless of the specific goals of care, the overarching requirement of palliative and hospice care is the relief and prevention of suffering.

OVERVIEW OF PAIN

When considering pain and how to prevent or relieve it, we need to start with the most commonly cited definition. According to the International Association for the Study of Pain, pain is "...an unpleasant sensory and emotional experience associated with actual or potential tissue damage, or described in terms of such damage. The inability to communicate verbally does not negate the possibility that an individual is experiencing pain and is in need of appropriate pain-relieving treatment."[4] The second half of this definition (which is, of course, the part of the definition most applicable to veterinary patients) was added several years after the first half of the definition was crafted.

An overview understanding of the physiology of pain allows the practitioner to make rational choices about how best to address an individual patient's pain management requirements. Chemical, thermal, mechanical, or electrical noxious stimuli at the periphery or on the viscera are transformed via transduction into electrical signals (action potentials) that are then carried by the afferent neurons to the dorsal horn of the spinal cord (transmission). In the dorsal horn of the spinal cord, incoming afferent signals are modified (modulation) and relayed (projected) up the spinal cord to the brainstem and brain (sensory cortex), where pain perception and memory occurs.[5] Ascending afferent signals may be blunted by descending inhibitory pathways modulated by activity in the periaqueductal gray matter (PAG) and rostral ventromedial medulla (RVM). The PAG and RVM have been shown to be involved in opiate analgesia.[6]

If the nervous system experiences an unrelenting afferent barrage, over time there are changes in the functional, chemical, and structural properties of primary sensory neurons as well as neurons in the dorsal horn and brain. This ability to change is called neuronal plasticity and is an essential component of pain perception.[7] The result of these changes in the face of painful stimuli is a state of peripheral and central sensitization in which the patient may suffer from one or all of the following phenomena:

- Allodynia: pain from a stimulus that does not normally cause pain
- Hyperesthesia: an increased sensitivity to sensation
- Hyperpathia: exaggerated pain response to a repetitive stimulus
- Neuropathic pain: spontaneous pain state resulting from damage to the peripheral or central nervous system (CNS).

Aberrant pain states seem to result from both enhanced/amplified afferent input coupled with the loss of inhibitory descending modulation as well as activation of glial cells (microglia).[7] Clifford Woolf[8] describes pain as a spectrum from adaptive (good pain) to maladaptive (bad pain) comprising 4 distinct pain types: nociceptive, inflammatory, neuropathic, and functional. Adaptive pain serves a protective purpose. Nociceptive pain is an example of adaptive pain and is the early warning mechanism of the nervous system (think about touching a hot stove and the subsequent reflexive withdrawal of the hand). Inflammatory pain, also considered adaptive pain, results from tissue damage and alerts the organism to behave in a way to support healing. On the other hand, maladaptive pain exists independent of noxious stimuli or healing of damaged tissues. Neuropathic pain results from damage to the nervous system (eg, amputation). Functional pain is the result of abnormal processing of afferent signals. Maladaptive pain does not serve a useful physiologic or protective purpose and is instead "pain as disease."[8]

Animal patients entering palliative and hospice care may experience any or all types of pain, encompassing the gamut from adaptive to maladaptive. For this reason it is imperative to review and understand the patient's medical history, both past and current, to be sensitive to any medical conditions that may contribute to pain (acute and/or chronic). Some possible sources/causes of pain in the palliative care or hospice patient include:

- trauma
- surgery
- osteoarthritis (OA)
- dental disease
- malignancy/cancer
- degenerative joint disease
- immune-mediated polyarthropathy
- congestive heart failure (difficulty breathing)
- pulmonary disease (difficulty breathing).

Pain, stress, and distress go hand in hand in the animal patient. Stress serves a protective role by focusing the animal's attention on avoiding or escaping the stressor. When the stressor is pain and the pain is ongoing or unmitigated, the pet cannot effectively escape or minimize that stress, leading to a state of distress in which biologic functions are disrupted. The adverse consequences of the pet's pain are determined by the severity and duration of the pain experience. Unrelieved distress results in suffering. There are physiologic consequences to unrelieved pain, including:

- altered behavior
- immunologic alterations
- metabolic disruptions
- neuroendocrine imbalances
- autonomic imbalance.[9]

PAIN ASSESSMENT IN THE PALLIATIVE CARE AND HOSPICE SETTING

Regardless of the root cause of the palliative care/hospice patient's pain, the practitioner must start with a careful pain assessment to determine all the uncomfortable areas on the body to create a pain management strategy that is as comprehensive as possible (**Fig. 1**).

One of the most important challenges facing the veterinary health care provider is the lack of a simple, objective, consistent tool with which to measure animal

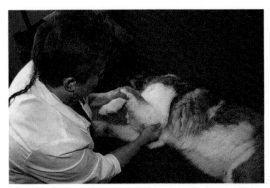

Fig. 1. Pain assessment via palpation. (*Courtesy of* Robin Downing, DVM, Windsor, CO.)

pain. In human pain medicine, pain is what the patient says it is (burning, aching, lancinating); for instance, an 8 of a possible 10. In veterinary medicine, pain is what the practitioner says it is. This situation places a huge responsibility on the practitioner's shoulders. When assessing the palliative care or hospice patient, the practitioner must include the pet owner's input in the pain equation at the first assessment, and at all subsequent reassessments. The pet owner is in the best position to provide input about the nuances of the pet's state of being and activity as well as its day-to-day comfort. It is critical for the veterinary health care provider to educate the client about behavior changes that may be seen as a result of pain. The behavioral signals that may indicate pain include (but are not limited to):

- changes in activity
- agitation
- aggression
- altered appetite
- altered interaction with family members
- posture
- changes in sleep pattern
- loss of house-training
- altered response to handling
- vocalizing
- facial expression
- lameness.[9]

(For a more comprehensive description of pain behaviors in dogs and cats please see Muir and Gaynor).[10]

When performing pain assessments on palliative care and hospice patients, there is no one right answer for evaluating animal pain. Animal pain assessment must involve more than simply observing the patient. There must be interaction with the pet. In addition, the evaluator must have some knowledge of the pet's normal behaviors to have a context within which to place the pain assessment parameters. Cancer pain (common in palliative care and hospice patients) often possesses characteristics associated with both acute and chronic pain. Assessment of cancer pain then carries with it unique challenges because both a pain scale appropriate for assessing acute pain and a pain scale best suited for chronic pain must be applied. A description and discussion of various pain scoring systems and pain scales that may be applied to animals experiencing both acute and chronic pain can be found in Mich and Hellyer (**Fig. 2**).[11]

In keeping with the recommendations in the American Animal Hospital Association/American Association of Feline Practitioners (AAHA/AAFP) *Pain Management Guidelines for Dogs and Cats*,[12] it is not so important which pain scale is chosen as it is to choose one (for the patient who has cancer, one for acute and one for chronic pain). Once acute and chronic pain scales are chosen, all members of the

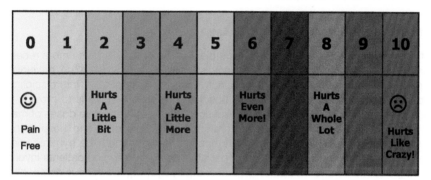

- Observe the patient's behavior, recognizing signs of pain
- Handle the patient, palpating the painful site and encourage the patient to move and respond to handling
- Record VAS value in the medical record
- Treat accordingly
- Recommend appropriate at home instructions, including the amount of exercise the patient should or should not receive
- Follow up with the same observer to determine the level of pain before and after treatment

Recognizing Pain Behaviors in Canines
- **Posture:** tail between legs, arched or hunched back, twisted body to protect painful site, drooped head, prolonged sitting position, tucked abdomen, lying in a flat, extended position
- **Temperament:** aggressive, clawing, attacking, biting, escaping
- **Vocalization:** barking, howling, moaning, whimpering
- **Locomotion:** reluctant to move, carrying one leg, lameness, unusual gait, unable to walk
- **Other:** unable to perform normal tasks, attacks other animals or people if painful area is touched, chewing painful areas, no interest in food or play

Recognizing Pain Behaviors in Felines
- **Posture:** tucked limbs, arched or hunched head and neck or back, tucked abdomen, lying flat, slumping of body, drooping of head
- **Temperament:** aggressive, biting, scratching, chewing, attacking, escaping, hiding
- **Vocalization:** crying, hissing, spitting, moaning, screaming
- **Locomotion:** reluctant to move, carrying one leg, lameness, unusual gait, unable to walk, inactive
- **Other:** unable to perform normal tasks, attacks if painful site is touched, failure to groom, chewing at painful site, "spacey" stare, no interest in food or play

Fig. 2. Visual analogue pain scale. (Copyright © The Downing Center for Animal Pain Management, LLC, Windsor, CO. Used with permission.)

veterinary health care team need to be briefed and trained in their use. Then it is up to the health care team to practice, practice, practice. Each patient who enters the veterinary practice should have a pain evaluation performed as a part of its physical examination. The acute pain scoring system can be practiced on surgical patients. The chronic pain scoring system can be applied to outpatients (no matter their presentation to the practice). In this scenario, all parties win. Surgical patients have their pain assessed and treated more consistently. Outpatients with pain are identified and therefore treated. Veterinary health care team members gain confidence in identifying both normal and painful pets. Palliative care and hospice patients benefit from greater expertise leveraged on their behalf to identify and treat both adaptive and maladaptive pain.

BUILDING THE PAIN MANAGEMENT PYRAMID

With our current understanding of the complex nature of pain, and the more recently illuminated mechanisms of pain that may specifically be targeted[8] in developing a pain management strategy, it is clear that a multimodal,[13] interdisciplinary approach best suits palliative care and hospice patients. The goal is to provide the patient with optimal comfort and pain relief using the lowest effective doses of medications. It may be useful to think of crafting a palliative care and hospice pain management strategy as building a pain management pyramid. The pyramid image is a reminder that managing the pain of palliative care and hospice patients involves layering treatments and modalities on one another, allowing the various components of the pain management plan to work synergistically. The broad base of the pyramid is comprised of the steps taken to lay a broad and strong foundation to support each addition piece/layer.

The foundation of the palliative care and hospice pain management plan contains elements that will be in place until the end of the pet's life. Most of the foundational pieces are common sense in focus. The key first step in any pain management strategy is to break the pain cycle, no matter the cause of the pain. Thus the broad base of the pain management pyramid includes essential pharmacologic elements. Because many patients with life-limiting disease that enter palliative care and hospice suffer maladaptive pain, targeted therapy that addresses multiple sites in both the peripheral and central nervous systems along the pain pathway provides the tools with which to initiate this process. It is worth keeping in mind the World Health Organization model for escalating pain management strategies as the patient's pain increases. As pain occurs nonopioids should be used. Then, as needed, mild opioids and adjuvant agents may be added, escalating to strong opioids as required until the patient is free of pain. Medications should be given by the clock rather than waiting until the patient is deemed to be painful. This is an approach that involves administering the right drug in the right dose at the right time (http://www.who.int/cancer/palliative/painladder/en/) (**Fig. 3**).

Although not all animal patients that need and deserve palliative care and hospice suffer from cancer, cancer is the leading cause of death among pets more than 8 years of age in the United States. Most of the pain management strategies in this article are applicable to all palliative care and hospice patients, whether or not they have cancer. However, some specific medications or techniques are typically restricted to patients with certain types of cancer. Cancer-related pain is often referred to as malignant pain and is emerging as its own subgroup within the human pain management community. Another consideration is that an animal patient nearing its death may experience multiple morbidities including cancer that are contributing to an ongoing pain state

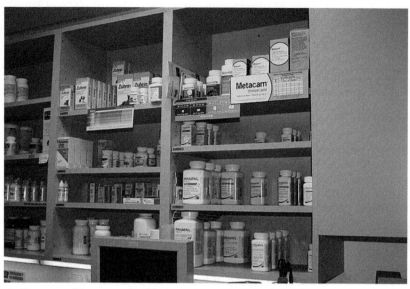

Fig. 3. Pharmacy. (*Courtesy of* Robin Downing, DVM, Windsor, CO.)

and overall compromise of quality of life. Regardless of cause, it is imperative to find pain in the pet's body wherever it resides, understand how to address the root cause whenever possible, recognize how to treat the symptoms when the root cause cannot be eliminated, and develop a comprehensive strategy to deliver the required elements that relieve suffering, provide comfort, and enhance quality of life.

PHARMACOLOGY IN PALLIATIVE CARE AND HOSPICE
NSAIDs

Approximately 20% of dogs and cats across all ages have OA. The older the pet, the higher the risk of OA. This observation means that the odds are good that patients with life-limiting disease have OA as part of their medical profile. For this reason, NSAIDs should play a role in the pain management pyramid, provided the patient does not have comorbidities that would preclude their use. The NSAIDs work by way of prostaglandin activity and are an important component of a balanced multimodal analgesic plan.[14] NSAIDS can play a role in dampening peripheral sensitization, and in addition, because of the presence of cyclooxygenase-2 (COX-2) expression in the CNS, COX-2–specific NSAIDS may assist in dampening central sensitization as well.[13] Multiple NSAIDS are currently labeled for use in dogs, so the practitioner is advised to review manufacturer's dosing guidelines. There is no compelling scientific or clinical evidence to suggest the superiority of one licensed NSAID versus another. The best NSAID for a particular patient is the NSAID that is the most effective for that patient while providing minimal or no adverse effects. An overview of NSAID use for pain is given by Budsberg.[15]

There are currently no NSAIDS labeled for long-term use in cats in the United States, although oral meloxicam is approved for feline use in Europe. The practitioner is advised to review the *International Society of Feline Medicine and AAFP Consensus Guidelines: Long-term Use of NSAIDs in Cats*[16] for guidance if a feline patient would benefit from an NSAID. The veterinarian must seek informed consent from the cat owner if NSAIDs are prescribed. Most of the medications recommended and used in the veterinary palliative care and hospice setting are not currently licensed for canine and feline use. Rather than paralyzing the practitioner to inaction, this lack merely reminds the veterinary professional of the importance of open, ongoing dialog with the pet owner to ensure and affirm informed consent.

Adjunctive Agents

As mentioned earlier, most animal patients entering palliative care and hospice are dealing with a maladaptive pain state (ie, pain that is not serving a useful physiologic function in the body). A maladaptive pain state may have multiple root causes, but the result is generally similar among individuals; these are animals whose life is an ongoing pain experience. Because a maladaptive pain state generally involves multiple areas of the nervous system in its perpetuation, it is reasonable to presume that an optimal outcome is best achieved through a strategy that targets various receptors in the nervous system. This approach allows multiple modalities targeting different nervous system components to work synergistically together more effectively than any single modality can by itself. Each additional agent is then, with rare exception, layered onto the last as the protocol evolves, taking us back to the pyramid analogy.

Adjuncts to the NSAIDs, then, are drugs that target specific receptors or areas of the nervous system to complement the action of any other agents the patient is taking.[17] The next sections address drugs commonly used for this purpose.

Gabapentin

Gabapentin is an analogue of γ-aminobutyric acid (GABA) and was first used as an antiseizure medication. However, it does not act at GABA receptors in the CNS. Gabapentin seems to bind to the α_2-δ ligand of calcium channels in the neurons of the dorsal horn of the spinal cord, thus altering calcium permeability. Its primary use in human pain medicine is in postherpetic neuralgia and painful diabetic peripheral neuropathy, although more recently it has been shown to reduce the need for opioids in the postoperative period in humans.[18] Gabapentin does not alter nociceptive threshold, so physiologic pain mechanisms and responses remain intact, but it does decrease allodynia and hyperalgesia. Although gabapentin can serve as a stand-alone agent for neuropathic pain, it seems to work most effectively as an adjunctive agent for most pain patients. Dosing of gabapentin for dogs and cats has been extrapolated from human medicine. Initial dosing ranges from 2.5 to 10 mg/kg by mouth twice or 3 times a day.[17] Pain practitioners have escalated gabapentin doses to more than 50 mg/kg by mouth 3 times a day to accommodate escalating pain in a patient. Sedation is the most common side effect of gabapentin, and generally a dose reduction is adequate to resolve this.

Gabapentin lends itself well to dose escalations as pain increases, with sedation and/or somnambulance remaining the dose-limiting side effect. Although clinical effects are seen within a day or two, maximal clinical effect typically occurs approximately two weeks after reaching therapeutic dose based on human studies.[19] Abrupt withdrawal of gabapentin can result in rebound pain in which the patient may become even more painful than before the initiation of gabapentin therapy. For this reason it is imperative to educate the client not to stop dosing gabapentin suddenly or without veterinary guidance. In patients with advanced renal disease, monitor for sedation caused by prolonged duration secondary to slower excretion. The dose may need to be reduced as renal failure advances.[20–22] This drug can be compounded for cats and small dogs.

Amantadine

Amantadine was initially used as an antiviral in humans and shows some efficacy for treating Parkinson disease. It is an N-methyl-D-aspartate (NMDA) receptor antagonist, which provides a specific target in managing maladaptive pain. The NMDA receptor has been implicated in the establishment of allodynia.[23] Amantadine may also allow for a lower dose of opioids in those patients who need them by increasing the analgesic effect of the opioid. Amantadine has been used for neuropathic pain in humans, and has been shown to be an effective adjunct to NSAIDS in canine patients with OA.[24] The dose used in dogs and cats is 3 to 5 mg/kg by mouth once daily. Amantadine does not cause sedation and seems to be well tolerated. Because it is excreted through the kidney, there is a potential for drug accumulation in patients with advanced renal disease. Monitor for anxiety, restlessness, and dry mouth, because these are signs of toxicity.[17] This drug can be compounded for cats and small dogs.

Tramadol

Tramadol is a synthetic codeine analogue analgesic. In addition to mild mu-receptor activity, tramadol inhibits norepinephrine and serotonin reuptake, much as an α_2 agonist. Because it has an exceptionally short half-life in the dog (about 1.7 hours), it must be dosed at least 3 times a day and is probably more efficacious at dosing 4 times a day. Dosing interval in the cat is reported to be every 12 hours.[25] Achieving a dosing schedule of 3 to 4 times a day may be challenging for a dog owner. For this reason, tramadol may lend itself best for use with breakthrough pain. Breakthrough pain has also been referred to as pain bursts. These are times during which the animal experiences brief escalations of pain that may or may not be related to an activity or injury. In this context, one would use tramadol as a periodic add-on during a time of increased discomfort. The dosing range for dogs is 1 to 5 mg/kg by mouth 3 to 4 times a day depending on pain intensity. Tramadol can cause sedation, and it can also cause dysphoria, especially in dogs who have experienced dysphoria with pure μ-agonists. In cats, dysphoria seems to be a common side effect of tramadol. Therefore, dosing in cats is recommended to be more conservative than in dogs: 1 to 2 mg/kg by mouth every 12 to 24 hours.[25] Because of its serotonin effects, tramadol must be used cautiously in patients taking other drugs that affect serotonin reuptake such as selegiline for cognitive dysfunction syndrome, selective serotonin reuptake inhibitors like fluoxetine for behavior issues, or tricyclic antidepressants (TCAs) for behavior issues or chronic maladaptive pain.

TCAs

TCAs may fill a role in the management of maladaptive pain at doses lower than are typically used for behavior issues. The analgesic effects of amitriptyline are hypothesized to be the result of inhibition of voltage-dependent sodium channels.[26] Amitriptyline also blocks the reuptake of serotonin and norepinephrine.[27] In addition, amitriptyline serves as an NMDA receptor antagonist, providing another dimension of antimaladaptive pain activity.[28] The recommended canine dose is 1 to 2 mg/kg every 12 to 24 hours, and the feline does is reported to be 2.5 to 12.5 mg per cat by mouth every 24 hours.[25]

Glucocorticoids

Glucocorticoids may play an important role in specific pain patients. They are potent antiinflammatory agents and may alleviate temporarily some of the adverse effects attributed to certain cancers. It is critical not to give corticosteroids concomitantly with NSAIDs. It is most appropriate to provide a several-day washout period between discontinuing an NSAID and beginning a corticosteroid. Prednisone/prednisolone administered orally is the most commonly applied glucocorticoid in the maladaptive pain end-of-life setting. The dosing range is enormous and depends on the condition being treated: 0.1 to 2 mg/kg by mouth once to twice daily. Glucocorticoids can be used in dogs and cats. Glucocorticoids may have an antitumor effect. It is important to be mindful of glucocorticoid side effects to alert the pet owner. Polyuria, polydypsia, and polyphagia are the most common side effects. Some side effects of long-term glucocorticoid use include muscle weakness and atrophy, development of cataracts, insulin resistance, immunosuppression, and hepatopathy.[29]

Bisphosphonates

Bisphosphonates play a special role in end-of-life care for dogs and cats with bone tumors (either primary or metastatic tumors). Most bone tumors cause osteolytic lesions. Bisphosphonates inhibit osteoclast-induced resorption, and can reduce pain in these patients. Alendronate can be used in dogs at 0.5 to 1.0 mg/kg by mouth once daily. Pamidronate is delivered intravenously over 2 to 4 hours at a dose of 1 to 2 mg/kg diluted in dogs and at a dose of 1 to 1.5 mg/kg diluted in cats. Pamidronate is delivered every 3 to 5 weeks for as long as it is effective.[27]

Opioids

Opioids are at the apex of the pain management pyramid. The opioids remain the gold standard for managing moderate to severe pain of multiple causes. This situation makes opioids an excellent choice, when needed, for helping palliative care and hospice patients. Opioids are most often described for use with cancer pain (also referred to as malignant pain), but opioids can also be used for chronic nonmalignant pain. Pure μ-agonists are given to effect, and do not have a ceiling effect; the more pain the pet has, the higher the dose that is needed and that may be given. Morphine is an effective opioid choice for dogs and cats receiving palliative and hospice care, for both short-term and long-term use. It is available in multiple formulations, including short-duration tablets and liquid as well as sustained-release tablets. In dogs, the starting oral dose of regular morphine is 1 mg/kg by mouth every 4 to 6 hours. In cats, the starting dose is 0.5 mg/kg twice to 3 times a day. Sustained-release morphine is used in dogs at 2 to 5 mg/kg by mouth twice a day.[27] When using sustained-release morphine, be sure to educate pet owners not to break or crush the tablets under any circumstances. Breaking or crushing turns sustained-release morphine into immediate-release and can result in overdose and death.

Oxycodone is an excellent oral analgesic in dogs at a dose of 0.1 to 0.3 mg/kg by mouth twice to 3 times a day. It seems to induce less sedation and dysphoria than morphine. There is not a dose described in cats.[27]

Buprenorphine is an injectable partial μ-agonist that can be delivered transmucosally with an effect nearly equivalent to intravenous dosing. It does not produce the same level of analgesia as morphine, and it does have a ceiling effect. The advantage to buprenorphine is a relatively long duration (6–12 hours) and there are good data to support its use in cats.[27,30] Because it is absorbed well transmucosally, it can be dosed easily at home by cat owners. Buprenorphine has been reported to suppress appetite in some cats with long-term use. The use of transmucosal buprenorphine in the dog is limited by the relatively dilute concentration of the available injectable solution, necessitating impractically high volumes of drug for effective delivery and absorption transmucosally. The starting dose in cats and small dogs is 0.02 mg/kg IV or transmucosally, and may be increased with escalating pain.[31]

In the past, butorphanol has been described for use in chronic maladaptive and malignant pain. The short duration of action, its effect of reversing morphine, and its lack of significant analgesia make it a poor pain management choice.[30]

Transdermal fentanyl patches have been suggested for use in cancer pain. Absorption from them is highly variable in dogs and cats, they are expensive, and they can be peeled off and ingested, which raises serious liability issues for the veterinarian. These challenges suggest that fentanyl patches may not make an effective or appropriate choice for controlling escalating pain in veterinary palliative care and hospice patients.[30]

Opioid considerations

When we add opioids to the top of the pain management pyramid, it is important to understand that liability issues may be involved. The most commonly abused drugs in the United States are not illicit drugs, but rather prescription pain medications. This situation raises serious concerns for the veterinary community in terms of the potential for drug diversion or abuse. The human pain management community is now faced with the evolution of risk evaluation and management strategies (REMS) by the US Food and Drug Administration. The goal of the REMS project is to decrease "abuse, misuse, addition and overdose deaths" from prescription opioids.[32] It is highly likely that the veterinary profession will eventually face a similar process as palliative and hospice care becomes more common and more veterinary patients receive the benefits of aggressive pharmacologic pain management. Some simple steps the veterinarian engaged in palliative care and hospice may choose to take to minimize risks in the face of opioid use include the following:

1. Follow Drug Enforcement Administration guidelines for schedule II drug use and handling to the letter at all times.
2. Conduct regular pill counts with clients to ensure that medications are being consumed at the prescribed/predicted rates.
3. Work with a limited member of pharmacists in prescribing opioids and communicate openly with them when prescriptions are written. This situation protects the veterinarian and the pharmacist by minimizing the risk of a pet owner seeking duplicate sources of opioids.
4. Become educated and remain alert to drug-seeking behaviors shown by pet owners.

DRUG DOSE ESCALATIONS AS DEATH APPROACHES

Eventually, animal patients receiving palliative and hospice care reach their time of death. As death nears, their pain may escalate. A 1995 study of human patients in an intensive care unit reported that 50% who were conscious and then subsequently died experienced moderate to severe pain during the final 3 days of life.[33] It is reasonable to presume that veterinary patients may be similarly affected. Veterinarians and their team members have a moral imperative to advocate on behalf of beings that cannot advocate for themselves. This imperative includes an ethical obligation to relieve and prevent pain and suffering. Excellent pain management is consistent with the veterinarian's oath. Extra vigilance to the presence of pain as death nears is appropriate. As palliative care and hospice patients experience escalating pain with the progression of their disease processes, they need and deserve to reap the benefit of escalating pain management strategies, including increased doses of opioids. If pain does increase, then it is reasonable to escalate doses of pain-relieving drugs to ease that pain, even if the result includes increased sedation or decreased interaction with human family members.

It is under these circumstances (increasing pain with an ongoing need to increase doses of pain-relieving medications) that a quality-of-life index/assessment serves its most important purpose.[34] When the effects of increased pain control result in the diminishing of life quality, or when pain cannot be relieved without inducing a state of unconsciousness, it is appropriate to expand discussion with the human family members to include euthanasia. Euthanasia remains the ultimate pain management strategy. Although there are pets who can be kept acceptably comfortable until they die on their own, there are many more for whom the act of living perpetuates unacceptable suffering. It is on behalf of these patients that the veterinary health care team must truly advocate to fulfill the obligation of the veterinarian's oath for "relief of animal suffering (see the article by Alice E. Villalobos elsewhere in this issue for further exploration of this topic)."

Although the doses of most of the analgesic medications used in the palliative care and hospice setting cannot be increased (eg, NSAIDs, TCAs), several medications used in this setting can be increased to meet the patient's needs as pain increases. Gabapentin is one example. As was mentioned earlier, sedation and somnambulance are the dose-limiting side effects. As an adjunct to the other medications that may be used in the palliative care and hospice setting, gabapentin serves a key role. As an example, if a painful patient receives 100 mg of gabapentin twice daily, and experiences a pain escalation as its disease progresses, gabapentin can be increased to 100 mg three times a day. If pain persists or escalates, the next step could be 200 mg twice daily. Ongoing dose increases may be accomplished by adding 50 to 100 mg per day to the total dose delivered. Patient pain reassessment should be conducted regularly, and dose adjustments are generally well tolerated even as frequently as weekly during an acute pain exacerbation. Once a patient in pain receiving gabapentin seems to be stable, the author conducts a follow-up pain assessment 2 to 3 weeks later to confirm that the patient is truly stable in its pain control.

It is critical for the veterinarian to remember that pure μ-opioids do not have a ceiling effect; they are dosed to match the patient's pain. More pain means a higher dose. Adverse effects of μ-agonists generally do not occur until or unless the dose exceeds the patient's needs. Using opioids effectively for end-of-life pain management mandates clear, open, honest, and ongoing communication with the client and all caregivers involved with a particular patient. Effectively relieving and preventing pain and suffering is one of the most rewarding activities available to the veterinary health care team.

NONPHARMACOLOGIC PAIN MANAGEMENT STRATEGIES IN PALLIATIVE CARE AND HOSPICE PATIENTS

Although breaking the maladaptive pain cycle of palliative care and hospice patients requires a multimodal pharmacologic component, the multimodal paradigm extends beyond drugs alone when building the pain management pyramid.

One important nonpharmacologic pain management tool for the patient who has cancer with primary or metastatic tumors in the bones is palliative radiation therapy. Curative radiation therapy is a rigorous process for the patient, involving anesthesia and irradiation daily or every other day. Palliative radiation is designed to provide a reasonable total dose of radiation condensed into a smaller number of doses, typically once weekly for 3 to 4 weeks. Many cancerous tumors are reasonably radiosensitive, making periodic irradiation a useful option for minimizing stress on the terminal patient and keeping tumor progression at bay. A radiation oncologist can assist in the decision making around a palliative care or hospice patient with cancer in determining whether palliative radiation is a reasonable choice.[35]

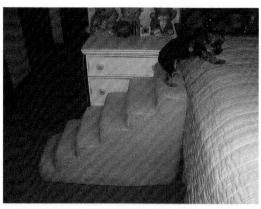

Fig. 4. Foam steps up to bed. (*Courtesy of* Robin Downing, DVM, Windsor, CO.)

Environmental management and modification provide some easy ways to enhance quality of life in the pet's everyday world. Adjusting the pet's home environment is an important foundational part of building the pain management pyramid, because these are team steps taken for the pet's comfort. Specific environmental modifications are unique to each palliative care and hospice patient, as well as unique to that pet's home environment (**Fig. 4**).

This is another example of the critical role played by open and ongoing communication between the client and the veterinary health care team. It is only through careful open-ended questioning and active listening that the pet owner and veterinary care providers can work together to make the pet's living space as comfortable as possible.

Comfort-driven home modifications are limited only by the imagination. The following list is by no means exhaustive, but provides a good foundation from which to begin:

- Cover slick floors (hardwood, tile, sheet vinyl) with nonskid surfaces (eg, rubber-backed/area rugs, permanent carpet, thin foam flooring like that found in gyms and weight rooms).
- Especially focus on nonskid additions at the top and bottom of stairs.

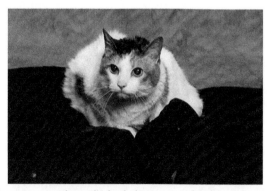

Fig. 5. Peikli resting on an orthopedic bed. (*Courtesy of* Robin Downing, DVM, Windsor, CO.)

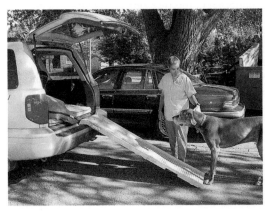

Fig. 6. Otis and ramp. (*Courtesy of* Robin Downing, DVM, Windsor, CO.)

- Block entrance to stairways (top and bottom) for pets that should negotiate stairs only with supervision.
- Provide an appropriate sleeping surface based on the pet's individual needs. Some dogs prefer orthopedic foam beds. Some dogs prefer a more plush surface. Move outdoor dogs indoors. Some cats like beds built like tents to facilitate hiding (**Fig. 5**).
- Provide a ramp for entry into and exit from the family vehicle for dogs (**Fig. 6**).
- Consider a ramp for short clusters of steps such as those leading into or out of the home.
- Raise food and water dishes to between shoulder and elbow height for animals that are still ambulatory (including cats) (**Fig. 7**).
- Consider an esophagostomy tube for those animals for which eating is itself difficult or painful or both. This is a relatively noninvasive technique that is not a heroic intervention when applied appropriately. It is amazing what a positive calorie balance can do (**Fig. 8**).
- Provide absorbent pads under pets with continence issues to wick moisture away from the body.
- Recommend absorbent pet diapers for ongoing incontinence (see article on hygiene by Downing and colleagues elsewhere in this issue).

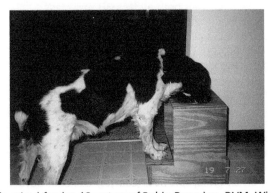

Fig. 7. Homemade raised feeder. (*Courtesy of* Robin Downing, DVM, Windsor, CO.)

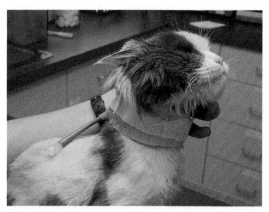

Fig. 8. Patches and her esophagostomy tube. (*Courtesy of* Robin Downing, DVM, Windsor, CO.)

- Recommend and facilitate using carts (also called wheelchairs) to maximize mobility for those pets still capable of using them. Look for a cart that is lightweight, custom-fit, and easy-on/easy-off (**Fig. 9**).

Dialog and brainstorm with the client to think through any additional strategies for helping the pet to be as comfortable and normal in its world as possible.

Physical medicine modalities as well as physiotherapy provide many additional steps that may be leveraged on the pet's behalf. Most of the physical medicine and physiotherapy modalities specifically address pain as well as movement, so they make excellent additions to the pain management pyramid. There are few limitations as to which physical therapy and other physical medicine modalities can be applied to pets in pain, including those patients receiving palliative and hospice care. Physical medicine modalities include, but are not limited to:

- Thermal therapy (heat and cold)
- Massage
- Therapeutic laser
- Therapeutic ultrasound
- Acupuncture
- Chiropractic adjustment
- Osteopathic manipulation

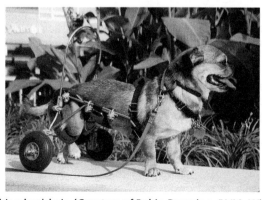

Fig. 9. Frankie in his wheelchair. (*Courtesy of* Robin Downing, DVM, Windsor, CO.)

- Passive, active, and active-assisted range of motion
- Tissue mobilization
- Stretching
- Controlled therapeutic exercise
- Myofascial trigger point release.

The reader is directed to the article by Robin Downing elsewhere in this issue dedicated to physical medicine, physiotherapy, and rehabilitation for palliative care and hospice patients.

SUMMARY

When negotiating with clients the challenges of end-of-life care for animal patients, veterinary health care providers must continually engage in ongoing evaluation of the pet's quality of life, as well as assessing (as accurately as possible) the client's quality of life to ensure that the best decisions possible are made at each step of the process. The veterinary profession's core competency is to advocate for what is in the best interest of the patient. As decisions are made about initiating a particular treatment with the intention of better managing pain, an important question that must be answered is "Do the anticipated benefits of the treatment/procedure/intervention outweigh the short-term discomfort (if any) to the patient and client?" If the answer is yes, then it is reasonable to proceed. It is important to establish fairly early in the palliative care scenario, the projected end point beyond which no additional treatment will be initiated. Although such an end point is never perfectly predictable, opening the discussion early in palliative care and hospice lays the foundation for ongoing dialog as disease progresses and the patient approaches the end of its life. It is critical for the veterinarian to remain focused on the medical risk/benefit ratio of each additional medication, treatment, or procedure so as not to create false or inappropriate outcome expectations.

The need for ongoing client education during palliative care and hospice cannot be overstated. Clear, concise summaries of each and every reassessment should be written both for the medical record and for the client. According to Edgar Dale, the US educationist who developed the cone of experience,[36] people retain only approximately 10% to 20% of what we hear (at best). However, that level of retention can be boosted to about 50% by combining reading, seeing, and hearing. In the palliative care and hospice setting, emotions tend to run high, as clients work through the process of anticipatory grief preparing for the inevitable loss of their beloved animal family member. It behooves veterinary health care providers to work together as a team with clients to assist in facing pain-related issues from as objective a perspective as possible, and that means both gathering and delivering lots of information. Encourage clients to record in a journal their day-to-day impressions of how the pet is doing overall, and how well the pet is engaging in the family's normal activities of daily living. Encourage clients to use a quality-of-life scoring system[34] to help them in their assessment and judgment of how well (or poorly) the pet is doing day to day.

By combining regular physical evaluations, including careful palpation to unmask pain, with open and honest dialog with the client about the pet's day-to-day reality, the partnership of pet owner and veterinary health care team can accept the challenge of anticipating, preventing, finding, and relieving pain in the veterinary palliative care and hospice patient. Dr James Giordano, the pain specialist famous for unlocking the role of the serotonin receptor in mediating pain, has stated that "...practicing pain medicine is an ongoing clinical experiment with an 'n' of one..." (James J. Giordano, PhD, personal conversation, 2007). His point is especially well taken within the context of the emerging practice of palliative care and hospice as applied to animal patients. Despite the uncertainties involved, helping a pet live until it dies is amazing, awe-inspiring, and humbling all at once. This is important and energizing work, and as pets continue to live longer, healthier lives, the demand increases for practitioners who are comfortable and well prepared to do the right things for the right reasons for these animals.

REFERENCES

1. Davis LE. Species differences in drug disposition as factors in alleviation of pain. In: Kitchell RL, Erickson HH, editors. Animal pain. Bethesda (MD): American Physiological Society; 1983. p. 175.
2. Kinzbrunner BM. Palliative care perspectives. In: Kuebler KK, Davis MP, Moore CD, editors. Palliative practices: an interdisciplinary approach. St Louis (MO): Elsevier Mosby; 2002. p. 3–7.
3. Forrow L, Smith HS. Pain management in end of life: palliative care. In: Warfield CA, Bajwa ZH, editors. Principles and practice of pain medicine. 2nd edition. New York: McGraw-Hill; 2004. p. 492–5.
4. IASP Task Force on Taxonomy. Part III: pain terms, a current list with definitions and notes on usage. In: Merskey H, Bogduk N, editors. Classification of chronic pain. 2nd edition. Seattle (WA): IASP Press; 1994. p. 210.
5. Muir WW. Physiology and pathophysiology of pain. In: Gaynor JS, Muir WW, editors. Handbook of veterinary pain management. 2nd edition. St Louis (MO): Mosby Elsevier; 2009. p. 14.
6. Faussett HJ. Anatomy and physiology of pain. In: Warfield CA, Bajwa ZH, editors. Principles and practice of pain medicine. 2nd edition. New York: McGraw-Hill; 2004. p. 32.
7. Woolf CJ, Salter MW. Plasticity and pain: the role of the dorsal horn. In: McMahon SB, Koltenburg M, editors. Wall and Melzack's textbook of pain. 5th edition. Philadelphia: Elsevier; 2006. p. 91, 99–101.
8. Woolf CJ. Pain: moving from symptom control toward mechanism-specific pharmacologic management. Ann Intern Med 2004;140:441–51.
9. Muir WW. Pain and stress. In: Gaynor JS, Muir WW, editors. Handbook of veterinary pain management. 2nd edition. St Louis (MO): Mosby Elsevier; 2009. p. 45–7.
10. Muir WW, Gaynor JS. Pain behaviors. In: Gaynor JS, Muir WW, editors. Handbook of veterinary pain management. 2nd edition. St Louis (MO): Mosby Elsevier; 2009. p. 62–77.
11. Mich PM, Hellyer PW. Objective, categoric methods for assessing pain and analgesia. In: Gaynor JS, Muir WW, editors. Handbook of veterinary pain management. 2nd edition. St Louis (MO): Mosby Elsevier; 2009. Chapter 6.
12. AAHA/AAFP Pain Management Guidelines Task Force. AAHA/AAFP Pain management guidelines for dogs & cats. J Am Anim Hosp Assoc 2007;43: 235–48.
13. Lamont LA. Multimodal pain management in veterinary medicine: the physiologic basis of pharmacologic therapies. Update on management of pain. Vet Clin North Am Small Anim Pract 2008;38(6):1173–86.

14. Loes MW. Acetaminophen and non-steroidal anti-inflammatory drugs. In: Wallace MS, Staats PS, editors. Pain medicine and management. New York: McGraw-Hill; 2005. p. 46–8.

15. Budsberg S. Nonsteroidal anti-inflammatory drugs. In: Gaynor JS, Muir WW, editors. Handbook of veterinary pain management. 2nd edition. St Louis (MO): Mosby Elsevier; 2009. p. 183–209.

16. Sparkes AH, Heiene R, Lascelles BD, et al. ISFM and AAFP consensus guidelines: long-term use of NSAIDs in cats. J Feline Med Surg 2010;12:521–38.

17. Gaynor JS. Other drugs used to treat pain. In: Gaynor JS, Muir WW, editors. Handbook of veterinary pain management. 2nd edition. St Louis (MO): Mosby Elsevier; 2009. p. 260–76.

18. Ho KY, Gan TJ, Habib AS. Gabapentin and postoperative pain–a systematic review of randomized controlled trials. Pain 2006;126:91–101.

19. de la Cruz MG, Bruera E. Pharmacological considerations in palliative care. In: Beaulieu P, Lussier D, Porreca F, et al, editors. Pharmacology of pain. Seattle (WA): IASP Press; 2010. p. 596.

20. Servin F. Pharmacology in special patient groups. In: Beaulieu P, Lussier D, Porreca F, et al, editors. Pharmacology of pain. Seattle (WA): IASP Press; 2010. p. 576.

21. McLean MJ. Clinical pharmacokinetics of gabapentin. Neurology 1994;44(6 Suppl 5): S17–22.

22. Radulovic LL, Türck D, von Hodenberg A, et al. Disposition of gabapentin in mice, rats, dogs, and monkeys. Drug Metab Dispos 1995;23(4):441–8.

23. Shiokawa H, Kaftan EJ, MacDermott AB, et al. NR2 subunits and NMDA receptors on lamina II inhibitory and excitatory interneurons of the mouse dorsal horn. Mol Pain 2010;6:26.

24. Lascelles BD, Gaynor JS, Smith SC, et al. Amantadine in a multimodal analgesic regimen for alleviation of refractory osteoarthritis pain in dogs. J Vet Intern Med 2008;22:53–9.

25. Mathews KA. Neuropathic pain in dogs and cats: if only they could tell us if they hurt. Update on management of pain. Vet Clin North Am Small Anim Pract 2008; 38(6):1400–2.

26. Cummins TR, Waxman SG. Sodium channels. In: Beaulieu P, Lussier D, Porreca F, et al, editors. Pharmacology of pain. Seattle (WA): IASP Press; 2010. p. 152.

27. Gaynor JS. Control of cancer pain in veterinary patients. Update on management of pain. Vet Clin North Am Small Anim Pract 2008;38(6):1434–6, 1440, 1441.

28. Watanabe HS, Abe K. Tricyclic antidepressants block NMDA receptor-mediated synaptic responses and induction of long-term potentiation in rat hippocampal slices. Neuropharmacology 1993;32(5):479–86.

29. Smith MO. Glucocorticoids. In: Gaynor JS, Muir WW, editors. Handbook of veterinary pain management. 2nd edition. St Louis (MO): Mosby Elsevier; 2009. p. 249–59.

30. Gaynor JS. Cancer pain management. In: Gaynor JS, Muir WW, editors. Handbook of veterinary pain management. 2nd edition. St Louis (MO): Mosby Elsevier; 2009. p. 406–7.

31. Robertson S. Pain management in the cat. In: Gaynor JS, Muir WW, editors. Handbook of veterinary pain management. 2nd edition. St Louis (MO): Mosby Elsevier; 2009. p. 421.

32. Food and Drug Administration. December 4, 2009, FDA/Industry Working Group (IWG) Public Meeting on Risk Evaluation and Mitigation Strategies (REMS) for Certain Opioids. 2009. Available at: http://www.fda.gov/Drugs/DrugSafety/InformationbyDrugClass/ucm193499.htm. Accessed October 15, 2010.

33. Lowenstein E. End of life ethics. In: Warfield CA, Bajwa ZH, editors. Principles and practice of pain medicine. 2nd edition. New York: McGraw-Hill; 2004. p. 860.

34. Villalobos A, Kaplan L. Palliative care: end of life "pawspice" care. In: Villalobos A, Kaplan L, editors. Canine and feline geriatric oncology: honoring the human-animal bond. Ames (IA): Blackwell Publishing; 2007. p. 303–6.

35. Villalobos A, Kaplan L. When and how to decide that a geriatric patient is terminal. In: Villalobos A, Kaplan L, editors. Canine and feline geriatric oncology: honoring the human-animal bond. Ames (IA): Blackwell Publishing; 2007. p. 289.

36. Dale Edgar. Audio-visual methods in teaching. 3rd edition. New York (NY): Holt, Rinehart, and Winston; 1969.

RECOMMENDED READINGS

AAHA/AAFP Pain Management Guidelines Task Force. AAHA/AAFP Pain management guidelines for dogs and cats. J Am Anim Hosp Assoc 2007;43:235–48.

Baldry PE. Acupuncture, trigger points and musculoskeletal pain. 3rd edition. Edinburgh (United Kingdom): Elsevier/Churchill Livingstone; 2005.

Berger AM, Portenoy RK, Weissman DE, editors. Principles & practice of palliative care & supportive oncology. 2nd edition. Philadelphia: Lippincott Williams & Wilkins; 2002.

Boswell MV, Cole BE, editors. Weiner's pain management: a practical guide for clinicians. 7th edition. Boca Raton (FL): Taylor & Francis Group; 2006.

Dommerholt J, Huijbregts P. Myofascial trigger points: pathophysiology and evidence-informed diagnosis and management. Boston: Jones and Bartlett Publishers; 2011.

Downing R. Pets living with cancer. Lakewood (CO): AAHA Press; 2000.

Mich PM, Hellyer PW. Clinical pain identification, assessment, and management. In: Ettinger SJ, Feldman EC, editors. Textbook of veterinary internal medicine: diseases of the dog and cat. 7th edition. St Louis (MO): Saunders, Elsevier; 2010. p. 48–63.

Filshie J, White A, editors. Medical acupuncture: a western scientific approach. Edinburgh (United Kingdom): Churchill Livingstone; 1998.

Fox SM. Chronic pain in small animal medicine. London: Manson Publishing LTD; 2010.

Gaynor JS, Muir WW. Handbook of veterinary pain management. 2nd edition. St Louis (MO): Mosby Elsevier; 2009.

Kuebler KK, Berry PH, Heidrich DE, editors. End of life care. Philadelphia: Saunders Elsevier; 2002.

Kuebler KK, Davis MP, Moore CD. Palliative practices: an interdisciplinary approach. St Louis (MO): Elsevier Mosby; 2005.

Ma Y, Ma M, Cho ZH. Biomedical acupuncture for pain management, an integrative approach. St Louis (MO): Elsevier Churchill Livingstone; 2005.

Marrelli TM. Hospice and palliative care handbook. St Louis (MO): Elsevier Mosby; 2005.

Mathews KA. Update on management of pain. Vet Clin North Am Small Anim Pract 2008;38(6):xi–xiii.

McMahon SB, Koltzenburg M, editors. Wall & Melzack's textbook of pain. 5th edition. Philadelphia: Elsevier; 2006.

Sluka KA, editor. Mechanisms and management of pain for the physical therapist. Seattle (WA): IASP Press; 2009.

Villalobos A, Kaplan L. Canine and feline geriatric oncology: honoring the human-animal bond. Ames (IA): Blackwell Publishing; 2007.

Wallace MS, Staats PS, editors. Pain medicine and management. New York: McGraw-Hill; 2005.

Warfield CA, Bajwa ZH, editors. Principles and practice of pain medicine. 2nd edition. New York: McGraw-Hill; 2004.

Woolf CJ. Pain: moving from symptom control toward mechanism-specific pharmacologic management. Ann Intern Med 2004;140:441–51.

Assessment and Treatment of Nonpain Conditions in Life-limiting Disease

Alice E. Villalobos, DVM, DPNAP[a,b,c,*]

KEYWORDS

- Pawspice • Quality of life • End of life • Sarcopenia
- Anorexia • Cachexia • Nausea • Decline

When a beloved pet exhibits age-related decline in vitality or is diagnosed with a terminal disease, the human-animal bond often grows stronger. Organ system failure leads as a major cause of death in older pets, whereas cancer claims 25% of dogs older than 2 years, 45% older than 10 years, and 32% of all cats.

Because the human-animal bond has become so powerful, veterinarians need to rethink how and when to recommend euthanasia. Despite the economic downturn, many families no longer accept early euthanasia of their pet as an option. Many of these same families cannot afford costly definitive or aggressive therapies and are wearier of overtreatment. Contemporary veterinarians are expected to knowingly reach for palliative care and adopt pet hospice into their option package.

The "Pawspice" philosophy, which the author introduced at the 2000 American Veterinary Medical Association meeting, focuses on *symptom* management along with a kinder, gentler, or modified approach to *standard* therapy. Many veterinarians have preconceived bias or ingrained beliefs about aging, serious illness, multiple comorbidities, and cancer, which may cause a negative or dismissive approach toward palliative treatment, especially in geriatric pets. Case by case, veterinarians and their v-teams must overcome this insensitive attitude about life-limiting disease. It would be ideal if every pet hospital would expand professional services to include palliative care or Pawspice, which easily transitions into hospice care at the final weeks, days, or hours of life.

Dr Steve Withrow of Colorado State University quoted Pogo, "*We face insurmountable opportunities*" in his keynote speech at the 2010 Veterinary Cancer Society

[a] Pawspice at VCA Coast Animal Hospital, Hermosa Beach, CA 90254, USA
[b] Pawspice at Beachside Animal Referral Center, Capistrano Beach, CA 92627, USA
[c] Animal Oncology Consultation Service at Animal Emergency and Care Center, Woodland Hills, CA 91364, USA
* Pawspice at VCA Coast Animal Hospital, Hermosa Beach, CA 90254.
E-mail address: pawspice@msn.com

Vet Clin Small Anim 41 (2011) 551–563
doi:10.1016/j.cvsm.2011.03.003
0195-5616/11/$ – see front matter © 2011 Published by Elsevier Inc.

meeting and ended with the comment, "Us old guys get stuck in our ways."[1] Yes, the time is now to dispel old negative notions. Fred J. Meyers, MD, of UC Davis, School of Medicine says, "Palliative care should not be the last resort...or about giving up. It's about increased Quality of Life and enhanced coordination of care. It is not about dying. It is about living with cancer [or terminal disease]. It's not about less care. It's more care."[2] This article describes assessment, treatment, and home management of some nonpainful life-limiting diseases, including cancer and age-related decline of vital functions in the Pawspice setting.

PRACTICAL CONSIDERATIONS

It is imperative to always speak to terminal pet caregivers in a tender, unhurried fashion because they are most likely under a tremendous amount of personal stress. They are struggling with logistics, finances of treatment, and their emotions, such as anticipatory grief, guilt, and pet loss. Each pet owner has their own personal lifestyle and tolerance considerations.[3,4] Some pet owners want to learn how to administer home care to their pets for convenience and needed financial savings, whereas others react with fear of medical procedures and needles. Some pet owners feel incapable of providing daily treatments. It might be stressful for some people to give pills to their fractious cat or stubborn dog or to give injections of insulin for a diabetic pet or to give subcutaneous (SQ) fluids to a cat or dog with failing kidneys or paraneoplastic hypercalcemia.

Placement of a feeding tube for a pet with anorexia or oral cancer may sound like heroics to one person and may make perfect sense to another. Home care for immobile pets or pets that need help to eliminate are tasks certain pet owners are willing to tackle, whereas others cannot imagine it. The v-team should provide pet owners with information to access support items, such as wound management materials, special harnesses, pet wheel chairs, ramps, egg crate mattresses, and portable oxygen tanks for pets with compromised respiration.[5]

Willingness is the most important ingredient to look for in oneself, in the v-team, and in the pet owner. Ask the clients to direct phone calls and concerns to a designated v-team member. Trained staff can handle most of the questions regarding home care procedures. A written daily treatment schedule or calendar helps keep pet owners and house call DVMs and nurses well organized. Clients should make notes on the treatment calendar regarding adverse events and responses. This practice provides attending doctors insight during recheck visits and helps to answer medical questions or adjust prescription medications. At each recheck, a quality-of-life (QoL) reassessment should be made. If the pet is in decline and scores poorly on the QoL scale, despite everyone's best efforts, it is time for the attending doctor to have a compassionate yet frank discussion about what to expect. This discussion helps the family to make plans for the final part of their Pawspice which transitions to hospice care. They can plan how and where they prefer euthanasia for their pet and make the decision for cremation or burial and other afterlife arrangements.

It is helpful to suggest a do-not-resuscitate (DNR) directive for all end-stage Pawspice patients. The DNR helps family members face reality and avoid unhelpful overtreatment in the event of a crisis. Using the quality-of-life scale (described in this author's article on Quality of Life Assessment) and the DNR directive guides the family to make the final call when it is time to give their pet the gift of euthanasia. These considerations and preparations play a role in every case discussed in this article to assure pet owners that their Pawspice pet will have good end-of-life care and a peaceful and painless passing.

ASSESSMENT OF CRITERIA

The most important criteria that pet owners need to assess and monitor are those that determine their pet's QoL. Objective use of the HHHHHMM QoL scale is discussed in great detail in the author's previous article. The acronym prompts these criteria: no Hurt, no Hunger, good Hydration, Hygiene, Happiness, Mobility, and More good days than bad days. Many end-of-life pets are readily able to experience great happiness and pleasure. They enjoy the increased love and attention and frequency of experiencing their favorite events. Happiness is important. For further information go to www.ivapm.org and review the Guidelines for Pain Management in Palliative and End-of-Life Care of Small Animals, Keri Jones, DVM, CVPP, Task Force Chair; Robin Downing, DVM, DAAPM; Tina Ellenbogen, DVM; Amir Shanan, DVM; Alice Villalobos, DVM, DPNAP, pending publication in 2011.

Clients should be forewarned that the ability to breathe properly holds priority above all other criterion. Some pet owners do not realize or recognize that their pet is experiencing respiratory distress yet this distress is ranked by humans as *the* most important QoL criterion. The v-team can train home caregivers to monitor their pets' respiration so they can deliver the care and attention that parallels the hospital. The v-team should periodically ask pet owners if they are satisfied with their Pawspice. It is important for the v-team to determine if it feels rewarding to help preserve the special human-animal bond between the clients and their beloved pets. If all of these necessary ingredients are present, then the Pawspice is a good experience to continue for all involved. The following suggestions regarding Pawspice care for nonpainful conditions automatically reflect all the considerations previously described.

PAWSPICE CARE FOR NONPAINFUL CONDITIONS

In addition to the major life-limiting diagnosis that initiated Pawspice care, many end-of-life pets have multiple concurrent conditions or comorbidities that may have slowly diminished the pet's overall QoL. If each condition can be improved by 30% to 60%, it is likely that QoL may be restored or improved and maintained during Pawspice until the pet's final fatal decline.

Aversion to Caregivers

End-of-life patients may show aversion to their caregiver for administering medications. If this problem is not solved, pet aversion to the caregiver may erode QoL at home, hurt the human-animal bond, and ruin the entire Pawspice experience. I experienced human-animal bond stress when Alaska, my dear, aging Great Pyrenees, started avoiding me during her 18-month Pawspice for degenerative myelopathy. Alaska no longer greeted me with her usual cheer. She would turn her head to avoid me when she knew that I might have a pill, a syringe, or some SQ fluids for her. What solved the problem? Lena Russell, one of our Pawspice nursing assistants, came every day to our home and gave Alaska her injections and SQ fluids. It only took 1 week for Alaska to be happy to greet me and be with me. Nursing house-call visits can and should be arranged for Pawspice patients that develop aversion to their family caregivers.

Sarcopenia

Sarcopenia is age-related decline of skeletal muscle mass and strength. As animals age, they generally eat less, which may also explain their weight loss. Reduced appetite may be from pain-related anorexia and other physiologic causes, such as poor oral or gastrointestinal health, sensory limitations, endocrine disease, and release of inflammatory cytokines. A pet's appetite might also be reduced by social isolation, stress, depression, cognitive syndrome, and other nonpainful diseases and comorbidities.

Immunonutrition

Dietary intervention for any Pawspice patient can be rewarding. Because most dogs and cats are on high-grain diets and almost one-third are overweight, it is easy to improve their nutritional status with the emerging knowledge of nutrigenomics, the study of how nutrients affect gene expression. The 2008 Nestle Purina Nutrition Symposium explained immunonutrition as an established scientific relationship on how diets interact with the innate immune system of the gut, which contains more than 65% of the immune cells in the body. Discussing immunonutrition as part of a pet's Pawspice program is inviting pet owners to elect a positive option. It may be the only treatment allowed by the pet owner when all versions of standard care are declined. It may be the only treatment feasible for a fragile pet's pawspice. The diet can be adjusted to minimize or exclude grains and to include carotenoids, antioxidants, flavonoids, beta glucans, omega (OM)-3 fatty acids, vitamins, glutathione, whey protein, and targeted nutraceuticals that have documented anticancer action or restorative function. If patients are obese, immunonutrition with caloric restriction may help weight loss to achieve lean body mass, which may benefit the pet's health, relieve symptoms of osteoarthritis, and extend lifespan.

Please accept the author's sincere advanced apologies because there are numerous good choices to provide a complete list of worthy agents for immunonutrition. Mainstay supplements used at the author's Pawspice practices are Platinum Performance Plus, Agaricus Bio (*Agaricus blazei*), Advanced Performance Drops (APF) drops, and inositol hexaphosphate. The author also places many older Pawspice patients on a new generation targeted nutraceutical, ageLocVitality (LifeGen/Pharmanex). LifeGen's patented technology, gene expression heat map profiling, was used to establish the unique ratio of extracts of *Panax* ginseng, Cordyceps Cs-4, and pomegranate, which composes the Vitality formula. It targets 92% of the 52 known genes in the youth gene cluster that codes for and restores mitochondrial numbers and function in brain, heart, and muscle tissue. The resulting increased cellular ATP, which is the fuel that drives multiple biologic functions, clinically counteracts age-related diminished cognition, sarcopenia, weakness, and decline.[6]

Chemoprevention and Metronomic Chemotherapy

Chemoprevention involves the use of natural or synthetic compounds that may reverse or suppress the process of carcinogenesis, metastasis, and recurrence.[7] Metronomic chemotherapy is the use of continuous low-dose agents to inhibit angiogenesis as well as affecting other mechanisms to inhibit neoplasia. These therapeutic modalities are kinder and gentler to the pet's body and generally cause no adverse events. Chemoprevention and metronomic chemotherapy are excellent palliative options for treated, untreated, or patients with terminal cancer in Pawspice care. Patients on these modalities may be given anticancer drugs, which require professional supervision and periodic evaluation of the complete blood count and organ function tests.

Patients with cancer that have received definitive surgery, chemotherapy, or radiation therapy remain at variable risk for recurrence. Dogs with hemangiosarcoma, osteosarcoma, adenocarcinoma, and lymphoma, and cats with breast cancer, vaccine associated sarcoma, lymphoma, inflammatory bowel disease, feline leukemia virus, and feline immunodeficiency virus all fall into the high-risk category. The majority of these treated pets are still expected to have recurrence or die of cancer within 2 to 12 months. Some of these animals may benefit with extended survival times using immunonutrition, chemoprevention, and metronomic chemotherapy. The judicious use of quality natural compounds that enhance cancer prevention and immunity can increase longevity and QoL in Pawspice programs at any veterinary practice.[8]

Anorexia, Cachexia

End-of-life dogs and cats with anorexia and cachexia may be coaxed to eat or be hand fed with tasty aromatic foods. Pet owners need v-team demonstrations to learn the best techniques to hand feed their ill pets properly and safely. Anorexia may be the key factor that drives pet owners to give up. Cats can be upset if force fed and it is discouraged in end-of-life care for felines if the cat remains disturbed and fearful. Cats like their food warmed to body temperature. They might be enticed to eat after a game or if petted and encouraged. Use appetite stimulants, such as mirtazipine (Remaron) at 1/8th of a 15 mg tablet every 48 hours or 1.25–2.5 mg per cat PO once every 72 hours. Dogs require mirtazipine daily for 4 to 5 days then every 48 hours by mouth. Mirtazipine is an antidepressant that increases norepinephrine, which increases the appetite but it may also cause sedation, hypotension, vocalization, tachycardia, and serotonin syndrome if given with monoamine oxidase inhibitors. A 30% dose reduction of mirtazipine is indicated for pets with cachexia, renal, or hepatic impairment. The author also uses megestrol acetate (Depo-Provera) injections at 2 mg/kg intramuscularly (IM) along with nandrolone injections 0.1 mL per 5 to 10 kg and prednisone to help dogs and cats that have malnutrition caused by persistent anorexia and cancer cachexia. When using appetite stimulants, caregivers should be instructed by the v-team to monitor their pet to determine if the pet is actually eating more food. Discontinue if there is no benefit.

Squamous cell carcinoma of the tongue in cats renders the tongue stiff and useless and causes early starvation and cachexia despite efforts to eat.[9] When a pet cannot or will not eat, consider placement of percutaneous esophageal (E) or gastrostomy feeding tubes. The E tube requires a short anesthetic with minimal risk. The procedure was initially described by CA Rawlings.[10] After the feeding tube is in place, the pet needs to be fed successfully several times in the hospital. It is essential that a v-team discharge appointment be scheduled to demonstrate how and what to feed the pet. Instruct the owner to call their demonstration nurse if they need further instructions during the first week using a feeding tube. It is best to use a blender to mix and liquefy the pet's diet, medications, and supplements with water or broth. This practice avoids clogging the tube. Use the calculations for resting energy requirement and a specialized diet, such as Hill's Canine/Feline anorexia diet or neoplasia diet for patients with cancer. This practice ensures that the Pawspice patient receives the proper ratio of protein, fat, calories, and liquid (50–100 mL/kg/24 h). The goal is to address abnormalities in carbohydrate, protein, and lipid metabolism associated with cachexia and to restore and maintain body weight.[11] If the feeding tube gets clogged, instruct the owner to use seltzer water or Sprite to dissolve the clog. Use a daily treatment calendar that clearly states the doses and scheduled times to give medications, supplements, fluids, feeding volumes, and so forth.

Refractory Nausea and Vomiting

Antiemetics given by SQ injection may be used at home to control refractory nausea and vomiting in Pawspice patients. Clients need demonstrations and education regarding SQ administration, dose and frequency, and adverse events. It is more convenient for clients if each dose of the injectable antiemetics is prepared in a separate syringe. Instruct the client to tightly place a new 27-gauge needle on each syringe before SQ administration. Use metoclopramide at 0.2 to 0.5 mg/kg SQ 3 times a day as a first-line antiemetic. Discontinue if the pet develops frenzied behavior, disorientation, or constipation. Maropitant (Cerenia) is an NK-1 receptor antagonist licensed for use in dogs and widely used in cats with an excellent margin of safety and minimal adverse reactions. Cats clear maropitant 4 times slower than dogs and respond to half the canine dose at 0.5 to 1.0 mg/kg SQ every 24 hours. The dog dose is 1 to 2 mg/kg SQ every 12 to 24 hours. Mirtazipine also possesses anti-nauseant and antiemetic effects by antagonizing 5HT and histamine (H-1) receptors at the doses given earlier for anorexia. Famotidine, ranitidine, and cimetidine are H-2 antagonists and act as adjunct antiemetics in dogs.[12]

Chronic Kidney Disease

Special modified diets, such as Hill's k/d or Select Balance, Modified Diet, may increase survival times and QoL. Pawspice care for chronic kidney disease includes SQ fluids, famotidine, vitamins, OM-3 fatty acids (marine fish oils), and Tumil-K and Amphogel when indicated. In addition, the author uses Azodyl, Epikitin, Renal Support, and Rubenol as supplements to support renal function. Regularly scheduled recheck profiles help monitor renal function, electrolytes, acidosis, and anemia. Erythropoietin (Epogen) may restore low hematocrit levels to normal; however, response is limited if patients develop antibodies. Famotidine, ranitidine, and cimetidine also act as antiemetics for uremic dogs and cats.[12] One 16-year-old cat, in the author's practice, survived 6 years with SQ fluids once a day at home until 22 years of age with a good QoL. If a cat resists SQ fluids, instruct pet owners to try using catnip, Liquid NutriCalm, Rescue Remedy, diazepam, HypnoClips, or a cat bag.

Diabetes

Some diabetic animals belong to reluctant, needle-shy owners. Clients need the option of trying oral hypoglycemic medications and in-home blood glucose monitoring. The author also uses APF drops that contain a formulation of Siberian ginseng, which has a glucose-lowering effect, and *A blazei,* which increases adiponectin, which stabilizes blood glucose by increasing insulin use.[13] One-third of patients with diabetes with negative ketonuria respond to oral medication and increasing protein in their diet. Patients with cancer also benefit because many have abnormal insulin use. This palliative approach may help the pet while prioritizing client concerns. If hyperglycemia persists after a trial with oral medications, the pet owner may be more accepting to use SQ insulin at home.

Feline Triad Disease

Some senior cats may develop *triad disease,* which is concurrent liver, pancreatic, and intestinal inflammatory disease. Palliative therapy includes SQ fluids, oral potassium gluconate, vitamin E, prednisolone, metronidazole, Clavamox, ursodiol (Actigall), pancreatic enzymes, l-carnitine, lactulose, S-adenosylmethionine, and SQ vitamin K-1. Feed small, frequent meals with Hill's Feline I/d or another palatable diet that contains L-carnitine and digestible protein to reduce hepatic workload.[14]

Liver Disease or Liver Cancer

Palliative therapy for pets with liver failure, hepatic encephalopathy, or liver cancer includes many of the previous recommendations. Feed 6 small meals daily. Use S-adenosyl-methionine (SAMe) and Hepato Support, which contains milk thistle (silymarin). Feed special diets that have a high-quality, easily digestible protein source (2.0–2.5 mg/kg),[15] such as egg, tofu, whey protein, cottage cheese, gluta-thione powder, quinoa, and Hill's l/d or k/d, which decreases the demands for hepatic function.

Refractory Seizures

Pets with brain tumors, insulinoma, liver disease, and poorly controlled epilepsy may develop refractory seizures. If patients with epilepsy had good control on an anticon-vulsant until recently, then a workup is indicated to determine if the seizures are caused by a newly acquired problem or a dose-related hepatotoxicity. Palliative care for refractory seizures may consist of using a loading dose of 600 mg/kg of potas-sium bromide divided into 4 doses per day for 36 hours or by giving 120 mg/kg once daily for 5 days. If possible, measure serum levels to achieve a 1.0- to 1.5-mg/mL target level. Some dogs will need more than 2.5 mg/kg for seizure control. If the pet was on phenobarbital or primidone, taper to a minimum level of 10 to 25 ug/mL for phenobarbital. If resistance develops on potassium bromide, the attending doctor may add phenobarbital or felbamate at 5 to 20 mg/kg 3 times a day or gabapentin at 25 to 50 mg/kg divided 4 times a day.[16] Pregaballan, a newer γ-aminobutyric acid analog, may improve control of refractory seizures at 2 mg/kg 3 times a day esca-lating to 3 to 4 mg/kg 3 times a day. In addition, the author sends home at least 3 to 6 syringes of diazepam injectable solution for clients to administer intranasally during or immediately after seizures. This practice keeps the Pawspice pet at home and emergency room costs down for the family. Advise hospitalization with the DNR direc-tive or euthanasia if the pet has more than 4 seizures a day.

Degenerative Myelopathy, Paresis, Paralysis

Disabled pets often require a wide range of resourceful home care items, such as ramps, hoisting slings, chest and rump lifts, wheel carts, and so forth. The Evans Mobility Cart (Jorvet, Loveland, CO, USA) is a canvass suspension hammock on wheels that helps pet caregivers to maintain QoL for their disabled Pawspice pets. Foot covers can be used to prevent wearing of digits and ulceration of metatarsals, metacarpals, and pads. Acupuncture, massage, and rehabilitation exercises may also palliate and improve QoL.

Decubital Ulcers and Hygiene Issues

Pressure sores and decubitus ulcers may be avoided in recumbent animals with frequent rotation of the body and thoughtful planning. Use soft pads, waterbeds, and egg crate mattresses with washable covers to prevent ulcers at pressure points. Frequent and complete examination of the pet's coat and skin is essential along with butt bathing if soiled with urine or feces. If the pet spends time outdoors, use repellents to prevent fly strike and maggots in wounds and body orifices espe-cially in longhair breeds. Treating the sores requires frequent cleaning, topical anti-biotics and relief of pressure, which might be facilitated with custom-designed cushion wraps.

Malignant Hypercalcemia

Sick polyuric and polydipsic pets and those approaching corrected serum calcium levels of 16 to 18 mg/dL require aggressive intravenous (IV) diuresis with 0.9% saline to stabilize and increase glomerular filtration rate. Once the pet is rehydrated, use furosemide at 1 to 4 mg/kg at 8- to 24-hour intervals to inhibit calcium absorption. After harvesting diagnostic samples to test for T-cell lymphoma, use prednisone orally at 1 mg/kg once or twice a day. If T-cell lymphoma is diagnosed, start induction therapy but avoid doxorubicin as T-cell lymphomas are resistant. Use IV vincristine at 0.55 to 0.7 mg/m^2 for week 1 and oral cyclophosphamide at 200 mg/m^2 divided over 2 days on week 2, repeat this sequence for weeks 3 and 4. On week 5 give IV vincristine and 3 to 4 days later, start lomustine at 60 mg/m^2 by mouth divided over 5 to 6 days. Recheck in 3 weeks and repeat. Recheck in complete blood count (CBC) each visit and check chemistry panels as needed. Serum calcium can be used as a tumor marker for recurrence. Anal sac tumors or other primary tumors require excision while maintaining diuresis and monitoring renal and cardiac function. If the family cannot afford the previous hospitalization and services and they want their pet to go home for hospice care, use a consent form that acknowledges the gravity of the pet's condition and release of your liability. Send the clients home with 0.9% saline for SQ use twice a day or 3 times a day and oral prednisone and furosemide on a specified schedule. Pawspice patients with chronic malignant hypercalcemia caused by resistant T-cell lymphoma or inoperable or recurrent tumors may be maintained at home with SQ 0.9% saline twice a day or 3 times a day, etidronate at 20 mg/kg/d in 3 to 4 divided doses, prednisone, furosemide, and gastroprotectants until their QoL scores drop lower than 35.

PAWSPICE CARE FOR NONPAINFUL MALIGNANCIES
Hemangiosarcoma

Unfortunately those who love German shepherds and golden and Labrador retrievers will be entering up to 20% of their pets into Pawspice programs for hemangiosarcoma (HSA). One in 5 golden retrievers develop HSA. Most are diagnosed following splenic rupture and collapse. On ultrasound, 75% of neoplastic lesions are found in the spleen as cavitated irregular nodules with variable echogenicity. Metastatic lesions are often identified in the liver, which might be confused with regenerative hyperplasia. Twenty-five percent of primary lesions occur in the right atrium. Splenectomy is the mainstay of treatment. With the exception of dermal, SQ, and IM HSAs, survival is quite short (20–60 days, with a 1-year survival of <10%) because of metastasis. Surgery plus chemotherapy yield slight increases in survival (141–179 days) with a 1-year survival of 10% or less.[17] The author's palliative protocol offers options, such as oral Yunan-Paio; metronomic chemotherapy, including HDAC inhibitors, masitinib, T-Cyte by SQ injections, or IV carboplatin every 21 days. Follow-up consists of CBC, panel with abdominal ultrasound, and chest radiographs every 2 months. Solar-induced dermal lesions are successfully treated with cryotherapy. We help families understand that visceral HSA is incurable and that Pawspice care may help extend life but will not cause harm. Some owners feel forced when given the either-or options of euthanasia versus splenectomy. However, a third and important option is pet hospice. This option is viable as some dogs may survive hemoabdomen with supportive care, pain management, belly wraps, and strict rest, which may allow resorption of red blood cells. Most doctors shun the idea of allowing a hemorrhaging dog in disseminated intravascular coagulation and shock to go home to die. However, the family has every right to request release of their pet to die at home with arrangements for home euthanasia. Use a client consent form that acknowledges that the pet is terminal and is going home with adequate pain control for pet hospice at the bequest of the family. The author has assisted families with HSA dogs that passed at home. Some dogs survive only hours, some a few days, occasionally some rally for 1 to 3 weeks after a near-death collapse. Sending the pet home gives their families a little more precious time for an extended farewell before the final gift of euthanasia.

Systemic Mast Cell Cancer

Mast cell tumors of the skin may become systemic and behave as hematopoietic malignancies (ie, lymphoma or leukemia). Most pets with systemic mast cell disease are evaluated because of lethargy, anorexia, vomiting, and weight loss, in association with splenomegaly, hepatomegaly, and pallor. Some have detectable skin tumors or a history of previously excised mast cell tumors. The CBC may show cytopenias with or without circulating mast cells. Mast cell tumors can release bioactive substances that may cause edema, erythema, or bruising of the affected area and intraoperative/postoperative bleeding and delayed wound healing. Gastrointestinal tract ulceration occurs in 80% of advanced cases caused by hyperhistaminemia. If requested, the attending doctor may release the terminal pet to the family for hospice care by using a signed consent form as previously discussed. The author's palliative Pawspice care protocol for home care initially includes sending home SQ injectable antiemetics, steroids, and famotidine on a specified schedule and transferring to oral medications when emesis is controlled. IV vinblastine might also be used along with masitinib or toceranib, which exhibits benefit as first-line therapy with or without prednisone in recurrent, resistant, and advanced stage disease.[18,19] Patients that experience complete remissions and continue therapy may sustain a good QoL during their Pawspice.

Brain Tumors

Brain tumors may cause seizures, nystagmus, nerve deficits, head tilt, ataxia, falling, circling, gait dysfunction, and nausea. Severe symptoms may be palliated with a single IV dose of mannitol at 1 g/kg. Most patients may be palliated with prednisone at 1 mg/kg by mouth every 24 hours. Omeprazole at 1 mg/kg by mouth every 24 hours and meclizine at 25 mg by mouth every 24 hours may also improve the pet's QoL.[20] The author uses valproic acid (VPA) at 15 mg/kg/d in divided doses with slow increases to 30 to 60 mg/kg/d for seizure control. VPA has histone deacetylase inhibition activity, which may have anticancer effects and antiheadache activity for QoL. Because VPA is protein bound, do not use with nonsteroidal antiinflammatory drugs (NSAIDs) or diazepam. Lomustine at 50 to 60 mg/M2 divided over 4 to 6 days every 21 days is used for dogs and every 40 days for cats. Oil of evening primrose at 2 capsules twice a day is given to cats as a source of linolenic acid. OM-3 fatty acids or 3 mL/kg of Hollywood safflower oil is given with a meal on 3 consecutive days per week (Monday, Tuesday, Wednesday) for dogs. This palliative brain tumor protocol has shown impressive clinical benefit and QoL with some cases surviving 6 to 12 months and one canine case in the author's practice survived 4 years.

Transitional Cell Carcinoma

Late diagnosis is typical for transitional cell carcinoma (TCC) because of owner delay and mimicry with cystitis. Surgery generally fails to prolong survival because of widespread seeding along the mucosal surface. Dogs and cats may live many months without surgery or treatment and up to 1 year with supportive care and piroxicam and chemotherapy using various protocols with mitoxantrone, vinblastine, and metronomic chlorambucil.[21,22] Use diapers for pets with pollakiuria and create easy and frequent access for eliminations. If hematuria causes severe blood loss anemia, place 3 mL of 1% formalin solution into to a bottle of Synotic topical ear solution, which contains dimethyl sulfoxide. Instill into the bladder via a urinary catheter. Keep the mixture in the bladder for 10 to 15 minutes. Then void and flush out the clots. Hematuria is reduced for 7 to 10 days. The procedure can be repeated as needed. If the tumor obstructs the trigone or urethra, a low-profile cystostomy tube (preferred by the author over stents) may be placed for owners who are willing to empty the bladder 2 to 3 times daily.[23] If hydronephrosis develops, surgery might be considered to reroute the ureters. The previously mentioned palliative measures do not arrest the cancer, so decision making is difficult in attempting to maintain QoL and provide relief for life-threatening dilemmas.

Prostate Cancer

Most dogs are diagnosed in advanced stages, which makes surgery other than stent placement for obstructions unhelpful. The prostate and prostatic urethra may also be invaded by TCC. Palliative and Pawspice therapy would be similar to suggestions for patients with TCC as previously described.[24] The author was surprised that palliative care for 2 cats with rare prostate cancer (one with an open cystostomy) on mitoxantrone and piroxicam, yielded 1-year survivals.

Nasal Passage Cancer

Nasal and sinus tumors may cause epistaxis, copious discharge, and night stridor, which may be palliated with IV carboplatin, NSAIDs, and nighttime sedation. Dogs have no trouble breathing when awake because they pant. Some dogs can be taught to sleep with a large toy, tennis ball, or bone in their mouth, which allows air to flow freely in and out of the trachea.

Oral Cancer

Pets with terminal primary or recurrent oral tumors require supportive palliative care. Oral and lingual tumors in cats lead to early dysphagia, weight loss and malnutrition. When a pet can't or won't eat, place a percutaneous esophageal feeding tube using a short anesthetic as referenced in the previous anorexia/cachexia section.[3,25,26] Cats with lingual tumors generally survive 3 to 4 months with esophageal feeding tubes that allow proper nutrition. Most cats with oral tumors start drooling malodorous saliva and require cleaning of legs and paws twice a day. The author uses a sponge soaked in a warmed dilute solution of lemon juice and white vinegar and instructs clients to gently swab the cat's cheeks, neck, face, and coat before cleaning the paws. Most cats gain pleasure from this ritual, sensing their caretaker is the mother tongue.

Lung Cancer

Caregivers can successfully maintain Pawspice for pets with primary or metastatic lung tumors as long as they are educated to recognize the early signs of dyspnea. Generally, pets are diagnosed with advanced pulmonary disease because the early signs are insidious. Opioids, antianxiety drugs, rotation of the body to sternal recumbency, and portable oxygen therapy may help pets with compromised respiration. If the pet develops pulmonary effusions, the client should monitor respiration rate and chest excursion to know when to bring the pet in for thoracocentesis. Chest tubes or palliative pleurodesis may be helpful for pets requiring multiple thoracocenteses. When QoL deteriorates, urge clients to increase the opioids, to enact DNR plans, and provide the gift of euthanasia for their pet.

SUPPORTIVE SERVICES
Nursing House Calls

Make arrangements for nursing support staff to visit clients who need help administering injections and fluids to their Pawspice pets at home. The home care nurse can educate the client with a list of side effects (adverse events) associated with poly pharmacy and use the QoL scale to help the family evaluate the current status of the Pawspice pet.[25] The nurse can also collect blood samples and vital signs for the supervising doctor to monitor the pet. The reception staff can keep a list of pets in the hospital's Pawspice program to be on alert and more responsive and compassionate when the owners call for help. Many house call veterinarians are eager for more referrals to provide palliative and Pawspice care.

Boarding and Daycare

Pawspice pets often require special boarding care or daycare with their local v-team for supervision, would care, hygiene, hand feeding, and so forth. This care can and should be willingly provided at the primary care veterinary hospital. This service may be the key to sustaining a Pawspice pet for working owners. Be sure to arrange convenient drop-off and pickup times that fit the client's working and travel schedule.[25]

Networking

It is important for some Pawspice caregivers to have another person to talk to who is in the same situation to share stories and give one another support. Get permission to share phone numbers or emails with clients who are providing similar Pawspice care for their pets. Dr Kathleen Carson and Christine Gray, both from the author's previous facility, have actively participated for many years in a chronic renal failure chat room for cats. It opens every Sunday evening at 5:00 PM PST on America Online. Networking is helpful and is a staff time saver. There are also several chat groups and blogs that offer support for specific cancers.

Group Sessions for Pet Loss

Group and private counseling can be helpful for caregivers who are suffering from anticipatory grief and for those who are depressed after their pet's death. Some pet owners will sink into the depression associated with maladaptive grief after they have lost a dear pet. It is important to introduce them to a professional pet loss counselor.

SUMMARY

Many Pawspice clients have confided to the author that their previous veterinarians dismissed them or seemed too quick to recommend euthanasia if they declined definitive care for their terminal pet. The either-or model is no longer acceptable. At times, their pet was dismissed or discharged by the either-or doctor without pain medications, despite being warned that their pet was suffering. Read the article by Robin Downing on palliative pain management. As long as the pet's best interests and QoL are respected, palliative Pawspice care can be rewarding for all involved. The majority of America's human cancer patients don't really die from their cancer. They actually die as their preexisting conditions worsen or they develop treatment-related complications that precipitate death. A matched study showed that aggressively treated lung cancer patients died 3 months sooner than palliative care patients.[27] This sad situation for people and pets can be avoided by adopting palliative care to support patients with cancer at the *start* of diagnosis, which is the Pawspice philosophy. It starts at diagnosis and focuses on symptom care and gives pets and their caretakers the option for a kinder, gentler approach to standard management of cancer, terminal disease, and aging to maintain the best possible QoL.[28]

REFERENCES

1. Withrow S. Keynote speaker. 30th Annual Conference of the Veterinary Cancer Society. San Diego (CA), October 31, 2010.
2. Meyers JF. Perspectives on palliative care: a chair of medicine viewpoint. J Palliat Med 1999Winter;2(4):371–5.
3. Lagoni L. Bond Centered Cancer Care: a applied approach to euthanasia and grief support for your clients, your staff and yourself. In: Withrow JS, Vail DM, editors. Withrow & MacEwen's small animal clinical oncology. St Louis (MO): Saunders/Elsevier; 2007. p. 333–46. Chapter 16d.
4. Choen SP, Fudin CE, editors. Animal illness and human emotion. Probl Vet Med 1991;3(1):1–37.
5. Downing R. Pets living with cancer: a pet owner's resource. Lakewood (CO): AAHA Press; 2000.
6. Park SK, Kim K, Page GP, et al. Gene expression profiling of aging in multiple mouse strains: identification of aging biomarkers and impact of dietary antioxidants. Aging Cell 2009;8(4):484–95.
7. Bergman P. Chemoprevention. Proceedings of ACVIM Forum. Chicago (IL), May 28–31, 1999.
8. Villalobos A, Kaplan L. Chemoprevention and immunonutrition for cancer patients. In: Canine and feline geriatric oncology: honoring the human-animal bond. Ames (IA): Blackwell Publishing; 2007. p. 195–204. Chapter 6.
9. Villalobos A. Oncology Outlook: those stubborn cats that won't eat. Irvine (CA): VPN; 1999.
10. Rawlings CA. Percutaneous placement of a midcervical esophagostomy tube: new technique and representative cases. J Am Anim Hosp Assoc 1993;29: 526–30.
11. Mauldin GE. Nutritional management of the cancer patient. In: Withrow SJ, Vail DM, editors. Withrow & MacEwen's small animal clinical oncology. 4th edition. St Louis (MO): Saunders/Elsevier; 2007. Chapter 16.
12. Allenspack K, Chan DL. Antiemetic therapy. In: August JR, editor, Consultations in feline internal medicine, vol. 6. St Louis (MO): Saunders/Elsevier; 2010. p. 232–9. Chapter 21.
13. Borchers AT, Stern JS, Hackman RM, et al. Mushrooms, tumors and immunity. Proc Soc Exp Biol Med 1999–2008;221:281–93.
14. Hoskins JD. Feline 'Triad Disease' not Breed or Sex Specific. North Olmstead (OH): DVM Practice Builder; 2000. p. 31–5.
15. Hoskins JD. The liver and exocrine pancreas. In: Geriatrics and gerontology of the dog and cat. St Louis (MO): Saunders/Elsevier; 2004. p. 189–204. Chapter 13.
16. Hoskins JD. The nervous system. In: Geriatrics and gerontology of the dog and cat. St Louis (MO): Saunders/Elsevier; 2004. p. 351–73. Chapter 22.
17. Thamm DH. Hemangiosarcoma. In: Withrow SJ, Vail DM, editors. Withrow & MacEwen's small animal clinical oncology. 4th edition. St Louis (MO): Saunders/Elsevier; 2007. p. 785–95. Chapter 32.
18. deVoss J. First line and rescue therapy with Masitinib Integrated Protocols for Canine MCT. Presented at Veterinary Cancer Society Proceedings. San Diego (CA), October 29 to November 1, 2010. p. 65.
19. Johannes C. Palladia year one clinical experience online case summary. Presented at Veterinary Cancer Society Proceedings. San Diego (CA), October 29 to November 1, 2010. p. 72.

20. Beasley MJ, Shores A, Hathcock JT. What is your neurologic diagnosis? J Am Vet Med Assoc 2009;234(6):744–5.
21. Arnold E, Childress M, Fourez L, et al. Phase II trial of vinblastine in dogs with Transitional cell carcinoma. Presented at Veterinary Cancer Society Proceedings. San Diego (CA), October 29 to November 1, 2010. p. 42.
22. Schremp D, Childress M, Moore G, et al. Phase II clinical trial of metronomic chlorambucil in dogs with transitional cell carcinoma of the urinary bladder. Presented at Veterinary Cancer Society Proceedings. San Diego (CA), October 29 to November 1, 2010. p. 43.
23. Stifler KS, McCrackin Stevenson MA, Cornell KK, et al. Clinical use of low profile cystostomy tubes in four dogs and a cat. J Am Vet Med Assoc 2003;223(3): 325–9.
24. Villalobos A. Oncology Outlook: on bladder and prostate cancer. Irvine (CA): VPN; 2000.
25. Shearer T. Hospice and palliative care. In: Gaynor J, Muir W, editors. Handbook of veterinary pain management. St Louis (MO): Mosby/Elsevier; 2008. p. 588–600. Chapter 30.
26. Villalobos A. Oncology outlook: pet hospice nurses the bond. Irvine (CA): VPN; 1999.
27. Temmel JS, Greer JA, Billings JA, et al. Early palliative care for patients with metastatic non small cell lung cancer. N Engl J Med 2010;363(8):733–42.
28. Villalobos A. Conceptualized end of life care: "Pawspice" Program for Pets. AVMA Proceedings. Salt Lake City, July 22–26, 2000. p. 322–27.

Clinical Signs and Management of Anxiety, Sleeplessness, and Cognitive Dysfunction in the Senior Pet

Gary M. Landsberg, DVM, MRCVS[a,b,*],
Theresa DePorter, DVM, MRCVS[c], Joseph A. Araujo, BSc[d,e]

KEYWORDS

- Anxiety • Behavior problems • Cognitive dysfunction • Fear
- Night waking • Senior pets

ASSESSING AND MAINTAINING COGNITIVE AND BEHAVIORAL WELL-BEING

Appreciation and compassion for welfare and quality of life, as well as emotional and physical well-being, is important at all stages of our patient's lives, but this becomes particularly complicated in the management of geriatric patients, especially those facing imminent end-of-life decisions. Patience and sensitivity for the pet's emotional state should be part of a comprehensive program for any patient; however, the geriatric hospice patient requires special consideration because changes in anxiety and cognitive function may be further compounded by other medical conditions, sensory perception, medications, and previous learning. For example, if the pet has learned to expect pain and uncomfortable restraint during previous experiences, then the debilitated or compromised pet will be more anxious, defensive, or even aggressive rather than

Disclosure: GL is an employee of, and JA is a consultant for, CanCog Technologies Inc, a contract research organization that provides cognitive and behavioral assessment of dogs and cats.
[a] North Toronto Animal Clinic, 99 Henderson Avenue, Thornhill, ON L3T 2K9, Canada
[b] CanCog Technologies Inc, 120 Carlton Street, Toronto, ON M5A 4K2, Canada
[c] Oakland Veterinary Referral Services, 1400 South Telegraph Road, Bloomfield Hills, MI, 48302, USA
[d] Department of Pharmacology, University of Toronto, 1 King's College Circle, Toronto, ON M5S 1A8, Canada
[e] CanCog Technologies Inc, 120 Carlton Street, Suite 204, Toronto, ON M5A 4K2, Canada
* Corresponding author. North Toronto Animal Clinic, 99 Henderson Avenue, Thornhill, ON L3T 2K9, Canada.
E-mail address: gmlandvm@aol.com

appreciative of even the most compassionate end-of-life care. Behavioral signs are often the first, or only, signs of pain, illness, and cognitive decline (**Table 1**). Therefore, family members need assistance in recognizing the significance of these changes and the importance of reporting these promptly to their veterinarian. Early detection of behavioral changes consistent with disease provides an opportunity for early diagnosis and treatment so that complications might be prevented, further decline might be slowed, longevity might be increased, and welfare issues can be promptly addressed.[1]

Both the American Hospital Association and American Association of Feline Practitioner Guidelines specifically refer to the importance of questioning pet owners at each visit as to any changes in health or behavior to improve early recognition of alterations

Table 1
Medical causes of behavioral signs

Medical Condition/Medical Presentation	Examples of Behavioral Signs
Neurologic: central (intracranial/extracranial), particularly if affecting forebrain, limbic/temporal, and hypothalamic; REM sleep disorders	Altered awareness, response to stimuli, loss of learned behaviors, house soiling, disorientation, confusion, altered activity levels, temporal disorientation, vocalization, soiling, change in temperament (fear, anxiety), altered appetite, altered sleep cycles, interrupted sleep
Partial seizures: temporal lobe epilepsy	Repetitive behaviors, self-traumatic disorders, chomping, staring, alterations in temperament (eg, intermittent states of fear or aggression), tremors, shaking, interrupted sleep
Sensory dysfunction	Altered response to stimuli, confusion, disorientation, irritability/aggression, vocalization, house soiling, altered sleep cycles
Endocrine: hyperthyroid or hypothyroid, hyperadrenocorticism or hypoadrenocorticism, insulinoma, diabetes, testicular or adrenal tumors	Altered emotional state, irritability/aggression, lethargy, decreased response to stimuli, anxiety, house soiling/marking, night waking, decreased or increased activity, altered appetite, mounting
Metabolic disorders: hepatic/renal	Signs associated with organ affected: may be anxiety, irritability, aggression, altered sleep, house soiling, mental dullness, decreased activity, restlessness, increase sleep, confusion
Pain	Altered response to stimuli, decreased activity, restless/unsettled, vocalization, house soiling, aggression/irritability, self-trauma, waking at night
Peripheral neuropathy	Self-mutilation, irritability/aggression, circling, hyperesthesia
Gastrointestinal	Licking, polyphagia, pica, coprophagia, fecal house soiling, wind sucking, tongue rolling, unsettled sleep, restlessness
Urogenital	House soiling (urine), polydypsia, waking at night
Dermatologic	Psychogenic alopecia (cats), acral lick dermatitis (dogs), nail biting, hyperesthesia, other self-trauma (chewing/biting/sucking/scratching)

Abbreviation: REM, rapid eye movement.

in physical or behavioral well-being.[2,3] In addition, ongoing monitoring of behavioral signs can aid in assessing the progress of disease as well as the pet's quality of life and emotional state.

The behavioral focus for pets of any age should be on (1) maintaining positive and healthy social relationships (while avoiding those that are unpleasant); (2) ensuring freedom from stress; (3) providing a sense of control to allow the pet to engage in pleasant, and avoid unpleasant, interactions; and (4) ensuring adequate mental stimulation.[4] Pets that are elderly, or ill, may be less interested or able to engage in mental, physical, and social stimulation, which could potentially lead to alterations in the type and frequency of activities and interactions that owners provide their pets. However, mental enrichment and physical activity are important in maintaining cognitive health in both humans and pets, and physical activity can be an important component of weight management and for improving mobility.[5,6] Therefore, a more case-specific approach for designing behavioral strategies may be required for pets that have physical, mental, or behavioral limitations. Interactions that support the human-animal bond are especially critical in pets that are aging and ill because owners need to be responsive and sensitive to their pet's subtle changes in behavior as indicators of pain, welfare, and quality of life. Positive and pleasant shared experiences provide caregivers a sense of accomplishment rather than anguish about their pet's illness.

BEHAVIORAL SIGNS IN SENIOR PETS: ANXIETY, SLEEP-WAKE DISTURBANCES, AND COGNITIVE DYSFUNCTION

Although most pet owners are likely to report more serious signs either because of their obvious health and welfare implications to the pet, or because of the effects they have on the owner-pet relationship, veterinarians must be proactive in asking owners about behavioral signs because those that tend to be more subtle or less problematic to the owners often go unreported.[7–10] Behavioral signs in geriatric pets that may have the most significance to the owner or the pet include those associated with anxiety, night waking, and cognitive dysfunction syndrome (CDS). Sleep-wake disturbances may be caused by CDS or anxiety, but also for many unrelated reasons, but it warrants special attention in the treatment and management of senior pets.

Prevalence of Behavior Problems Reported by Owners of Senior Pets

Several studies have examined the prevalence of behavioral signs in senior pets (**Tables 2** and **3**).[11–13] In a Spanish study of 270 dogs more than 7 years of age presented for behavior problems, 74%, 19.8%, 4.6%, and 1.3% of the owners detected at least 1, 2, 3, and 4 behavior problems, respectively.[11] In this same study, although 16% were diagnosed with CDS, the most common signs were related to aggression (53%) and, to a lesser extent, those consistent with fear and anxiety.[11] Similarly, when examining the distribution of 103 senior dogs referred to a veterinary behaviorist in another study, in which 7% were diagnosed with CDS, most cases displayed aggression (34%) or signs of fear and anxiety (39%) (see **Table 2**).[12] In 83 senior cats referred for behavioral consultations, most cats displayed signs of marking or soiling (73%); however, cases of aggression (16%), vocalization (6%), and restlessness (6%) were also serious enough to require referral (see **Table 3**).[12] To further examine the distribution of problems reported by owners in senior dogs and cats, the Veterinary Information Network (VIN) database was searched for behavior problems of 50 senior dogs (aged 9–17 years) and 100 senior cats (aged 12–22 years). In the 50 canine cases reviewed from VIN boards, 31 dogs (62%) had signs consistent

Table 2
Canine behavior problem distribution reported by senior dog owner

Behavior Referral Practice (n = 103 Dogs) >7 y[12] (%)	Spanish Study (n = 270 Dogs) >7 y)[11] (%)	VIN[a] Boards (n = 50 Dogs) (%)
Separation anxiety 30	Aggression family member 32	Anxiety (fear, vocal, salivate, hypervigilant) 74
Aggression to people 27	Cognitive dysfunction 16	Cognitive dysfunction 62
Aggression to animals 17	Aggression to family dogs 16	Separation anxiety 36
Compulsive disorders 8	Barking 9	Wandering 26
Cognitive dysfunction 7	Separation anxiety 8	Night anxiety/waking 22
Phobias 5	Disorientation 6	Noise phobias 18
Anxiety 4	Aggression unfamiliar people 5	Vocalization 14
House soiling 3	House soiling 4	Stereotypic behavior 4
Vocalization 1	Destructive 4 Compulsive 4 Noise fears and phobias 3	Aggression 2

[a] Veterinary Information Network (www.VIN.com).

with CDS, but most of the dogs had signs related to anxiety, including night waking and vocalization (see **Table 2**). In the 100 feline cases reviewed from VIN boards, 27% of the complaints were related to elimination problems, and the most common complaints were vocalization (61%), especially at night, and other signs associated with anxiety (see **Table 3**). Although many of these signs could be caused by underlying medical problems (see **Table 1**), in many of these cases, all possible medical causes were reported to have been ruled out.

Prevalence of Behavior Problems Solicited by Veterinary Inquiry

Although studies on the prevalence of behavior problems reported by owners may be representative of those problems that are serious enough for the owners to seek behavioral guidance, many of the most common behavioral signs that arise in senior pets require a more proactive approach on the part of the practitioner because they often go unreported.

Table 3
Feline behavior problem distribution reported by senior cat owner

Behavior Referral Practices n = 83[a] >10 y (%)	VIN Boards n = 100, Aged 12 to 22 y (%)
House soiling (elimination and marking) 73	Excessive vocalization 61 (night vocal 31)
Intercat aggression 10	House soiling (elimination and marking) 27
Aggression to humans 6	Disorientation 22
Excessive vocalization 6	Aimless wandering 19
Restlessness 6	Restlessness/night waking 18
Overgrooming 4	Irritable/aggressive 6 Fear/hiding 4 Clingy (attachment) 3

[a] Cases recruited from behavior referral practices Landsberg (n = 25), Horwitz (n = 33), Chapman, Voith (n = 25).
Data from Chapman BL, Voith VL. Geriatric behavior problems not always related to age. DVM 1987;18:32.

In one study of dogs aged 11 to 16 years that had no medical signs, 28% of dogs aged 11 to 12 years and 68% of dogs aged 15 to 16 years showed at least 1 sign consistent with CDS.[8] In a study of 14 dogs with CDS, all dogs visited the veterinarian for a routine annual checkup and the owners reported no behavioral complaints until actively questioned by the veterinarian.[9] In another recent study, 124 dogs more than 7 years of age were evaluated and 22 were eliminated because of possible medical factors.[10] Of the remaining dogs, 42 had alterations in 1 category and 33 had signs in 2 or more categories associated with CDS.[10] In a recent Spanish study that examined the prevalence and risk factors for age-related cognitive impairment in a population of 325 dogs more than 9 years of age, 22.5% of geriatric dogs were affected.[13] Females and neutered males were significantly more affected than males and entire dogs, and the prevalence and severity increased with age.[13] In this study, social interactions and house training were the most impaired categories.[13] The possible relationship between gonadectomy and an increased prevalence in CDS was previously described.[14] In a large-scale epidemiologic study using Internet survey responses regarding 497 dogs ranging in age from 8 to 19 years, the estimated prevalence of CDS was 14.2%. However, only 1.9% of these dogs were diagnosed with CDS by their veterinarian, exemplifying that CDS is severely underdiagnosed.[7] In a Hills Market Research study, 75% of owners of dogs more than 7 years of age indicated that their pet had 1 or more signs consistent with CDS when asked, but only 12% had previously reported the signs to their veterinarian (Hills Pet Nutrition. US Market Research Survey, Omnibus study on aging pets. Topeka [KS]: Hills Pet Nutrition; 2000, data on file). In one study of aged cats presented to veterinary clinics for routine annual care, 154 owners of cats aged 11 years and older were asked to report any signs of CDS. After eliminating 19 cats with medical problems, 35% of the cats were diagnosed with possible CDS, and this increased with age: 28% of 95 cats aged 11 to 15 years, and 50% of 46 cats more than 15 years of age, were diagnosed with possible CDS.[15,16]

CLIENT EDUCATION AND SCREENING

Given the prevalence and underdiagnosis of behavioral problems in senior pets, monitoring and assessing behavioral signs is a critical component of every veterinary visit. The earlier a diagnosis can be made, the greater the opportunity to implement interventions that can positively affect the pet's health, comfort, and perhaps even longevity. Veterinarians and staff must inform clients of the potential health and welfare implications for the pet if these signs go unrecognized or unreported. Specific recommendations for monitoring might also be required based on previously diagnosed health issues and any medications being used. Handouts and web links can be used to further educate owners about the value of regular geriatric evaluations. The use of a questionnaire can be particularly effective in quickly and comprehensively screening for changes in both health and behavior.

HOW HEALTH MAY AFFECT BEHAVIOR AND BEHAVIOR MAY AFFECT HEALTH

Although the presence of gastrointestinal, neurologic, or dermatologic signs, polyuria or polydypsia, altered mobility, or declining sensory function may indicate an underlying medical problem, it is common for behavioral signs to be the first, or only, indication of medical problems (see **Table 1**). Sickness behaviors that may manifest as lethargy and inappetance are usually considered to be passive and in response to debilitation or weakness; this may be a well-organized adaptive process that diverts energy to the immune system to enhance disease resistance and facilitate recovery.[17]

When senior pets are presented with a recent onset of a change in behavior, such as house soiling; alterations in social interactions; altered responses to stimuli; changes in activity levels (whether increased or decreased); night waking; excessive vocalization; or an increase in fear, anxiety, or phobias, then possible medical causes of these signs must first be ruled out.

In senior pets, especially those receiving palliative care for previously diagnosed health issues, the practitioner must be cognizant that multiple health and behavior issues may coexist. Although a physical examination and diagnostic tests are invaluable in diagnosing and monitoring many medical conditions, the potential for pain and neurologic diseases, including sensory dysfunction and CDS, to contribute to the pet's behavioral signs must also be evaluated. In addition, for pets that are on medication for existing health or behavioral problems, all potential behavioral effects of the medications must also be considered. Pain and illness further contribute to stress and anxiety, just as stress and anxiety can contribute to pain and illness. If a medical cause is diagnosed or suspected, a therapeutic trial may help to confirm the cause by monitoring the pet's behavioral response. Therefore, identifying signs of stress and anxiety (**Box 1**) are critical in the monitoring of both behavioral and medical health as well as animal welfare.

The Effects of Health on Behavior

Any disease that affects the central nervous system or its circulation (eg, cardiac, anemia, hypertension) can affect behavior (see **Table 1**). Both intracranial (eg, degenerative, tumor) and extracranial causes (eg, organ failure, immune diseases, endocrinopathies, circulatory, respiratory) become increasingly common in older pets. A change in personality or mood, awareness, inability to recognize or respond appropriately to stimuli, and loss of previously learned behavior might indicate forebrain or brainstem involvement. Altered responsiveness to stimuli can also arise from sensory or motor dysfunction, as well as pain. Episodic changes in conscious response may be

---

Box 1
Signs of stress and anxiety

Alteration/change from normal behavior

Reduced activity ←-------→ Increased activity (restlessness)

Increased sleeping ←-------→ Increased nighttime waking

Avoidance of social interaction ←-------→ Increased attention seeking

Reduced feeding and/or drinking

Increased huddling or shivering

Alterations in vocalization (whining, barking, or howling)

Increased irritability and aggression ←-------→ Apathy or reduced response to stimuli

Increased sensitivity or reactivity to stimuli

Depression

Elimination in home

Decreased interest in toys or social play

Increased sensitivity to stimuli including phobia and separation anxiety

Physiologic changes (heart rate, respiratory rate, blood pressure, panting, salivation, other autonomic signs, eg, dilated pupils)

caused by neurologic conditions such as seizures or other clinical conditions such as syncope, acute vestibular dysfunction, tremors, narcolepsy/cataplexy, rapid eye movement (REM) disorder, and movement disorders, all of which may mimic anxiety attacks and result in nighttime waking and which are particularly challenging to distinguish. These disorders must be differentiated by history and, if possible, video recordings of episodic anxiety and especially night waking behaviors.

Any disease that alters hormone levels (thyroid, adrenal, reproductive organs) can also affect behavior. For example, in elderly felines, hyperthyroidism (which can also contribute to behavioral signs of hypertension including vocalization, restlessness, and night waking) can be associated with behavioral signs ranging from appetite stimulation to increased irritability, anxiety, and urine marking.

Self-traumatic disorders including biting, chewing, scratching, licking, or excessive barbering lead to skin lesions and alopecia. Although self-traumatic disorders can have a behavioral cause, when dermatologic diagnostics do not identify a medical cause, hypersensitivity reactions and neuropathic pain must first be ruled out.[18]

Pain can be identified by both behavioral and physical signs. Studies have shown that behavioral measures are an accurate means of measuring pain, and pain assessment scoring systems have been developed for both veterinarians and pet owners.[19–21] Pain can be a contributing factor to many of the behavioral signs associated with CDS, self-traumatic disorders, and anxiety disorders.

Unusual oral behaviors including licking, sucking, pica, smacking lips, and gulping might arise because of partial complex seizures or gastrointestinal disorders. In a recent study of dogs with excessive licking of surfaces, gastrointestinal disorders were identified as a cause in at least half of the dogs.[22]

House soiling is often considered a behavior problem but is often precipitated by medical problems. In a retrospective study of cats with problem elimination behavior, 60% of the cats had a history of feline urological syndrome/feline lower urinary tract disease.[23] Inappropriate elimination can be caused by any medical problem, or in response to medications, that causes an increased volume of urine or stool, increased discomfort during elimination, decreased control, or diseases that affect cortical control.

Consider all medications the pet is taking and possible side effects or interactions, because these effects may influence behavior. For example, steroids may cause irritability and pain medications may cause sedation. Conversely, the conditions these medications alleviate may lead to an improvement in the behaviors associated with the medical condition. Monitoring behavioral signs may be a critical component in monitoring drug efficacy.

CDS (discussed later) is generally a slowly progressive disorder that cannot be definitively diagnosed and early symptoms are easily overlooked. Patients undergoing palliative and end-of-life care may have undiagnosed CDS. The challenge for the clinician is to identify evidence of early CDS and distinguish these from signs of illness or medication side effects, because diagnosis of cognitive dysfunction is based on exclusion and confirmed only by characteristic deterioration of cognitive function and the associated progression of symptoms.

The Effects of Stress on Health and Mental Well-being

Although it is common to consider the effects of disease on behavior, acute and chronic stress can also have an impact on both health and behavior.[24] Stress is an altered state of homeostasis that can be caused by physical or emotional factors that trigger psychological, behavioral, endocrine, and immune effects that are designed to handle stress.[25] In the aging or ill pet, there is a general deterioration in physical condition; tissue hypoxia; alterations in cell membranes; increased production and decreased clearance of reactive oxygen species; a decline in organ, sensory, and mental function; a gradual deterioration of the immune system; and decreased ability to cope with change. Thus, the senior pet in particular is less able to respond to stress and maintain homeostatic balance.

In humans, there may be a correlation between stress and poor health, including poor immune function, cardiovascular disease, skin disease, asthma, gastrointestinal disorders, and cellular aging. Similarly, in pets, stress may alter immune function, and has been shown to be a contributing or aggravating factor in gastrointestinal diseases, urinary tract disorders in cats, dermatologic conditions, respiratory and cardiac conditions, behavioral disorders, and a shortened lifespan.[26] For example, cats with interstitial cystitis (FIC) may have altered bladder permeability and an increase in plasma noradrenaline, whereas cats receiving environmental modification had a significant reduction in FIC, respiratory disease, fearfulness, nervousness, inflammatory bowel disease, and aggression.[27–29] Fear, anxiety, and stress can also contribute to gastrointestinal signs including anorexia, vomiting, diarrhea, and colitis.

Although stress leads to an immune response intended to enhance defense mechanisms, in some individuals, stressors may contribute to inflammatory dermatoses and endocrinoimmunologic factors, which, in situations of stress, may play a role in the pathogenesis of dermatoses such as atopic dermatitis, psoriasis, and urticaria.[30–32] An increased severity and frequency of skin disorders in dogs with nonsocial fear and separation anxiety has been identified.[26] Chronic anxiety, stress, conflict, and frustration may lead to behavioral disorders in humans, including panic disorders, separation anxiety, social and other phobias, obsessive-compulsive disorders, generalized anxiety disorders, posttraumatic stress disorders, impulse control disorders, and sleep disorders, all of which may have animal correlates.[33] Pets that are physically or mentally impaired may find it difficult to deal with the effects of stress. Aging pets may have difficulty with forgetfulness, just as described in people, and the pet may appear confused or stubborn as a result of impaired short-term memory or reduced cognitive abilities. Therefore, although enrichment (discussed later) may have beneficial effects in helping to maintain both physical and mental health, changes in the pet's household or schedule should be made slowly to help the pet cope. When changes must be made, pet owners should pay particular attention to the pet's emotional and behavioral state, as well as its appetite, sleep, and elimination, to gauge whether additional support in the form of behavior therapy or drugs might be warranted.

AGING AND ITS EFFECT ON THE BRAIN

In dogs, frontal volume decreases, ventricular size increases, and there is evidence of meningeal calcification, demyelination, increased lipofuscin and apoptic bodies, neuroaxonal degeneration, and a reduction in neurons.[34,35] Although not as well defined, similar changes including neuronal loss, cerebral atrophy, widening of the sulci, and an increase in ventricular size are also reported in cats.[16,36] Perivascular changes including microhemorrhage or infarcts in periventricular vessels have been reported in senior dogs and cats, which may be responsible for some of the signs of cognitive dysfunction.[16,34,35,37–40] With increasing age, there is also an increase in reactive oxygen species leading to oxidative damage in dogs, which is speculated to also be a factor in aged cats.[16,41] There may also be a depletion of catecholamines and an increase in monoamine oxidase B (MAOB) activity in dogs.[42] A decline in the cholinergic system has also been identified in dogs and cats, which may contribute to cognitive decline and, possibly, alterations in motor function, as well as alterations in REM sleep.[36,42–45] In dogs, cats, and humans, there is an increased accumulation of diffuse amyloid-β (Aβ) plaques and perivascular infiltrates of Aβ.[16,37–39] Furthermore, increased Aβ is positively correlated with cognitive impairment in dogs.[38,39,46] Aβ plaques in cats older than 10 years are more diffuse than those seen in humans and dogs.[16,37,40,47,48] The link between CDS and Aβ disorders in the cat is inconsistent because some studies found a positive link,[37,47] whereas others show no correlation.[47,48] Nonetheless, the overall similarity in brain aging among various mammalian species suggests that some level of dementia, and other age-related behavioral changes including anxiety, memory loss (forgetfulness) and sleeplessness, occurs with aging across many species. A video example of a cat performing a memory task in a laboratory model may be viewed online (within this article at www.vetsmall.theclinics.com, May 2011 issue). In this video, the cat is performing a delayed non–matching to position (DNMP) task, which tests memory. Initially, the cat is presented with an object over 1 of 2 possible food wells. The cat must displace the object to retrieve a food reward beneath. After responding, the tray is removed from the cat's view and a delay is initiated (in this case, there is a delay of 90 seconds, but this is sped up in the video). After the delay, the cat is presented with duplicates of the object from the previous presentation. The correct choice, leading to a food reward, is the object in the position not used previously (ie, the nonmatch). To prevent the use of olfactory-based responding, the incorrect object is baited with an unattainable food reward. By increasing the delay between the 2 presentations, memory can effectively be tested by assessing the cat's ability to make the right choice, which is rewarded by food. A long the delay between the first and second presentation results in a poorer performance, which means the cat has an increased incidence of forgetting. Consequently, cats (or dogs) with cognitive impairment score poorly on a memory test, relative degrees of loss or decline in short-term memory may be assessed, and interventions intended to reduce the short-term memory loss effects of cognitive impairment may be assessed in this laboratory model (Video 1).

CLINICAL SIGNS
Anxiety, Stress, and Distress

Signs related to anxiety may indicate impaired cognitive function, compromised health, or pain. Therefore, the recognition of pain, anxiety, memory loss, and stress in pets requires curiosity and sensitivity because these may occur without overt signs, particularly because pets are instinctually driven to avoid revealing obvious signs of stress or vulnerability (see **Box 1; Box 2**). Furthermore, species, breed, and individual differences in both the perception and display of anxiety further confounds the problem of accurate assessment. Physiologic monitors may indicate pain so that assessments of changes in heart rate, respiratory rate, and blood pressure are important indicators in pain management, particularly in hospitalized pets. However, these physiologic indicators are not unique to pain and may also be influenced by fear or anxiety. However, more subjective measures are required for pet owners to evaluate pain in the home environment, which needs to be differentiated from other causes of fear and anxiety.[19–21]

Animals may display anxiety in an array of manifestations but generally these reflect either the absence of normal behaviors or the expression of abnormal or atypical response for the individual animal. An appreciation for the pet's normal display of behaviors provides the foundation for the assessment. New behaviors such as vocalizing, pacing, eliminating in the home, or even panting are readily observed by the attentive caregiver. However, the absence or muted expression of normal behaviors

Box 2
Canine communication: gradient of expression of anxiety

Subtle low-level anxiety signs:

    Sniffing ground, scratching, urination, or defecation

    Yawning, blinking

    Nose licking or tongue flicking

    Diverting eyes

Low-level anxiety, conflict signs:

    Turning head away,

    So-called wet dog shake (when not wet)

    Momentary lack of motion

    Cowering or crouching

Moderate-level anxiety, conflict signs:

    Freezing (holding still, sitting)

    Turning body away

    Pawing or attention seeking

    Snatching or grabbing offered food

    Quiver of lip

    Tail down or motionless

    Submissive urination

Medium-level anxiety, conflict signs:

    Walking away, retreating

    Weight shifted back

    Creeping

    Ears back

Intense or aroused signs of anxiety, conflict

    So-called whale eye (sideways glance shows white of eye)

    Hackles raised on back

    Tail tucked, body lowered, or crouching

    Lip lift

Reactive signs of anxiety, conflict:

    Staring, orienting toward rather than away

    Weight shifted forward

    Stiffening of body, tightening of muscles

    Snarl or lip lift with teeth exposed

Reactive signs of anxiety, conflict; may include aggression:

    Staring, orienting toward rather than away

    Weight shifted forward

    Stiffening of body, tightening of muscles

    Snarl or lip lift with teeth exposed

Growl

Vicious barking

Lunging forward

Erect, tall stance (tail may be in motion)

Bite (may range from single inhibited bites to multiple or uninhibited bites)

requires keen observation. The dog that fails to bark when someone comes to the door may be suffering from severe pain, memory loss, anxiety, or poor health. Moreover, clients rarely complain when their dog ceases to steal food off the counter, jump up during greeting, or chase the family cat, and the absence of these undesirable behaviors may be important determinants in an accurate diagnosis. Although the onset and progression of signs of fear or anxiety may be immediate when the stimulus approaches quickly or appears unexpectedly, most pets begin expressing subtle signs of anxiety such as yawning, nose licking, or momentary immobilization (see **Box 2**). If the threat either increases in intensity or persists, the pet may show signs of increased anxiety that may lead to avoidance and retreat or could escalate to threats (growling) or defensive aggression (fight or flight). Pain, illness, and cognitive dysfunction may also result in reduced tolerance and an increase in avoidance or aggression; however, pets that are ill or painful may be more likely to maintain their position (especially a resting or hiding location) and use aggression rather than avoidance as a strategy to remove the threat. Reduction of anxiety, along with pain control, should reduce the frequency and intensity of aggressive displays. **Box 2** shows a gradient of anxiety expression beginning with mild responses, escalating to aggression.[49]

Behaviors to consider when assessing anxiety include posture, facial expression, ability/willingness to walk or move around, tendency to lie down and sleep, position when in its bed or crate, locations of rest or sleep, appetite, demeanor, mental status, greeting behavior, and vocalization. Specifically, alterations in social interactions including decreased play with family members or other pets, decreased interest in chase or tug games, hiding or seeking seclusion, increased sleep or altered quality of sleep, and decreased interest in play toys (**Fig. 1**) may indicate pain or an underlying medical concern. Pain, illness, changes in sensory perception, and unfamiliar contexts may all reduce a pet's tolerance and thus result in an incremental increase in the expression of intense conflict-based or anxiety-based signs. If the underlying health problem can be managed or resolved, there may be a return to normalcy. However, because many conditions in the patient in palliative care cannot be resolved, monitoring for improvement in signs is an important component of assessing response to therapy and patient welfare.

Cognitive Dysfunction Syndrome

Cognitive dysfunction is a neurodegenerative disorder of senior dogs and cats that is characterized by gradual cognitive decline and increasing brain disorders.[1,16,34,35,37–39,50–53] The development and validation of neuropsychological tests for assessing canine cognitive function in a laboratory setting, including discrimination learning, oddity discrimination learning, reversal learning, and spatial memory, has been instrumental in documenting age-related cognitive differences (**Fig. 2**).[1,5,34,35,50–52] Recently, the canine test apparatus and protocols have been modified for use in cats. Preliminary data show age differences, with senior cats being impaired relative to normal adults.[15,53] This feline battery should also prove

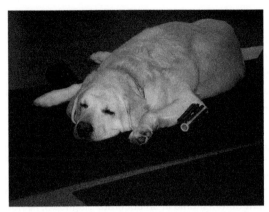

Fig. 1. This dog has lost interest in manipulating food toys; the cognitive, social, and exploratory changes in behavior with cognitive impairment may depend on observing the absence of normal activities. (*Courtesy of* Theresa DePorter, DVM, Bloomfield Hills, MI.)

instrumental in determining the relationship between brain disorders and CDS in cats as well as in the development of therapeutic interventions.

Based on clinical signs alone, CDS has been traditionally diagnosed in dogs 11 years of age and older. However, dogs show impairment in the spatial memory task as early as 6 to 8 years of age.[51] Laboratory studies have identified altered sleep-wake cycles, increased stereotypy, and decreased social contact with humans in dogs with cognitive impairment.[54] In cats, based on more limited data, cognitive and motor performance seem to decline starting at approximately 10 to 11 years of age, but functional change in the neurons of the caudate nucleus have been seen by 6 to 7 years of age.[55–57]

To diagnose CDS, veterinarians must rely on owner history. Only with careful questioning is it likely that signs will be detectable in the earliest stages of development. The diagnosis was initially based on the following clinical signs: (1) disorientation, (2) altered interactions with people or other pets, (3) altered sleep-wake cycles, and (4)

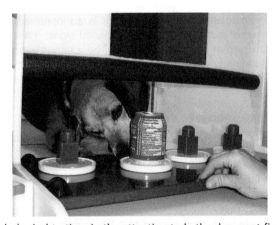

Fig. 2. Neuropsychological testing. In the attention task, the dog must find the food under the correct (different) object when 0, 1, 2, or 3 incorrect objects (distracters) are presented concurrently. (*Courtesy of* CanCog Technologies Inc., Toronto, ON; with permission.)

house soiling, which are represented by the acronym DISH. In addition, because activity may decline, increase, or become repetitive (stereotypical) in pets with CDS, an A for activity has been added to DISH (DISHA).[1] Although age-related impairments in learning and memory are arguably the most important hallmark of cognitive decline, the average pet may appear minimally challenged as its learning and memory declines, currently limiting the use of this measure in a clinically meaningful way; by contrast, neuropsychological testing can show changes many years earlier than behavioral questionnaires and may provide an important measure in the future if it can be adopted for use with the average pet. In addition, anxiety seems to be associated with brain aging and cognitive decline. In humans with Alzheimer disease and other age-related dementias, anxiety, troubled sleep, and agitation may be associated with cognitive decline and frontal lobe dysfunction.[58,59]

Clinically, a questionnaire is generally used to assess whether a pet may have signs consistent with CDS (**Table 4**).[1] However, further work is ongoing to develop standardized and validated questionnaires for the assessment of CDS in dogs and cats. One recent publication based primarily on an Internet questionnaire of 957 dogs produced a standardized rating scale that measured both severity for confusion (staring blankly, getting stuck), repetitive activity, recognition of familiar people and pets, avoidance of patting, and ability to find food, as well as changes in the previous 6 months in recognition of people, confusion, activity, and finding food.[60] Another scale, the Age-related Cognitive and Affective Disorders (ARCAD) scale, has been developed in France.[1] In cats, clinicians tend to assume that CDS has parallel signs to those seen in a dog, which requires additional research to confirm. Once potential CDS signs are identified, any medical condition that might cause or contribute to the signs must first be ruled out. Because senior pets often have multiple health issues, the diagnosis of a medical problem does not rule out the possibility of concurrent CDS. The clinician is required to use best judgment in an attempt to determine the contribution of medical or drug factors to the behavioral signs.

MANAGEMENT AND TREATMENT OPTIONS
Management of Nighttime Waking and Anxiety

Many of the common behavioral presenting complaints in senior pets are related to anxiety, including an increased prevalence of separation anxiety, phobias, excessive vocalization, aggression, and waking at nights. Because disruption of nighttime rest is detrimental to the elderly and debilitated patient and to the family caring for their pet, it is one of the most common presenting complaints for behavior problems in senior dogs and cats (see **Table 1**).

For night waking in dogs and cats, CDS and neurologic diseases, pain, an increased need to eliminate, sensory decline, hypertension, and the behavioral effects of drugs are some of the more common contributing factors. In addition, when signs of anxiety, fears, and phobias are exhibited at night, then the added sleep disruption for the owner can severely affect the owner's level of tolerance and the bond between pet and owner. Further compounding the problem is that, even if the underlying cause can be identified and controlled or resolved, once the pet's sleep cycle is altered, a combination of medical therapeutics, cognitive therapeutics, behavioral modification, and environmental management, as well as drugs (discussed later and in **Table 5**), to reduce anxiety and help reestablish normal sleep cycles may all be required concurrently.

It is important to determine the precise pattern of aberrant nighttime waking. Some pets may be slow to settle and go to sleep compared with others that go to sleep and

Table 4
Cognitive dysfunction screening checklist

	Age First Noticed	Score: None, 0; Mild, 1; Moderate, 2; Severe, 3
Confusion – awareness – spatial orientation		
Gets stuck or cannot get around objects		
Stares blankly at walls or floor		
Decreased recognition of familiar people/pets		
Goes into wrong side of door; walks into door/ walls		
Relationships – social interactions		
Decreased interest in petting/avoids contact		
Decreased greeting behavior		
In need of constant contact, overdependent, clingy		
Altered relationship with other household pets – less social		
Altered relationship with other household pets – fear/anxiety		
Aggression – family members – unfamiliar people –		
Family pets – unfamiliar pets – other:		
Response to stimuli		
Decreased response to auditory stimuli (sounds)		
Increased response, fear, phobia to auditory stimuli		
Decreased response to visual stimuli (sights)		
Increased response, fear, phobia to visual stimuli		
Decreased responsiveness to food/odor		
Activity/anxiety – increased/repetitive		
Pacing/wanders aimlessly		
Anaps at air/licks air		
Licking owners – household objects –		
Vocalization		
Increased appetite (eats quicker or more food)		
Restless/agitation		
Activity – apathy/depressed		
Decreased interest in food/treats		
Decreased exploration/activity		
Decreased interest in social interactions/play		
Decreased self-care (hygiene)		
Sleep-wake cycles; reversed day/night schedule		
Restless sleep/waking at nights		
Increased daytime sleep		
Learning and memory – House soiling		
Indoor elimination at sites previously trained		

(continued on next page)

Table 4 (continued)		
	Age First Noticed	Score: None, 0; Mild, 1; Moderate, 2; Severe, 3
Decrease/loss of signaling		
Goes outdoors, then returns indoors and eliminates		
Elimination in crate or sleeping area		
Learning and memory – work, tasks, commands		
Impaired working ability – decreased ability to perform task		
Decreased responsiveness to familiar commands and tricks		
Inability/slow to learn new tasks		

Adapted from Landsberg GM, Hunthausen W, Ackerman L. The effects of aging on the behavior of senior pets. Handbook of behavior problems of the dog and cat. 2nd edition. Saunders; 2003. p. 273; with permission.

then wake multiple times a night. Although rare, some pets may be unable to settle for the entire night. It is also important to determine the dogs daily routine: some dogs sleep more during the day or early morning or throughout the evening but then keep family members awake at night. Cats are naturally more active at night, especially around dawn, so nighttime waking is not necessarily an abnormal behavior in the cat. However, a change in previously established sleep patterns, increased activity, disorientation, and vocalization may be related to abnormal conditions, such as medical conditions, pain, or cognitive dysfunction. Furthermore, cats may be territorially reactive to activities by felines outside the home. Noise phobias may occur all the time but be more problematic at night, presumably because of reduced ambient noise, which may lead to an apparent random or unpredictable pattern of nighttime waking when the stimulus is not audible to the people. When nighttime waking is mentioned by families, it is important to regard this as an immediate and serious concern; it is essential to resume normal nighttime sleeping patterns promptly to assure the welfare of family and pets.

Consideration of the pet's medical health issues, the pet's daily routine, and the pattern of nighttime waking, aids in both diagnosis and the development of treatment recommendations. For example, if a dog is not waking up the family until 5 AM, then modifications to the bedtime routine are not likely to be helpful and may be counterproductive. Pets that cannot settle, but then eventually sleep all night and into the morning, may benefit from changes to prebedtime routine. It is important to inquire about the desired sleeping pattern for family members because variations or unusual patterns in their routine will affect the timing of recommendations.

Basic recommendations begin with a consistent and predictable bedtime routine. Use family habits or the dog's previous sleeping patterns as a guide. For dogs, massage or gentle petting while the pet is resting in desired sleeping area may promote the atmosphere and routine essential for sleeping. Turn off the TV and at least dim the lights, though some elderly pets benefit from a night light as their vision deteriorates. Recommend a pheromone collar or a pheromone diffuser in the sleeping area of the dog or cat, respectively. Provide a comfortable place to sleep; again, first consider the pet's previous pattern of rest before making recommendations. Most

Table 5
Drug doses for behavior therapy

	Dog	Cat
Alprazolam[a]	0.02–0.1 mg/kg twice to 4 times a day	0.125–0.25 mg/cat once to 3 times a day
Diazepam[a]	0.5–2 mg/kg once to 4 times a day	0.2–0.5 mg/kg twice a day to 3 times a day
Oxazepam[a]	0.2–1 mg/kg once to twice a day	0.2–0.5 mg/kg once to twice a day
Clonazepam[a]	0.1–1.0 mg/kg twice to 3 times a day	0.02–0.2 mg/kg once to twice a day
Lorazepam[a]	0.025–0.2 mg/kg once to 3 times a day	0.025–0.05 mg/kg once to twice a day
Melatonin	3–9 mg/dog	1.5–6 mg/cat
Diphenhydramine[a]	2–4 mg/kg	1–4 mg/kg
Fluoxetine	1.0–2.0 mg/kg once a day	0.5–1 mg/kg once a day
Sertraline	1–5 mg/kg once a day or 2.5 mg/kg divided twice a day	0.5–1.5 mg/kg once a day
Buspirone	0.5–2.0 mg/kg once to 3 times a day	0.5 to 1 mg/kg twice a day
Trazodone	2–5 mg/kg as needed up to 8–10 mg/kg twice to 3 times a day	Not determined
Phenobarbital[b]	2.5–5 mg/kg twice a day	2.5 mg/kg twice a day
Gabapentin[b]	10–30 mg/kg twice to 3 times a day	5–10 mg/kg once to 3 times a day
Potassium bromide[b]	10–35 mg/kg daily or divided twice a day	Not recommended
Selegiline	0.5–1 mg/kg once a day in the morning	0.5–1 mg/kg once a day in the morning
Memantine	0.3–1 mg/kg once a day	Not determined
Amantadine	1.25–4 mg/kg by mouth once to twice a day	3 mg/kg by mouth once a day

[a] Use single dosing before sleep or anxiety-evoking event, up to maximum daily dosing for control of ongoing anxiety.
[b] Doses are for seizure control: dose and frequency may need to be adjusted when used for other applications (pain management, behavior therapy) or if combined with other drugs.

pets benefit from a specific preferred resting area; for dogs this may be near family members such as in the bedroom, with a crate or tether or with the door closed (if the dog tends to wander or soil at night). Some dogs select another location removed from family members. Provision of a heated bed may ease pain and sensory discomfort caused by cold.

Advise families that punishment or scolding will not ease nighttime waking but will contribute to the pet's anxiety and confusion. However, unless the dog's medical needs require that it be attended to during the night, giving any form of attention (feeding, walks, allowing onto the family bed, or even scolding) may further reinforce the behavior. For dogs with extreme difficulty sleeping accompanied by increased activity at night, tethering or crating the pet might be considered. A head halter may help a dog settle if it has been trained to it already. Comfort wraps such as the Anxiety Wrap (Animals Plus, LLC) or Thundershirt (Thundershirt) may reduce agitation and allow rest. The Calming Cap (Premier Pet Products) may be useful to help a dog settle, but some form of confinement should be used to prevent wandering because the dog's visual ability is reduced. In the morning, open blinds to allow natural sunlight early in the morning and consider the benefits of getting the pet outdoors. Exposure to natural light may help maintain a night-day cycle. The long walks the family took when the pet was healthy could be replaced by quiet time together in the outdoors; quality time on park benches or picnic blankets should replace long, strenuous walks in dogs with weakness or pain. Increased daytime enrichment with several quality interactive sessions, feeding toys (as demonstrated by a senior cat and a dog on videos online (within this article at www.vetsmall.theclinics.com, May 2011 issue); (Videos 2 and 3) and a final interactive play session before bedtime may help encourage better nighttime sleep while promoting the human-animal bond. Further discussion of drugs or natural alternatives to reduce anxiety and help reestablish nighttime sleep are discussed later.

Management of CDS

Although both environmental enrichment and therapeutic options are useful in improving the signs, and perhaps slowing the decline, of CDS, the first consideration is the treatment of any other concurrent medical problems, including the management of pain and discomfort. Any medications that are essential in the treatment of the pet's medical health need to be considered in the use and selection of therapeutic agents for CDS. Because it is increasingly likely that geriatric and palliative care patients will require multiple medications or supplements, the veterinarian should take responsibility to advise owners of potential interactions (both beneficial or harmful) of those medications and supplements dispensed as well as those that the owner may obtain from other sources.

Maintaining a regular, predictable daily routine and providing the pet with control to engage in pleasant, and avoid unpleasant, interactions may help to reduce stress and anxiety and maintain temporal orientation.[2] Canine studies have also shown that, not only is mental stimulation an essential component in maintaining quality of life, but that continued enrichment in the form of training, play, exercise, and novel toys can help to maintain cognitive function and perhaps slow cognitive decline.[5] This is analogous to human studies in which education, brain exercise, and physical exercise have been found to delay the onset of dementia. Concurrent use of diets and supplements for improving cognitive function may help the pet better engage in enrichment activities as well as, perhaps, provide some level of neuroprotective effect.

Because medical problems may preclude the pet from engaging in some forms of enrichment, owners should find alternative forms of social activities (eg, short walks, tug toys, find-and-seek games, reward training) and various forms of object play (eg, food manipulation toys, chew toys) that are within the pet's physical and mental capabilities (**Figs. 3** and **4**). A video of the cat in **Fig. 3** is available online (within this article at www.vetsmall.theclinics.com, May 2011 issue) that illustrates play in a senior cat (Video 4). Owners should also have realistic expectations, or be advised, as to the limitations that might be achieved in improving the behavior of a senior pet based on the pet's physical health and cognitive function. Accommodations may also need to be made to the owner's schedule or the pet's environment to address such needs. For example, dogs may require more frequent trips outdoors, a dog walker, or an indoor elimination area if they have medical conditions leading to polyuria or incontinence, whereas ramps and physical support devices may be required to help address mobility issues. For cats, more litterboxes, or more frequent cleaning, may be required to treat house soiling caused by polyuria, whereas ramps, litterboxes with lower sides, larger litter boxes, or relocation of litterboxes may be required for cats with mobility problems. Provision of nonslip surfaces or rugs may provide stability and avoid an

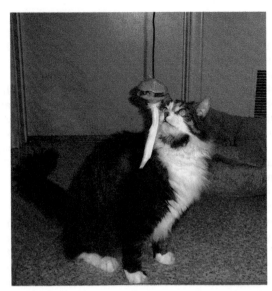

Fig. 3. A food-filled toy, hanging from the doorway, can be used to encourage and stimulate both physical and mental activity to acquire food. (*Courtesy of* Gary Landsberg, DVM, MRCVS, Thornhill, Ontario, Canada.)

anxiety-causing event such as falling or slipping. As sensory acuity, sensory processing, and cognitive function decline, adding new odor, tactile, and sound cues (provided there is some residual hearing) might help the pet better navigate its environment and maintain some degree of environmental familiarity and comfort.

Therapeutic Options for Sleeplessness and Anxiety

In addition to the control of medical problems including CDS, and the use of behavior modification and environmental management, pharmacologic or natural therapeutics

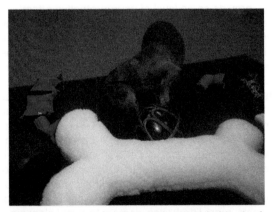

Fig. 4. Mental enrichment for the senior pet may be provided in the form of food puzzle toys. Manipulation of the toy by oral or physical means allows release of the food, which immediately rewards the exploratory behavior of a novel item. (*Courtesy of* Theresa DePorter, DVM, Bloomfield Hills, MI.)

may be required to reduce anxiety and aid in reestablishing normal sleep-wake cycles (see **Table 5**). Melatonin, although not sedating, may be useful as part of a bedtime routine ritual and may be best given 30 minutes before bedtime; melatonin should not be redosed at other times of day when used to establish nighttime sleeping patterns. Some medications, such as diphenhydramine, phenobarbital, or trazodone, which may be given for other indications or solely for sleep support, may provide useful sedation if dosed before bedtime provided they do not cause excessive sedation or incoordination that lasts into the daytime. For the dog or cat that has difficulty settling at night but then sleeps well, situational use of anxiolytics that may promote sleep may be beneficial as adjunctive therapy to behavior modification. Benzodiazepines maybe useful because of rapid onset of short-acting anxiolytic and sedative effects. In senior pets, especially if liver function might be compromised, clonazepam, lorazepam, or oxazepam might be preferable to alprazolam or diazepam because they have no active intermediate metabolites. Because pain may contribute to unsettled sleep or night waking, consider pain management products. Gabapentin might be a consideration as an adjunctive therapy for pain management as well as for its behavioral calming effects.

For senior pets with generalized anxiety, noise phobias, or separation anxiety that is not restricted to nighttime anxiety, consider drugs with fewer side effects, such as buspirone and selective serotonin reuptake inhibitors such as fluoxetine and sertraline. Paroxetine and tricyclic antidepressants have varying degrees of anticholinergic effects and may therefore be less desirable. Natural compounds that have been shown to be beneficial in reducing anxiety and perhaps help pets to settle at night include suntheanine (Anxitane, Virbac), honokiol and berberine extracts (Harmonease, VPL), α-casein (Zylkene Intervet/Schering-Plough Animal Health), pheromones (DAP and Feliway, CEVA Animal Health), and lavender essential oils.[61]

Drug Therapy for CDS

There are many medications available for treatment of cognitive dysfunction but data to support efficacy is variable and in some cases minimal (see **Table 5**). Selegiline (Anipryl, Pfizer Animal Health) was the first product approved for the treatment of CDS in dogs. Selegiline (which is also licensed in Europe under the brand name Selgian, CEVA Animal Health) is a selective and irreversible inhibitor of MAOB in the dog.[62] It may act by enhancing dopamine and other catecholamines in the cortex and hippocampus and has been shown both in the laboratory and clinical setting to improve signs related to CDS. Selegiline is considered to be neuroprotective, potentially by increasing efficiency of superoxide dismutase and catalase for improved free radical scavenging, which may decrease nerve damage/degeneration.[63] Selegiline is not licensed in cats; however, it has been used off label at the same dose with anecdotal reports of improvement in CDS-like signs.[64] Selegiline may require from 2 to 6 weeks of administration to show clinical improvement. It should not be used concurrently with other monoamine oxidase (MAO) inhibitors including amitraz (Mitaban, Upjohn, Preventic Allerderm/Virbac), selective serotonin reuptake inhibitors, tricyclic antidepressants, narcotics, and dextromethorphan. Selegiline should be used cautiously with drugs that might enhance serotonin transmission, such as buspirone, trazodone, and tramadol.

Propentofylline (Vivitonin, Intervet/Schering-Plough Animal Health) is licensed in some European countries for the treatment of dullness, lethargy, and depressed demeanor in old dogs. Propentofylline may increase blood flow to the heart, skeletal muscles, and brain. It inhibits platelet aggregation, inhibits thrombus formation, has bronchodilator action, and improves the flow properties of erythrocytes. It has a direct effect on the heart and reduces peripheral vascular resistance, thereby lowering cardiac load. Although not licensed in cats, it has been anecdotally reported to be useful.[16]

Drugs that may enhance the noradrenergic system, such as adrafinil and modafinil, might be useful in older dogs to improve alertness and help maintain normal sleep-wake cycles (by increasing daytime exploration and activity).[65,66] However, dose and efficacy in dogs has not been established. Other new treatment strategies may include the N-methyl-D-aspartate receptor antagonist memantine or hormone replacement therapy.[67]

Because the elderly are particularly susceptible to the effects of anticholinergic drugs, it is prudent to consider therapies with less anticholinergic effects and those that are less sedating for both dogs and cats; however, although drugs that enhance cholinergic transmission might be beneficial for senior dogs, there is limited evidence available for dose schedule recommendations.[68]

Nutritional and Dietary Therapy for CDS

Another strategy in the treatment of CDS is to use dietary supplements to improve antioxidant defense and reduce the toxic effects of free radicals. In humans, several studies have found that dietary management may reduce the risk, or delay the onset, of dementia. For example, a high intake of fruits and vegetables, nuts, whole grains, and vitamins E and C may decrease the risk for cognitive decline and dementia.[69,70] In dogs, a senior diet (Canine b/d, Hills Pet Nutrition) has been shown to improve the signs and slow the progress of cognitive decline. It is supplemented with a combination of fatty acids, antioxidants (vitamins C and E, β-carotene, selenium, flavonoids, and carotenoids), as well as DL-α-lipoic diet and L-carnitine, which are intended to enhance mitochondrial function.[5,71,72] The diet improved performance on several cognitive tasks when compared with a nonsupplemented diet, beginning as early as to 2 to 8 weeks after the onset of therapy. After 2 years, a control group (no enrichment, control diet) showed a dramatic decline in cognitive function, whereas those in either the enriched diet or the environmental enrichment group continued to do better than controls.[71,72] However, the combined effect of the enriched diet plus the enriched environment provided the greatest improvement.[5] More recently, Purina One Vibrant Maturity 7+ Formula (Nestlé Purina PetCare), a diet that uses botanic oils containing medium-chain triglycerides (MCT) to provide ketone bodies as an alternate source of energy for aging neurons, has also been shown to significantly improve cognitive function in senior dogs.[73] Supplementation with MCTs has been shown to improve mitochondrial function, increase polyunsaturated fatty acids, and decrease amyloid precursor protein in the parietal cortex of aged dogs.[74,75] Cognitive diets for cats have not yet been developed, although canine cognitive diets are generally nutritionally sound for cats.

Several clinical trials have shown improvements in clinical signs associated with CDS in dogs using dietary supplements containing phosphatidylserine, a membrane phospholipid.[10,76,77] One product, Senilife (CEVA Animal Health) was tested on dogs using a memory task after administration of 60 days of either a placebo or the product.[78] An example of a cat performing a memory task in a laboratory model may be viewed online (within this article at www.vetsmall.theclinics.com, May 2011 issue) and is discussed earlier (see Video 1).

There is also a video online (within this article at www.vetsmall.theclinics.com, May 2011 issue) showing a dog performing the variable-object discrimination test, which examines selective attention. In this task, the correct object is presented with 0 to 3

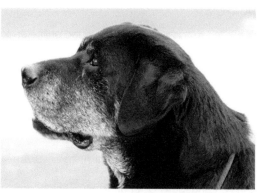

Fig. 5. Senior pets may show profound physical changes such as graying of hair around the face and muzzle that can be recognized effortlessly as a sign of aging, but the cognitive changes are more subtle and oblige our intuitive and thoughtful compassion for our aging pets. (*Courtesy of* Theresa DePorter, DVM, Bloomfield Hills, MI.)

identical incorrect objects (distracters). Performance declines as distracter number increases (Video 5).

Performance accuracy was improved in the treated group compared with baseline, and dogs receiving the supplement in the first portion of the study maintained their improved performance.[78] The product also contains *Gingko biloba*, an MAO inhibitor and free radical scavenger, vitamin B6 (pyridoxine), vitamin E, and resveratrol, which may protect against oxidative damage and reduce β-amyloid secretion. The tested product was an earlier formulation excluding resveratrol.

S-Adenosyl-L-methionine (SAMe; Novifit, Virbac), is found in all living cells and is formed from methionine and ATP. SAMe may help to maintain cell membrane fluidity, receptor function, and the turnover of monoamine transmitters, as well as increase the production of glutathione.[79] In a recent placebo-controlled trial, greater improvement in activity and awareness was reported in the SAMe group after 8 weeks.[80] Both Seni-life and SAMe have label claims for use in cats, but there are no published studies to support their efficacy in improving signs of CDS in cats.

SUMMARY

The assessment and consideration of the senior dog's and cat's quality of life is complicated by age-related changes in health and behavioral signs. Physical signs of old age may be obvious (**Fig. 5**), but mental and cognitive changes require more careful observation. Changes in behavior may represent the earliest indications of medical problems, or disorders of the central nervous system, and these may be bidirectional. Moreover, diagnoses of CDS and other age-related behavioral problems are underdiagnosed and affect a substantial portion of aged companion animals. Therefore, the primary caregiver must establish the contribution of medical problems, as well as the effects of concurrent medications and pain, to behavioral signs consistent with age-related behavioral problems such as CDS, sleep disturbances, and anxiety. This article describes potential treatment regimens to address age-related behavioral problems, as well as a framework for investigating differential diagnoses. Overall, early identification of changes in behavior are essential for the adequate treatment and management of both medical and behavioral problems, as well as for monitoring outcomes.

SUPPLEMENTARY DATA

Supplementary data related to this article can be found online at doi:10.1016/j.cvsm.2011.03.017.

REFERENCES

1. Landsberg GM, Hunthausen W, Ackerman L. The effects of aging on the behavior of senior pets. Handbook of behavior problems of the dog and cat. 2nd edition. Philadelphia: Saunders; 2003. p. 269–304.
2. McMillan FD. Maximizing quality of life in ill animals. J Am Anim Hosp Assoc 2003;39(3):227–35.
3. Epstein M, Kuehn N, Landsberg G, et al. AAHA senior care guidelines for dogs and cats. J Am Anim Hosp Assoc 2005;41(2):81–91.
4. American Association of Feline Practitioners Senior Care Guidelines. December 2008. Available at: http://www.catvets.com/professionals/guidelines/publications/?Id=398. Accessed June 22, 2010.
5. Milgram NW, Head EA, Zicker SC, et al. Long term treatment with antioxidants and a program of behavioral enrichment reduces age-dependant impairment in discrimination and reversal learning in beagle dogs. Exp Gerontol 2004; 39(5):753–65.
6. Barak Y, Aizenberg D. Is dementia preventable? Focus on Alzheimer's disease. Expert Rev Neurother 2010;10(11):1689–98.
7. Salvin HE, McGreevy PD, Sachev PS, et al. Under diagnosis of canine cognitive dysfunction; a cross-sectional survey of older companion dogs. Vet J 2010; 184(3):277–81.
8. Nielson JC, Hart BL, Cliff KD, et al. Prevalence of behavioral changes associated with age-related cognitive impairment in dogs. J Am Vet Med Assoc 2001; 218(11):1787–91.
9. Golini L, Colangeli R, Tranquillo V, et al. Association between neurologic and cognitive dysfunction signs in a sample of aging dogs. J Vet Behav 2009;4(1): 25–30.
10. Osella MC, Re G, Odore R, et al. Canine cognitive dysfunction syndrome: Prevalence, clinical signs and treatment with a neuroprotective nutraceutical. Appl Anim Behav Sci 2007;105(4):297–310.
11. Mariotti VM, Landucci M, Lippi I, et al. Epidemiological study of behavioural disorders in elderly dogs [abstract]. In: Heath S, editor. Proceedings 7th International Meeting of Veterinary Behaviour Medicine. Belgium: ESVCE; 2009. p. 241–43.
12. Horwitz D. Dealing with common behavior problems in senior dogs. Vet Med 2001;96(11):869–87.
13. Azkona G, Garcia-Beleguer S, Chacon G, et al. Prevalence and risk factors of behavioral changes associated with age-related cognitive impairment in geriatric dogs. J Small Anim Pract 2009;50(2):87–91.
14. Hart BL. Effect of gonadectomy on subsequent development of age-related cognitive impairment in dogs. J Am Vet Med Assoc 2001;219(1):51–6.
15. Landsberg G, Denenberg S, Araujo J. Cognitive dysfunction in cats. A syndrome we used to dismiss as old age. J Feline Med Surg 2010;12(11):837–48.
16. Gunn-Moore D, Moffat K, Christie LA, et al. Cognitive dysfunction and the neurobiology of ageing in cats. J Small Anim Pract 2007;48(10):546–53.
17. Johnson RW. The concept of sickness behavior: a brief chronological account of four key discoveries. Vet Immunol Immunopathol 2002;87(3-4):443–50.

18. Waisglass SE, Landsberg GM, Yager JA, et al. Underlying medical conditions in cats with presumptive psychogenic alopecia. J Am Vet Med Assoc 2006;228(11): 1705–9.
19. Hielm Bjorkman AK, Kuusela E, Liman A, et al. Evaluation of methods for assessment of pain associated with chronic osteoarthritis in dogs. J Am Vet Med Assoc 2003;222(11):1552–8.
20. Hellyer P, Rodan I, Brunt J, et al. AAHA/AAFP Pain Management Guidelines for dogs and cats. J Feline Med Surg 2007;9(6):466–80.
21. Lascelles D. Robertson SA DJD-associated pain in cats. What can we do to promote patient comfort? J Feline Med Surg 2010;12(3):200–12.
22. Bécuwe V, Bélanger MC, Frank D, et al. Gastrointestinal disease in dogs with excessive licking of surfaces [abstract #173]. J Vet Intern Med 2009;23:736.
23. Horwitz D. Behavioral and environmental factors associated with elimination behavior problems in cats: a retrospective study. Appl Anim Behav Sci 1997; 52(1):129–37.
24. Berteselli GV, Servidaq F, DallAra P, et al. Evaluation of the immunological, stress and behavioral parameters in dogs (Canis familiaris) with anxiety-related disorders. In: Mills D, Levine E, Landsberg G, et al, editors. Current issues and research in veterinary behavioral medicine. West Lafayette (IN): Purdue Press; 2005. p. 18–22.
25. Riva J, Bondiolotti G, Micelazzi M, et al. Anxiety related behavioural disorders and neurotransmitters in dogs. Appl Anim Behav Sci 2008;114(1):168–81.
26. Dreschel NA. Anxiety, fear, disease and lifespan in domestic dogs. J Vet Behav 2009;4(6):249–50.
27. Weistropp JL, Kass PH, Buffington CAT. Evaluation of the effects of stress in cats with Idiopathic cystitis. Am J Vet Res 2006;67(4):731–6.
28. Buffington CAT, Pacak K. Increased plasma norepinephrine concentration in cats with interstitial cystitis. J Urol 2001;165(6 part 1):2051–4.
29. Buffington CAT, Westropp JL, Chew DJ, et al. Clinical evaluation of multimodal environmental modification (MEMO) in the management of cats with idiopathic cystitis. J Feline Med Surg 2006;8(4):261–8.
30. Virga V. Behavioral dermatology. Vet Clin North Am 2003;33(2):231–51.
31. Nagata M, Shibata K. Importance of psychogenic factors in canine recurrent pyoderma. Vet Dermatol 2004;15(s1):42.
32. Nagata M, Shibata K, Irimajiri M, et al. Importance of psychogenic dermatoses in dogs with pruritic behavior. Vet Dermatol 2002;13(4):211–9.
33. Overall KL. Dogs as "natural" models of human psychiatric disorders: assessing validity and understanding mechanism. Prog Neuropsychopharmacol Biol Psychiatry 2000;24(5):727–76.
34. Borras D, Ferrer I, Pumarola M. Age related changes in the brain of the dog. Vet Pathol 1999;36(3):202–11.
35. Tapp PD, Siwak CT, Gao FQ, et al. Frontal lobe volume, function, and beta-amyloid pathology in a canine model of aging. J Neurosci 2004;24(38):8205–13.
36. Zhang C, Hua T, Zhu Z, et al. Age related changes of structures in cerebellar cortex of cat. J Biosci 2006;31(1):55–60.
37. Cummings BJ, Satou T, Head E, et al. Diffuse plaques contain c-terminal AB42 and not AB40: evidence from cats and dogs. Neurobiol Aging 1996;17(4):653–9.
38. Cummings BJ, Head E, Afagh AJ, et al. B-Amyloid accumulation correlates with cognitive dysfunction in the aged canine. Neurobiol Learn Mem 1996;66(1):11–23.
39. Colle MA, Hauw JJ, Crespau F, et al. Vascular and parenchymal beta-amyloid deposition in the aging dog: correlation with behavior. Neurobiol Aging 2000; 21(5):695–704.

40. Nakamura S, Nakayama H, Kiatipattanasakul W, et al. Senile plaques in very aged cats. Acta Neuropathol 1996;91(4):437–9.

41. Head E, Liu J, Hagen TM, et al. Oxidative damage increases with age in a canine model of human brain aging. J Neurochem 2002;82(2):375–81.

42. Araujo JA, Studzinski CM, Milgram NW, et al. Further evidence for the cholinergic hypothesis of aging and dementia from the canine model of aging. Prog Neuro-psychopharmacol Biol Psychiatry 2005;29(3):411–22.

43. Araujo JA, Chan AD, Winka LL, et al. Dose-specific effects of scopolamine on canine cognition: impairment of visuospatial memory, but not visuospatial discrimination. Psychopharmacology 2004;175(1):92–8.

44. Pugliese M, Cangitano C, Ceccariglia S, et al. Canine cognitive dysfunction and the cerebellum: acetylcholinesterase reduction, neuronal and glial changes. Brain Res 2007;1139:85–94.

45. Zhang JH, Sampogna S, Morales FR, et al. Age-related changes in cholinergic neurons in the laterodorsal and the pedunculo-pontine tegmental nuclei of cats: a combined light and electron microscopic study. Brain Res 2005;1052: 47–55.

46. Head E, McCleary R, Hahn FF, et al. Region-specific age at onset of beta-amyloid in dogs. Neurobiol Aging 2000;21(1):89–96.

47. Gunn-Moore DA, McVee J, Bradshaw JM, et al. β-Amyloid and hyper-phosphorylated tau deposition in cat brains. J Feline Med Surg 2006;8(4): 234–42.

48. Head E, Moffat K, Das P, et al. Beta-amyloid deposition and tau phosphorylation in clinically characterized aged cats. Neurobiol Aging 2005;26(5):749–63.

49. Shepherd K. Behavioural medicine as an integral part of veterinary practice. In: Horwitz D, Mills D, Heath S, editors. BSAVA Manual of Canine and Feline Behav-ioural Medicine. 2nd edition. Gloucester (UK): British Small Animal Veterinary Association; 2010. p. 10–23.

50. Tapp PD, Siwak CT, Estrada J, et al. Size and reversal learning in the beagle dog as a measure of executive function and inhibitory control in aging. Learn Mem 2003;10(1):64–73.

51. Studzinski CM, Christie L-A, Araujo JA, et al. Visuospatial function in the beagle dog: an early marker of cognitive decline in a model of human cognitive aging and dementia. Neurobiol Learn Mem 2006;86(2):197–204.

52. Milgram NW, Head E, Weiner E, et al. Cognitive functions and aging in the dog: acquisition of nonspatial visual tasks. Behav Neurosci 1994;108(1):57–68.

53. Milgram NW. Neuropsychological function and aging in cats. Proceedings of Canine Cognition and Aging 15th Annual Conference. Laguna Beach, November 11, 12, 2010.

54. Siwak CT, Tapp PD, Milgram NW. Effect of age and level of cognitive function on spontaneous and exploratory behaviors in the beagle dog. Learn Mem 2001;8(6): 65–70.

55. Harrison J, Buchwald J. Eyeblink conditioning deficits in the old cat. Neurobiol Aging 1983;4(1):45–51.

56. Levine MS, Lloyd RL, Fisher RS, et al. Sensory, motor and cognitive alterations in aged cats. Neurobiol Aging 1987;8(3):253–63.

57. Levine MS, Lloyd RL, Hull CD, et al. Neurophysiological alterations in caudate neurons in aged cats. Brain Res 1987;401(2):213–30.

58. Senanarong V, Cummings JL, Fairbanks L, et al. Agitation in Alzheimer's disease is a manifestation of frontal lobe dysfunction. Dement Geriatr Cogn Disord 2004; 17(1–2):14–20.

59. McCurry SM, Gibbons LE, Logsdon RG, et al. Anxiety and nighttime behavioral disturbances. Awakenings in patients with Alzheimer's disease. J Gerontol Nurs 2004;30(1):12–20.
60. Salvin HE, McGreevy PD, Sachdev PS, et al. The canine cognition dysfunction rating scale (CCDR): A data driven and ecologically relevant assessment tool. Vet J 2010. DOI: 10.1016/j.tvjl.2010.05.014.
61. Wells DL. Aromatherapy for travel-induced excitement in dogs. J Am Vet Med Assoc 2006;229(6):964–7.
62. Milgram NW, Ivy GO, Head E, et al. The effect of L-deprenyl on behavior, cognitive function, and biogenic amines in the dog. Neurochem Res 1993;18(12):1211–9.
63. Carillo MC, Ivy GO, Milgram NW, et al. Deprenyl increases activity of superoxide dismutase in striatum of dog brain. Life Sci 1994;54:1483–9.
64. Landsberg G. Therapeutic options for cognitive decline in senior pets. J Am Anim Hosp Assoc 2006;42(6):407–13.
65. Siwak CT, Gruet P, Woehrle F, et al. Behavioral activating effects of adrafinil in aged canines. Pharmacol Biochem Behav 2000;66(2):293–300.
66. Siwak CT, Gruet P, Woehrle F, et al. Comparison of the effects of adrafinil, propentofylline and nicergoline on behavior in aged dogs. Am J Vet Res 2000;61(11): 1410–4.
67. Martinez-Coria H, Green KN, Billings LM, et al. Memantine improves cognition and reduces Alzheimer's-like neuropathology in transgenic mice. Am J Pathol 2010;176(2):870–80.
68. Studzinski CM, Araujo JA, Milgram NW. The canine model of human cognitive aging and dementia: Pharmacological validity of the model for assessment of human cognitive-enhancing drugs. Prog Neuropsychopharmacol Biol Psychiatry 2005;29(3):489–98.
69. Joseph JA, Shukitt-Hale B, Denisova NA, et al. Long-term dietary strawberry, spinach, or vitamin E supplementation retards the onset of age-related neuronal signal transduction and cognitive behavioral deficits. J Neurosci 1998;18(19): 8047–55.
70. Barberger-Gateau P, Raffaitin C, Letenneur L, et al. Dietary Patterns and Risk of Dementia: a three-city cohort study. Neurology 2007;69(20):1921–30.
71. Milgram NW, Zicker SC, Head E, et al. Dietary enrichment counteracts age-associated cognitive dysfunction in canines. Neurobiol Aging 2002;23(5):737–45.
72. Araujo JA, Studzinski CM, Head E, et al. Assessment of nutritional interventions for modification of age-associated cognitive decline using a canine model of human aging. Age 2005;27(1):27–37.
73. Pan Y, Larson B, Araujo JA, et al. Dietary supplementation with medium-chain TAG has long-lasting cognition-enhancing effects in aged dogs. Br J Nutr 2010;103(12):1746–54.
74. Taha AY, Henderson ST, Burnham WM. Dietary enrichment with medium chain-triglycerides (AC-1203) elevates polyunsaturated fatty acids in the parietal cortex of aged dogs; implications for treating age-related cognitive decline. Neurochem Res 2009;34(9):1619–25.
75. Studzinski CM, MacKay WA, Beckett TL, et al. Induction of ketosis may improve mitochondrial function and decrease steady-state amyloid-beta precursor protein (APP) levels in the aged dog. Brain Res 2008;1226:209–17.
76. Cena F, Colangeli R, Fassola F, et al. Effect of a combination of phosphatidylserine, Gingko biloba, vitamin E and pyridoxine on clinical signs of brain ageing; a pilot multicentric study. In: Beata C, Heath S, Pageat P, editors. Behaviour and internal medicine. Marseille: ESVCE; 2005. p. 127–35.

77. Heath SE, Barabas S, Craze PG. Nutritional supplementation in cases of canine cognitive dysfunction - a clinical trial. Appl Anim Behav Sci 2007;105(4):274–83.
78. Araujo JA, Landsberg GM, Milgram NW, et al. Improvement of short-term memory performance in aged beagles by a nutraceutical supplement containing phosphatidylserine, *Ginkgo biloba*, vitamin E and pyridoxine. Can Vet J 2008;49(4): 379–85.
79. Bottiglieri T. *S*-Adenosyl-L-methionine (SAMe): from the bench to the bedside-molecular basis of a pleiotrophic molecule. Am J Clin Nutr 2002;76(suppl): 1151S–7S.
80. Rème CA, Dramard V, Kern L, et al. Effect of *S*-adenosylmethionine tablets on the reduction of age-related mental decline in dogs: a double-blind placebo-controlled trial. Vet Ther 2008;9(2):69–82.

The Role of Physical Medicine and Rehabilitation for Patients in Palliative and Hospice Care

Robin Downing, DVM, CCRP, CPE

KEYWORDS

- Physical medicine • Physiotherapy • Mobility • End of life

The most common recipients of veterinary physical medicine, physiotherapy, and rehabilitation are animal patients who are recovering from surgery or an injury. It is time to expand consideration of who can benefit from these modalities to include patients in palliative and hospice care. Veterinary patients in palliative and hospice care are animals approaching the end of their lives and for whom aggressive treatment of their disease processes is no longer considered appropriate. Palliative care shifts the focus from curing disease to managing symptoms to maximize comfort and function. Well-designed palliative care is said to allow the pet to live until it dies, enjoying its time with its human family and vice versa. By definition, veterinary patients in palliative and hospice care experience progressive medical diseases, and these are patients who can benefit from physical medicine and rehabilitation.[1] If this application is considered palliative rehabilitation, there are ample opportunities to improve and sustain function and comfort, thus contributing to overall quality of life. Palliative rehabilitation focuses on long-term impairments, working within the patient's illness-dependent limitations to enable participation in as many activities of daily living (ADLs) as possible.[1]

Physical medicine and rehabilitation for the patient in palliative and hospice care acknowledges the adage *use it or lose it*. Chronically ill patients, particularly patients experiencing chronic, maladaptive pain, are generally less active than their nonpainful counterparts. Prolonged inactivity leads to a state of deconditioning in which muscle strength is lost, endurance declines, muscles may contract leading to decreased range of motion (ROM), and bones may become osteopenic.[1] For the immobile patient, or one that spends most of its time recumbent, the weight of the body over boney

The author has nothing to disclose.

The Downing Center for Animal Pain Management, LLC, 415 Main Street, Windsor, CO 80550, USA

E-mail address: drrobin@downingcenter.com

Vet Clin Small Anim 41 (2011) 591–608

doi:10.1016/j.cvsm.2011.03.011

vetsmall.theclinics.com

prominences may lead to pressure necrosis: bed sores. Physical medicine and rehabilitation provide a strategy for preventing such negative consequences while offering a framework within which to engage the pet and the family in ongoing interaction.

Physical medicine and rehabilitation techniques lend themselves well to application both in the veterinary practice and in the home. Practitioners are generally limited only by their imagination in developing a reasonable physical medicine and rehabilitation program for the patient in palliative and hospice care. Many of the practices and techniques that are considered to be palliative rehabilitation can be taught to the client so that they may be performed each day. Specific activities, procedures, and techniques may be performed as tolerated[1] to avoid compromising pain management or overly fatiguing the patient. Physical medicine and rehabilitation provide nonpharmacologic interventions and tools used to enhance care of the patient in palliative and hospice care (**Fig. 1**).

The benefits of applying physical medicine and rehabilitation techniques include maintaining and/or enhancing circulation, preventing joint freezing, keeping the patient mentally engaged, as well as enhancing the patient's sense of well-being. Many physical medicine and rehabilitation techniques are useful adjuncts to help manage pain, although painful patients need and deserve to reap the benefits of comprehensive pain management, including a pharmacologic component. The reader is directed to the appropriate article by Robin Downing elsewhere in this issue. Every plan for applying physical medicine and rehabilitation to a specific veterinary patient in hospice or palliative care must be created individually; tailored to meet the needs of that particular patient, and reevaluated on a regular basis to be modified as the patient's condition changes.

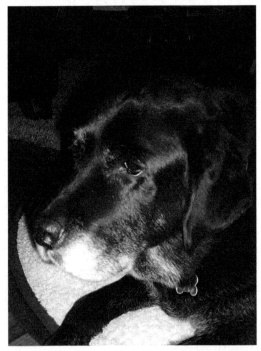

Fig. 1. Rascal is ready for his medical massage. (*Courtesy of* Robin Downing, DVM, Windsor, CO.)

Physical medicine and rehabilitation have formally been applied to pets only recently. Consequently, the body of evidence for veterinary rehabilitation is growing but still limited. The compassionate and progressive practitioner must therefore extrapolate from the evidence in human medicine that supports the application of various physical medicine and rehabilitation techniques to veterinary patients. A good fundamental understanding of anatomy, biomechanics, and neurology makes such extrapolation reasonable. Formal training is now available for veterinarians and other members of the extended veterinary health care team in physiotherapy, rehabilitation, animal chiropractic, acupuncture, and canine medical massage, with other expanded offerings sure to follow as new information and clinically relevant data become available.

This article provides an overview of the physical medicine and therapeutic techniques that are commonly applied to pets and that may be beneficial to the veterinary patient in palliative and hospice care. Applying these techniques provides an interdisciplinary approach to patients in palliative and hospice care, with all parties working together toward the common goal of maximal comfort and maximal function of the patient. As previously stated, many physical medicine and rehabilitation techniques can be taught to the pet owner for everyday application at home.

The most commonly applied physical medicine and rehabilitation techniques that lend themselves well to the hospice and palliative care setting include:

- Thermal modalities (cold/heat/therapeutic ultrasound)
- Massage
- ROM
- Stretching
- Chiropractic
- Joint mobilization
- Acupuncture
- Myofascial trigger point release
- Therapeutic laser
- Electrical stimulation
- Targeted pulsed electromagnetic field therapy (tPEMF)
- Therapeutic exercise.

THERMAL MODALITIES

Superficial thermal therapies have long been a staple of pain relief and physiotherapy, and they achieve their effects by changing tissue temperature, which alters cellular and physiologic function.[2] The depth of penetration for most thermal modalities is approximately 1 to 2 cm^3 and these techniques transfer energy by conduction. Both heat and cold have been shown to increase pain thresholds (**Fig. 2**).

The rate of heat transfer when applying superficial cold depends on several factors including the temperature difference between the body and the modality, the heat storage capacity of the cold modality, the area of the body in contact with the modality, the application duration, and individual variability.[3] Cold therapy causes various physiologic effects including vasoconstriction, which decreases blood flow; reduced cellular metabolism; decreased nerve conduction velocity; and decreased muscle spasm. Application of cold may be accomplished by ice pack (place a thin damp cloth between the ice pack and skin), commercial cold pack, or cold-compression units.[3] In addition, ice massage provides a focused application of cold to a targeted area of the body. Generally, cold therapy is applied for 5 to 10 minutes

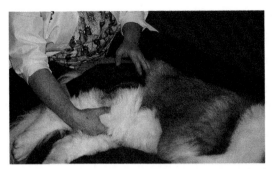

Fig. 2. Applying heat to thigh muscles before stretching. (*Courtesy of* Robin Downing, DVM, Windsor, CO.)

at a time, and may be applied following increased activity or exercise to decrease reactive swelling or pain.[3] Avoid using cold therapy in animals that are sensitive to cold, over insensate areas, or over areas with poor circulation.

Heat may be applied either superficially or deeply. Superficial heat is typically applied by conductive agents (eg, hot pack), radiant heat (eg, infrared lamp), or a combination of conduction and convection (eg, whirlpool). Superficial heat decreases blood pressure and muscle spasm, and increases local circulation, muscle relaxation, and tissue elasticity.[4] Superficial heat is generally applied for 15 to 30 minutes unless skin color changes. Deep heat is delivered via therapeutic ultrasound. The technology of ultrasound involves passage of an electrical current through a crystal to cause vibration and sound waves. This technique produces a piezoelectric effect.[5] The depth of penetration depends on the frequency in therapeutic ultrasound: 1 MHz penetrates to approximately 5 cm, whereas 3 MHz only penetrates to approximately 1 cm.[5] Ultrasound needs a liquid medium for transfer of sound waves to the tissue. In addition, hair coat interferes with sound wave transfer, which means shaving the treated area on the pet and using ultrasound gel as a transfer medium. Although ultrasound affects tissue distensibility, there is no evidence that ultrasound can relieve pain.[5] For veterinary patients in palliative and hospice care, therapeutic ultrasound may have a role in improving tissue mobility once pain is well managed. Use of therapeutic ultrasound has risks, so contraindications should be carefully reviewed.

MASSAGE/ROM/STRETCHING

Massage is the purposeful manipulation of the soft tissues of the body and has been used throughout history as a part of the art of medicine. It has origins in Chinese folk medicine and figured prominently in the writings of the ancient physicians Hippocrates and Asclepiades.[6] Massage is a well-established component of physical medicine and is commonly incorporated alongside medical management of human patients for both prevention and treatment of pain. It is often included in a general category called therapeutic touch. Chiropractic and osteopathic physicians, as well as physical therapists, often include massage techniques among the manual therapies they provide. Animals use touch to relieve pain, respond to injury, and for comfort[6] by licking or rubbing the affected area of the body. Human interaction with animal companions centers on touch, which brings comfort to both parties. It is a natural extension of that close physical contact to include massage in a palliative care and hospice plan for pets.

Massage as a form of therapeutic touch is directed toward a specific purpose targeting physiologic change and providing psychological benefit[7] Massage has mechanical effects on the soft tissues as well as reflexive or involuntary effects that influence the nervous and endocrine systems.[6] Massage can increase lymphatic flow as well as the exchange of fluid between the vascular and interstitial space. The increased exchange and movement of fluids throughout the soft tissues helps the body remove metabolites and chemical irritants from muscles, which may help to reduce chronic pain.[7] Massage also moves tissue and, by doing so, stimulates both sensory and autonomic nerves affecting the nervous system and the circulation. The physiologic effects of massage include the release of endorphins (the body's natural narcotic), which contributes to relaxation. Other neuroendocrine chemicals that are influenced by massage and may positively affect the patient in palliative and hospice care include serotonin, norepinephrine, adrenaline, and cortisol.[6] These chemicals in the body influence the pain experience. Massage, therefore, has the potential to supplement a pharmacologic approach to pain management during end-of-life care (**Fig. 3**).

Massage lends itself well to incorporating the client in the day-to-day palliative care strategy. Typically, multiple treatments over time are needed to see sustained benefits from massage. Also, the patient in palliative and hospice care is usually dealing with 1 or more disease processes that will progress with time. Daily (or several times per week) massage may help mitigate the adverse effects of progressive degenerative disease and enhance the animal's sense of well-being and overall comfort. Massage typically combines several different movements of the hands that have various effects on the tissues. The most commonly combined techniques include[7]:

- Stroking (long movements)
  - medium pressure to introduce touch and relax the patient
- Effleurage (the most common massage technique)
  - increases venous and lymphatic movement
  - moderate to deep pressure, depending on patient comfort
- Compressions and wringing (effective on larger muscles)
  - large contact area with pressure
  - wringing involves the right and left hand moving in opposite directions while in close proximately
- Percussion (tapping the tissue with a cupped or open hand)
  - stimulates circulation
  - can be used over the chest with a cupped hand (coupage) to help move lung secretions and improve breathing.

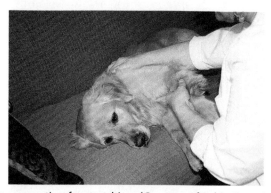

Fig. 3. Massage in preparation for stretching. (*Courtesy of* Robin Downing, DVM, Windsor, CO.)

Deeper massage techniques used to release adhesions or work through scar tissue may not be appropriate for patients at the end of life because of the discomfort they induce.

ROM and stretching are techniques that are related to massage and may easily be incorporated into the application of massage to patients in palliative and hospice care. Typically, stretch is best applied to warm muscles, so providing massage before stretching increases patient comfort and allows the stretches to be more effective. Another way to warm muscles before stretching or ROM is with hot packs; preferably moist heat. Stretching and ROM are often performed together to improve joint flexibility and sustain the extensibility of muscles and tendons.[8] Patients in palliative and hospice care tend to be less active than they once were. Downtime and decreased purposeful movement can lead to shortening of tissues and muscle weakness, and can ultimately lead to contracture of the soft tissues, interfering with simple mobility and ADLs (**Fig. 4**).

Skin, muscle, tendons, ligaments, and joint capsule all respond differently to stretching.[8] Muscle tissue is the most distensible, and for this reason it makes the most sense to focus stretching exercises and activities on the muscles. Although ROM exercises focus on moving joints and tissues through the available ROM, stretching moves tissues beyond the available ROM without causing trauma or damage. Although humans can stretch their own tissues, selectively contracting and relaxing specific muscles, veterinary patients are stretched passively by the practitioner or pet owner. The individual performing the stretches must be careful to avoid stretching too quickly to prevent a reflex contraction of the muscle being stretched. Once the muscle groups to be stretched are identified, a stretching plan and schedule can be developed. For patients in palliative and hospice care who are minimally mobile, daily stretching to prevent tissue contracture is most appropriate. For patients

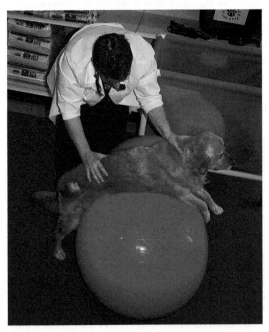

Fig. 4. Stretching on a physioroll. (*Courtesy of* Robin Downing, DVM, Windsor, CO.)

who remain mobile, stretching 3 to 5 times per week gives the best opportunity to improve and sustain flexibility. Once stiffness is reduced and activity increases, it is reasonable to rely less on stretching and more on active mobility for maintaining normal tissue ROM and function (**Fig. 5**).

As stated earlier, stretching and ROM are generally performed together, and are best accomplished once muscles are slightly warmed and enjoying increased blood flow. This condition may be accomplished by hot packing for 5 to 10 minutes, by massage, or by having the pet engage in a short period of activity such as a short walk. Before stretching, take the limb through its available ROM to determine the starting point of the stretches both into extension and flexion. The limb above the joint involved in the stretch is stabilized with one hand, and the other hand grasps and moves the bone below the joint. Slowly and steadily the joint is flexed, and, once restriction is felt, the stretch is held for 30 to 90 seconds.[9] Then the limb is moved, extending the joint to the point of restriction and holding the stretch for 30 to 90 seconds. Plan for 2 to 5 repetitions of each stretch during a stretching session. In no circumstance should stretching precipitate a pain reaction, vocalizing, or an attempt to bite. Any adverse patient reaction indicates that the stretching is inappropriately aggressive.

Pets experiencing palliative care and hospice who have limited mobility seem to enjoy and appreciate the tissue stimulation and interaction involved in massage, ROM exercises, and stretching. It is easy for these techniques to be combined. Likewise, it is easy to teach pet owners how to apply these techniques at home to maximize the pet's comfort, to enhance tissue function and mobility, and to reinforce the human-animal bond. We all pet our pets; these activities may be considered purposeful petting. Pets can and do enjoy structured physical contact, so these are specific strategies for them to enjoy that contact right up to the end of life.

ROM (also referred to as passive ROM) exercises are often combined with massage[8] and stretching to enhance and maintain function and mobility. ROM relies on external force to move the joint without muscle contraction. Taking joints through their normal ROM helps maintain joint health,[10] increase flexibility, prevent adhesions between soft tissue and bone, and enhance tissue extensibility. Ideally, each joint of the appendicular skeleton should be moved through flexion and extension slowly and gently 10 to 20 times per session. It is important to remember the digits of the feet. In no circumstance should the pet give a pain reaction, vocalize, or attempt to bite during ROM. Depending on the patient's level of comfort and mobility, it may

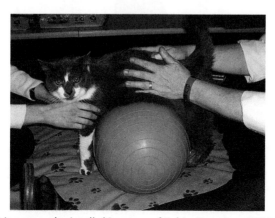

Fig. 5. Cat stretching on a physioroll. (*Courtesy of* Robin Downing, DVM, Windsor, CO.)

be possible to combine multiple joints, or even the entire limb, in ROM movements (eg, bicycle movement of the rear limb).

ROM does not prevent muscle atrophy, increase strength, or improve circulation, but it may help calm an anxious patient.[8] As for stretching, working with warmed muscles (either via hot packs or mild exercise) may improve both comfort and the pet's ability and willingness to relax. It is easy to move from ROM into stretching or back into massage depending on the desire of the practitioner and the attitude/preference of the patient (**Fig. 6**).

CHIROPRACTIC

Chiropractic is a system of medical care founded by Daniel David Palmer in the 1890s, and developed by his son, Bartlett Joshua (BJ) Palmer during the first half of the twentieth century.[11] The chiropractic paradigm emphasizes the relationship between the skeleton and the nervous system, and focuses on the interaction between the structure and function of the body. At its core, chiropractic considers the nervous system to be the master system of the body, and emphasizes that health is the natural state as the body strives to regulate and heal itself.[11] The manifestation of disease within the chiropractic context is called a vertebral subluxation complex (VSC).[12] The VSC describes a situation in which 2 adjacent vertebrae, the joints that link them, the supportive ligaments between them, and the skeletal muscles that move the joints are not interacting with optimal mobility within the normal ROM. This hypomobility is described as a fixation,[12] and this fixation is the focus of the chiropractic treatment.

The goal of restoring normal movement at a VSC and eliminating fixation is accomplished by an adjustment.[13] A chiropractic adjustment is accomplished by applying a high-velocity, low-amplitude thrust (also called a dynamic thrust) using a specific osseous contact point and a specific line of correction to move the affected joint beyond what is accessible through active and passive movements to restore its normal ROM. The VSC is classically identified via a motion palpation that identifies the specific spinal segments that are affected as well as the direction in which the motion is restricted. Each spinal segment of the dog and cat enjoys vectors of motion that include extension and flexion, lateral bending, dorsoventral shear, and rotation.

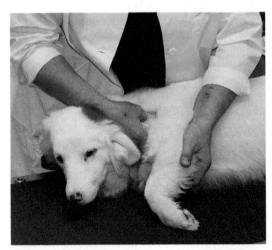

Fig. 6. Teaching range-of-motion exercise. (*Courtesy of* Robin Downing, DVM, Windsor, CO.)

The amount of movement in each of these directions is determined by the anatomy and biomechanics of the particular location along the spine.

Pain relief is critical to the discipline of chiropractic and is the primary reason humans seek chiropractic care. It is therefore reasonable to consider using chiropractic adjustment for the benefit of veterinary patients in palliative and hospice care. Because a VSC involves restricted movement of a spinal segment through its normal ROM, that altered function may have an impact on the normal anatomy surrounding the spinal nerves as they exit the intervertebral foramina as well as the nociceptors in the tissues comprising the spinal segment. The adjustment that restores normal movement at a particular spinal segment may act to normalize afferent and efferent nervous activity at that level.

It is critical to have a complete and accurate diagnosis of any patient in palliative care or hospice to determine whether chiropractic is an appropriate modality for that patient. Contraindications for chiropractic adjustment at specific spinal segments include an actively inflamed intervertebral disc, tumor disease in or near the spine, an infected or open wound, significant or generalized maladaptive pain, and osteoporosis or osteopenia increasing the risk of pathologic fracture. In a significantly painful patient, once the pain cycle is adequately managed pharmacologically, chiropractic may be an effective adjunct.

Currently in the United States, 210 contact hours of training (minimum) specific to the application of chiropractic theory and techniques to animals is the entry-level requirement for DVMs and DCs (Doctors of Chiropractic) to practice chiropractic medicine on animals. DCs trained in animal chiropractic must work on animals only in conjunction and cooperation with a primary veterinary care provider. There are several programs available in North America that provide instruction for both DVMs and DCs. There is not yet evidence for the effectiveness of chiropractic for animals; however, the literature for humans offers evidence for the benefits of chiropractic for functional spinal pain.

JOINT MOBILIZATION

Most dogs and cats enjoy being touched. Touch is often described as healing. Patients in palliative and hospice care often experience loss of motion secondary to their progressing disease processes. Joint mobilization is a manual therapy technique intended to improve tissue extensibility, increase ROM, induce relaxation, modulate pain, and reduce tissue restriction.[14] Mobilizations are passive movements performed by the practitioner and may be either oscillatory or involve a sustained stretch. The nature of mobilizations is such that the patient can prevent the motion. Manual therapy complements other strategies[15] for maximizing patient comfort in the palliative care and hospice setting. Mobilizations are typically performed within the available ROM[14] and involve the rhythmical oscillatory application of movement at a comfortable speed (**Fig. 7**).

It is important to understand the relationship between ROM and pain. When evaluating ROM in preparation for joint mobilization, if pain occurs before resistance is felt, then pain is the primary problem and should be addressed before mobilizations are performed. If pain occurs at the same time that resistance is felt, then the primary problem is restriction of joint movement.[14] In any case, mobilizations should only be used if they can assist the patient in feeling better and moving more easily.

Joint mobilization should be planned with specific grades of mobilizations in mind. The grade of the mobilization is defined by the range through which it is applied and the point in the range at which it is applied. Grade I mobilizations are small-amplitude

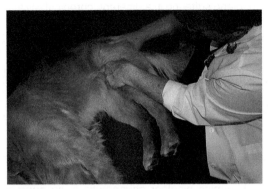

Fig. 7. Mobilizing the coxofemoral joint into extension. (*Courtesy of* Robin Downing, DVM, Windsor, CO.)

movements that avoid the end range of the joint ROM delivered at a rate of 3 to 4 oscillations per second. There should be no pain during grade I mobilizations. Grade II mobilizations are large-amplitude movements that also avoid end range. They are performed at a rate of 3 to 4 oscillations per second and should cause no pain. Grades III and IV mobilizations are large-amplitude and small-amplitude oscillations respectively that may cause discomfort to the patient.[14] Patients in palliative and hospice care need to be protected from pain, so, for this reason, grades III and IV mobilizations should probably be avoided. Joint mobilizations involve various types of movements including convex on concave, distraction, accessory glide, extension, flexion, and compressions. The reader is directed to the work of Saunders and colleagues[14] for a detailed description of joint mobilization as applied to animal patients.

ACUPUNCTURE AND MYOFASCIAL TRIGGER POINT RELEASE

Within the context of comfort care for veterinary patients in palliative and hospice care, acupuncture can serve as an important addition to a comprehensive care plan, particularly for those patients facing pain issues. Although acupuncture is not a panacea for pain, it has held up well to scrutiny.[16] Acupuncture may be used alone for managing musculoskeletal pain, but, if applied in conjunction with more conventional pain management modalities, it provides a synergistic effect.[17] Acupuncture treatment generally involves the insertion of very fine sterile needles into specific anatomically located sites that are heavily innervated. The needles may be used alone or the practitioner may add heat or electricity to the needles; the latter is called electroacupuncture. Electroacupuncture often augments the analgesic effects of acupuncture.[18]

Acupuncture originated in China in prehistory. The first textbook of acupuncture is acknowledged to be the Huang Di Nei Jing (*Yellow Emperor's Classic of Internal Medicine*). Beginning in the 1970s, acupuncture became a focus of medical attention in the United States, and, in 1997, the National Institutes of Health published a consensus statement that reported favorable findings for the application of acupuncture in several conditions.[19] As interest in acupuncture has grown, so has the research to explore and articulate how it works. However, designing rigorous randomized clinical trials to examine the outcome effects of acupuncture has proved challenging. In spite of these challenges, information about how acupuncture affects the body, and the nervous system, in particular, has been revealed (**Fig. 8**).

Acupuncture exerts its effects in the body primarily via neuromodulation. When an acupuncture needle pierces a nerve-rich acupuncture point, there is a cascade of

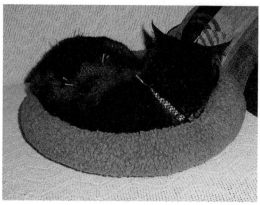

Fig. 8. Feline acupuncture. (*Courtesy of* Robin Downing, DVM, Windsor, CO.)

neural responses in the peripheral, autonomic, and central nervous systems.[20] Acupuncture increases endorphin levels in the body that contribute to the attenuation of pain by way of opioid receptors. In addition, acupuncture stimulation can result in nonopioid analgesia by way of γ-aminobutyric acid (GABA) receptors, δ-receptors, and κ-receptors.[21] Autonomic effects of acupuncture include decreased sympathetic tone and increased blood flow to the treated area that may benefit patients with chronic pain.[18] The most common conditions treated by acupuncture in animal patients include the following:

- paralysis, paresis, pain from trauma
- paralysis and/or paresis from type II intervertebral disk protrusion, degenerative myelopathy, and spondylosis
- pain from degenerative joint disease.[17]

Veterinary patients in palliative and hospice care are commonly afflicted with degenerative disease processes (often more than one) that result in various degrees of disability, loss of mobility, and pain. Managing these patients to allow them to live until they die means enhancing their life quality by any means possible. Within the context of a comprehensive pain management and comfort care strategy, acupuncture provides an excellent tool to leverage on their behalf. Although there is still a need for ongoing rigorous research into the effects of acupuncture, strong evidence exists to support its use for pain conditions, particularly musculoskeletal pain. For instance, acupuncture is efficacious for low back pain.[22] In the author's experience, most patients with chronic pain exhibit sensitivity in the caudal torso on palpation of the longissimus muscle, the lateral lumbar musculature, and the iliopsoas muscles (the equivalent of the human low back). Likewise, the spine itself provides many potential structural sources of neck and back pain in cats and dogs,[18] many of which may be present in the patient in palliative and hospice care. Examples include the following:

- intervertebral disk
- facet joint capsule
- dorsal root ganglia
- muscles attached to or supporting the neck and spine.

Tender points in the soft tissue are of particular interest from an acupuncture and pain management perspective. These areas of increased sensitivity were described and defined by Simons and colleagues[23] as "myofascial trigger points" that contain a sensory component, a motor component, and an autonomic component. Clinically, trigger points produce pain, restrict movement, and can cause muscle weakness.[21] Comparing charts of accepted acupuncture points with charts of commonly encountered trigger points, it makes intuitive sense to see the high degree of overlap. Although the precise physiology of trigger points has yet to be illuminated, treatment recommendations share common elements. Needling with acupuncture needles may be combined with massage, stretching, and exercise to release the tight area in the muscle often associated with a trigger point.[21]

Identifying tender points in the muscles of veterinary patients in palliative and hospice care provides an opportunity for the veterinarian to perform an empiric approach to acupuncture treatment by focusing on the specific areas of discomfort. Acupuncture treatment is best accomplished within the context of a thorough understanding of musculoskeletal anatomy as well as neuroanatomy to target therapy to achieve optimal results. That said, with currently available references and resources, it is possible to incorporate basic acupuncture techniques into a comprehensive comfort care strategy for pets receiving end-of-life care.

THERAPEUTIC LASER, TRANSCUTANEOUS ELECTRICAL NERVE STIMULATION, AND TPEMF

Therapeutic laser therapy (also referred to as low-level laser) uses light of a single wavelength to deliver photons (packets of light energy) to the tissue to induce a photobiologic/photochemical response in cells. The light energy is absorbed into the mitochondria, upregulating metabolism resulting in a net increase in ATP production, as well as increased synthesis of DNA and RNA. Laser also modulates levels of nitric oxide and prostaglandins. Therapeutic laser is gaining popularity in physiotherapy to speed healing after surgery and after injury, as well as for pain control. Within the palliative care and hospice setting, therapeutic laser is applied primarily as part of a comprehensive pain management strategy. In vivo, therapeutic laser has been shown to increase circulation and decrease inflammation, and human patients report decreased pain. Therapeutic lasers are recognized to have both direct effects and indirect effects on the tissues (**Fig. 9**).

In therapeutic laser, depth of penetration is a function primarily of wavelength but also of power output. In general, longer wavelengths penetrate to a greater depth,

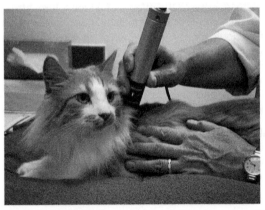

Fig. 9. Feline therapeutic laser, class IIIB. (*Courtesy of* Robin Downing, DVM, Windsor, CO.)

and therapeutic lasers have typically used wavelengths ranging from 600 nm to 1000 nm, with 600 nm penetrating to approximately 1 cm and 1000 nm to a depth of 2 to 3 cm. Lasers are divided into 4 major classes (class 1 to class 4[24]) and most therapeutic lasers currently in use are either class 3B or class 4. Class 3 lasers have an output ranging from 5 to 500 mW. Class 4 therapeutic lasers typically have output of 1 W or greater. The light energy delivered by therapeutic lasers is measured in joules, which is watts/s. For instance, a 1 W laser delivers 1 J of energy in 1 second. The dose of light energy delivered to the patient is expressed as J/cm^2 of surface area of the patient. The optimal number of joules to treat various conditions in veterinary patients has yet to be determined; however, therapeutic laser studies have revealed an antinociceptive effect in a rat model,[2] and many clinicians dose between 5 and 20 J/cm^2 at the surface. When using a therapeutic laser, the handheld probe is directed perpendicular to the tissue and is moved over the entire surface to be treated in a grid fashion.[25] It is important to provide protective eyewear rated to the appropriate wavelength of the laser to the client as well as the veterinary health care worker who is delivering the treatment. Avoid using laser over the patient's eyes, over malignancies, or over photosensitive areas of the skin (**Fig. 10**).

In the author's experience with both a class 3B and class 4 therapeutic laser, the class 4 provides for a much shorter treatment time. In a recently published meta-analysis of the use of therapeutic laser for neck pain, the treated group had a statistically significant improvement compared with the placebo group.[26] It is the author's experience, based on palpation examination before and after therapeutic laser treatment, that painful veterinary patients experience a nearly immediate reduction in their pain score, implying analgesic effects.

Electrical therapies have been used for generations in the treatment of various medical ailments.[27] By the late 1800s, US physicians were using electricity to treat pain regularly, despite the lack of scientific data to support its use.[27] Transcutaneous electrical neuromuscular stimulation (TENS), as defined by the American Physical Therapy Association (Sluka and Walsh[29]), is the application of electricity to the skin specifically for pain control, and it provides analgesia by several potential mechanisms of action. Peripheral stimulation with electrical impulses activates large unmyelinated afferent Aβ nerve fibers in the skin and inhibits small unmyelinated C fibers within the dorsal horn of the spinal cord.[28] There is also release of endogenous opioids in response to TENS. The frequency range commonly used for acute pain is 80 to 150 Hz (cycles per second), whereas lower settings (2–10 Hz) are commonly used for chronic pain.[24] The

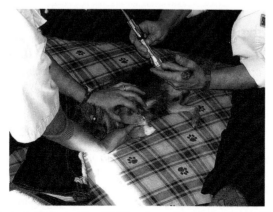

Fig. 10. Canine therapeutic laser, class IV. (*Courtesy of* Robin Downing, DVM, Windsor, CO.)

electrical impulse is delivered via electrodes placed on the skin, which most often means shaving the pet in the appropriate areas. In pets with short hair, water-soluble electrode gel may be adequate to provide good contact with the skin.

Electrode placement in TENS can be along nerve roots, over the painful area, or along dermatomes of respective nerves.[27] Different TENS frequencies may mitigate pain via different neurotransmitter systems. For instance, low-frequency TENS activates serotonin and μ-opioid receptors, whereas higher frequency TENS activates δ-opioid receptors.[28] Pulse duration and the intensity of the stimulus also influence the effectiveness of TENS. Greater intensity stimulation provides a higher level of analgesia, however increasing the intensity or pulse duration must be balanced with the patient's comfort level. Although the evidence in human studies to support TENS use for chronic pain is overall inconclusive,[29] TENS remains a popular noninvasive way to address pain that is otherwise challenging to treat. Although optimal treatment times and frequencies in animals are as yet unclear, most practitioners believe that TENS should be applied in the target areas for 30 minutes per treatment, 3 to 7 times per week.[28] TENS for pain relief lends itself well to the palliative care setting because of its noninvasive nature. A protocol can be defined and pet owners can easily be taught how to do the treatments at home, on their own, once the animal is used to the sensations generated during treatment.

One emerging technology in the management of animal pain is tPEMF therapy. The principle behind its use is that, if an electromagnetic current is pulsed near tissue, this induces current flow within the tissue. It is thought that this induction of electrical current within the tissue provides the therapeutic effect of tPEMF. tPEMF seems to enhance production of nitric oxide (NO), a key antiinflammatory molecule that reduces pain, improves blood flow, and reduces edema. Human studies suggest that tPEMF may play a role for both acute postoperative pain as well as chronic osteoarthritis (OA) pain. Studies on cartilage suggest that tPEMF may slow the progression of OA in addition to providing pain relief.[30] The potential advantages of tPEMF for veterinary patients in palliative and hospice care are many. First, tPEMF can be easily applied at home by the pet owner. Most practitioners prescribe 2 treatments of 15 minutes per day over the painful area. Second, tPEMF promises in preliminary studies to be as effective in some painful patients as nonsteroidal antiinflammatory drugs. When tPEMF works well, this can decrease the patient's need for pharmacologic pain relief. More research needs to be performed, but preliminary data suggest that tPEMF will quickly become a staple for enhancing comfort in painful patients in palliative and hospice care.

MISCELLANEOUS PHYSICAL MEDICINE TECHNIQUES

Keeping veterinary patients in palliative and hospice care active and engaged in their surroundings can present challenges. As their disease conditions progress, these animals experience increasing mobility challenges. They may become bedridden. They may lose interest in their surroundings because they are no longer able to move about on their own. For pets who lose their strength and mobility, there are some simple techniques for helping them remain engaged in their ADLs, even though those activities may need to be modified.

For those animals who are still able to stand and walk, strength and balance may be sustained by engaging in therapeutic exercises like sit-to-stand and weight-shifting activities, walking (with support) on an uneven surface such as a large piece of memory foam or a partially inflated air mattress, and engaging in hydrotherapy. The sit-to-stand activity is the dog equivalent of crunches. Weight shifting may be accomplished by picking up and holding each foot in sequence for 5 to 30 seconds. For instance, the focus may be the rear legs, in which case the right rear foot would be picked up and held a few inches off the ground, challenging the pet to shift weight to the 3 remaining feet. Once the right rear foot is placed on the ground, the left rear foot is picked up and held. This sequence can be repeated 3 to 10 times per set. Uneven surfaces challenge proprioception and balance, so walking on these surfaces sustains proprioceptive input into the nervous system. Another strategy for building balance and proprioception involves the use of balance boards and wobble boards. Because of the proprioceptive challenges presented by such activities, it is wise to consider protecting the pet from falling by using assistive devices such as a sling or vest. Short sessions scheduled at various times of the day help to prevent these activities from becoming tedious for the pet.

Hydrotherapy offers another strategy for sustaining balance, mobility, and strength. Hydrotherapy may involve walking in an underwater treadmill or working in a pool with a personal flotation device (PFD) (**Figs. 11** and **12**).

In an underwater treadmill, the higher the water, the less the influence of gravity, allowing the pet to pattern its legs through walking without having to work as hard as it would on dry land. In addition to balance and strength improvements, hydrotherapy can also improve and sustain cardiovascular health.

The reader is directed to the article by Tamara Shearer elsewhere in this issue for ideas of how to keep patients in palliative and hospice care moving.

Once a pet is bedridden, it becomes critical to prevent the body's tissues from devitalizing because of disuse. The biggest worry for a bedridden veterinary palliative care

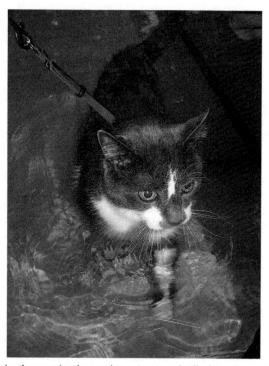

Fig. 11. Feline hydrotherapy in the underwater treadmill. (*Courtesy of* Robin Downing, DVM, Windsor, CO.)

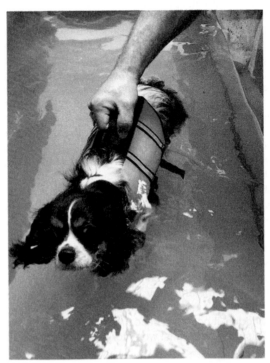

Fig. 12. Hydrotherapy using a PFD. (*Courtesy of* Robin Downing, DVM, Windsor, CO.)

or hospice patient is the pressure sore or decubitus ulcer (bed sores in humans). Pressure sores are easier to prevent than treat, so regular turning of the patient is important. It is also important to consider the body posture and strategic positioning of the patient to maximize comfort and interaction. The pet may reach a point at which sternal recumbency can only be maintained by propping the animal up with towels or pillows. It is important to maintain a schedule of turning the patient periodically to prevent consolidation in dependent lung lobes. As these patients lose their ability to stand and walk on their own, the simple act of standing with the help of an assistive device like a sling may give the pets the mental and physical stimulation they need to boost their mood.

Physical manipulation, physical medicine, and physiotherapy provide excellent strategies for improving the quality of life for the veterinary patient in palliative and hospice care, as that animal approaches the end of its life. In addition, those techniques that can be provided at home day to day by the pet owner serve not only to maximize the pet's quality of life but also to reinforce and strengthen the human-animal bond.

SUMMARY

Veterinary patients in palliative and hospice care comprise a unique population of pets with progressive and often degenerative diseases that can cause pain as well as loss of function and decreased quality of life. The patient with a progressive disease can often benefit from the application of physical medicine and rehabilitation techniques, not with the intention of curing the issue at hand, or necessarily reversing the disease process, but rather to maximize both comfort and function. Comfortable animals are more likely to continue to engage in normal, expected ADLs. In addition, comfortable animals maintain their relationships with their human companions. Thus, a more subjective benefit of applying physical medicine and rehabilitation techniques in the palliative care and hospice setting, particularly if pet owners are trained by the veterinary health care team to participate by delivering care at home, is a strengthening of the human-animal bond.

Physical medicine and rehabilitation are most effective in the veterinary palliative care and hospice context as adjuncts to a pharmacologically-driven pain management strategy. The reader is again directed to the article elsewhere in this issue for medication strategies to use with these patients. Physical medicine and rehabilitation can decrease the doses of analgesics required to keep these patients comfortable. The blend of physical and pharmacologic medicine allows the practitioner and family to work together to achieve a balance between maximum comfort and maximum mentation. It is this balance that empowers the patient to live until it dies: truly the goal in any end-of-life scenario.

REFERENCES

1. Tinkel RS, Lachmann EA. Rehabilitative medicine. In: Berger AM, Portenoy RK, Weissman DE, editors. Principles and practice of palliative care and supportive Oncology. 2nd edition. Philadelphia: Lippincott William & Wilkins; 2002. p. 968–70.
2. Baxter GD, Basford JR. Electrotherapeutic and thermal agents. In: Sluka KA, editor. Mechanisms and management of pain for the physical therapist. Seattle (WA): IASP Press; 2009. p. 194, 199.
3. Heinrichs K. Superficial thermal modalities. In: Millis D, Levine D, Taylor R, editors. Canine rehabilitation and physical therapy. St Louis (MO): Saunders Elsevier; 2004. p. 278–9, 282–5.
4. Steiss JE, Levine D. Physical agent modalities. Update on management of pain. Vet Clin North Am Small Anim Pract 2005;35(6):1321–2.
5. Schram-Bloodworth D, Gabois M. Physical medicine and rehabilitation. In: Warfield CA, Bajwa ZH, editors. Principles and practice of pain management. 2nd edition. New York: McGraw-Hill; 2004. p. 798.
6. Fritz S. Mosby's fundamentals of therapeutic massage. 3rd edition. St Louis (MO): Mosby Elsevier; 2004. p. 11, 14, 128–32.
7. Sutton A. Massage. In: Millis D, Levine D, Taylor R, editors. Canine rehabilitation and physical therapy. St Louis (MO): Saunders Elsevier; 2004. p. 303, 305, 316–20.
8. Millis DL, Lewelling A, Siri H. Range of motion and stretching exercises. In: Millis D, Levine D, Taylor R, editors. Canine rehabilitation and physical therapy. St Louis (MO): Saunders Elsevier; 2004. p. 228, 229, 236.
9. Bockstahler B, Levine D, Millis DL. Essential facts of physiotherapy in dogs and cats. Babenhausen (Germany): BE VetVerlag; 2004. p. 58.
10. Olby N, Halling KB, Glick TR. Rehabilitation for the neurologic patient. Rehabilitation and physical therapy. Vet Clin North Am Small Anim Pract 2005; 35(6):1401.
11. Wiese G. Major themes in chiropractic history. In: Redwood D, Cleveland CS, editors. Fundamentals of chiropractic. St Louis (MO): Mosby Elsevier; 2003. p. 21, 30–31.
12. Cleveland CS. Vertebral subluxation. In: Redwood D, Cleveland CS, editors. Fundamentals of chiropractic. St Louis (MO): Mosby Elsevier; 2003. p. 129, 137.

13. Scarunge JG, Cooperstein R. Chiropractic manual procedures. In: Redwood D, Cleveland CS, editors. Fundamentals of chiropractic. St Louis (MO): Mosby Elsevier; 2003. p. 258–60.
14. Saunders DG, Walker JR, Levine D. Joint mobilization. Rehabilitation and physical therapy. Vet Clin North Am Small Anim Pract 2005;35(6):1287,1290, 1292–3.
15. Goff L, Jull G. Manual therapy. In: McGowan C, Goff L, Stubbs N, editors. Animal physiotherapy: assessment, treatment, and rehabilitation of animals. Ames (IA): Blackwell Publishing; 2007. p. 164.
16. Audette J. Acupuncture. In: Warfield CA, Bajwa ZH, editors. Principles and practice of pain medicine. 2nd edition. New York: McGraw-Hill; 2004. p. 785.
17. McCauley L, Glinski MH. Acupuncture for veterinary rehabilitation. In: Millis D, Levine D, Taylor R, editors. Canine rehabilitation and physical therapy. St Louis (MO): Saunders Elsevier; 2004. p. 337, 341–2.
18. Robinson NG. Complementary and alternative medicine. In: Gaynor JS, Muir WW, editors. Handbook of veterinary pain management. 2nd edition. St Louis (MO): Mosby Elsevier; 2009. p. 303–5, 313.
19. Williams JE. Acupuncture and traditional Chinese medicine. In: Boswell MV, Cole BE, editors. Weiner's pain management. 7th edition. Boca Raton (FL): Taylor & Francis; 2006. p. 1121.
20. Staud R, Price DD. Mechanisms of acupuncture analgesia for clinical and experimental pain. Expert Rev Neurother 2006;6(5):661–7.
21. Sourlis T. Acupuncture and trigger points. In: McGowen C, Goff L, Stubbs N, editors. Animal physiotherapy: assessment, treatment, and rehabilitation of animals. Ames (IA): Blackwell Publishing; 2007. p. 201–4.
22. Manheimer E, White A, Berman B, et al. Meta-analysis: acupuncture for low back pain. Ann Intern Med 2005;142:651–63.
23. Simons DG, Travell JG, Simons LS. Travell and Simons' myofascial pain and dysfunction, the trigger point manual. The upper half of body, vol. 1. 2nd edition. Baltimore (MD): Lippincott Williams & Wilkins; 1999.
24. Canapp DA. Select modalities. Clin Tech Small Anim Pract 2007;20(4):163–5, 182.
25. Millis DL, Francis D, Adamson C. Emerging modalities in veterinary rehabilitation. Rehabilitation and physical therapy. Vet Clin North Am Small Anim Pract 2005; 35(6):1344.
26. Chow RT, Johnson MI, Lopes-Martins RA, et al. Efficacy of low-level laser therapy in the management of neck pain: a systematic review and meta-analysis of randomized placebo or active-treatment controlled trials. Lancet 2009;374:1897–908.
27. Sva S, Kashi AR. Electromedicine. In: Boswell MV, Cole BE, editors. Weiner's pain management: a practical guide for clinicians. 7th edition. Boca Raton (FL): Taylor & Francis; 2006. p. 1221, 1224.
28. Millis DL. Physical therapy and rehabilitation in dogs. In: Gaynor JS, Muir WW, editors. Handbook of veterinary pain management. 2nd edition. St Louis (MO): Mosby Elsevier; 2009. p. 526, 528.
29. Sluka KA, Walsh DM. TENS and IFT. In: Sluka KA, editor. Mechanisms and management of pain for the physical therapist. Seattle (WA): IASP Press; 2009. p. 182.
30. Ciombor D, Aaron RK, Wang S, et al. Modification of osteoarthritis by pulsed electromagnetic field – morphological study. Osteoarthritis Cartilage 2003;11:455–62.

Managing Mobility Challenges in Palliative and Hospice Care Patients

Tamara S. Shearer, DVM, CCRP[a,b,*]

KEYWORDS

- Paralysis • Ataxia • Mobility • Hospice • Palliative
- Assistive devices

Some pet owners may have more difficulty managing a pet's mobility challenges than any other disorder. This problem is especially frustrating because the pet is often otherwise healthy. The decline in mobility is also connected to many disease processes, such as the neuropathies seen in poorly regulated diabetes and the weakness associated with degenerative myelopathy. As death nears, a decline in mobility toward becoming recumbent or moribund is expected. The progression of the mobility disorder will vary according to the disease process. As the pet's mobility declines, the burden of care will increase.

Unlike other symptoms of disease, mobility challenges with pets pose several unique problems that can disrupt the relationship between a pet and the caretaker. Relationships are disrupted when a pet is no longer able to share a walk with the pet owner or engage in play, such as a game of fetch. Mobility challenges often require a pet owner to provide extra care for maintaining good hygiene. For medium to large dogs, mobility changes are physically demanding, but even small dogs and cats can pose a problem for pet owners who are not physically capable of bending and lifting. Pets that are heavier than 30 kg are especially challenging for even physically fit individuals.

Managing a mobility challenge can also be emotionally demanding because of the responsibilities in caring for the pet. Caretakers must expend a lot of effort to prevent or manage the progression of the disorder and to maintain a good quality of life for their pet. Some mobility changes require 24-hour care to preserve comfort.

Veterinarians are faced with four common types of mobility challenges in palliative and hospice care. The first is an acute mobility change often associated with a serious

---

The author has nothing to disclose.

[a] Shearer Pet Health Hospital, 1054 Haywood Road, Sylva, NC 28779, USA
[b] Pet Hospice and Education Center, 16111 State Route, 37 Sunbury, OH 43074, USA
* Shearer Pet Health Hospital, 1054 Haywood Road, Sylva, NC 28779.
E-mail address: tshearer5@frontier.com

injury. The second is a chronic condition in which the problem has stabilized or is slowly progressing. Examples of this type of disorder are osteoarthritis, myopathies, and neuropathies, which may cause pain and mechanical dysfunction. The third type of mobility challenge is secondary to weakness associated with the specific disease. For example, low potassium resulting from several disease processes may lead to weakness. Lastly, the final mobility change is associated with the end stage of dying when the pet becomes moribund.

A thorough orthopedic and neurologic examination will help determine the seriousness of the mobility change. Once a mobility change has been identified and has little hope for improvement or is confirmed to be irreversible, immediate enrollment in a palliative care plan is of the utmost importance, especially if the disorder is interfering with the routine of the pet or long-term intensive care is needed. Consideration of this program is important because it helps to keep the pet comfortable, lends emotional support to the pet owner, may prevent the disorder from progressing, and sometimes prevents injury to pet owners.

An important part of the evaluation should include information about the pet's living conditions and activities of daily life. Owners should be asked questions such as whether the pet is an indoor or outdoor pet. If the pet is indoors, does the home have steps that the pet must navigate? Does the pet sleep in the owner's bed? Does the pet travel in the car? What type of flooring is in the house, and what type of terrain is outside? Questionnaires regarding mobility and activities of daily living will help determine how much care the pet may need to maintain quality of life (**Boxes 1** and **2**).

After a detailed history and an evaluation are performed, the pet should be placed in a category that defines its ability to support itself. These categories range from mild

---

Box 1
Mobility questionnaire

Owners should assign a grade to each question based on the rating scale.
Rating System: 0 = none; 1 = mild; 2 = moderate; 3 = severe

Difficulty with walking: 0, 1, 2, 3

Difficulty to move from lying down to stand: 0, 1, 2, 3

Difficulty to move from stand to lying down: 0, 1, 2, 3

Difficulty to move from sit to stand: 0, 1, 2, 3

Difficulty to move from stand to sit: 0, 1, 2, 3

Difficulty to hold posture to defecate: 0, 1, 2, 3

Difficulty to hold posture to urinate: 0, 1, 2, 3

Difficulty ascending stairs: 0, 1, 2, 3

Difficulty descending stairs: 0, 1, 2, 3

Difficulty with jumping: 0, 1, 2, 3

Difficulty with running: 0, 1, 2, 3

Difficulty with climbing inclines: 0, 1, 2, 3

Difficulty with losing weight: 0, 1, 2, 3

Difficulty with gaining weight: 0, 1, 2, 3

Difficulty with endurance: 0, 1, 2, 3

Box 2
Questionnaire on activities of daily living
Is the pet an indoor or outdoor pet?
What type of terrain is outside? Rugged, inclines, flat?
What type of flooring is in the house?
Does the pet have steps to climb? How many and where?
Does the pet sleep in the pet owner's bed?
Does the pet travel in the car?
What activities does the pet participate in?

changes to the absence of purposeful movement. Through categorizing the mobility disorder, the type and amount of care needed to ensure the best quality of life will be defined. Additionally, progression of disease can be followed through monitoring changes in the categories of disability (**Box 3**).

In all cases, facilitating a referral to a specialist in pet rehabilitation or pain management is highly recommended to ensure that the pet owner is aware of all aspects of care that may improve a pet's quality of life. Many pets benefit from physical rehabilitation and pain management. A veterinarian should look for facilities that have Certified Canine Rehabilitation Practitioners or Certified Canine Rehabilitation Therapists for advanced care for mobility impaired pets. A referral to a veterinarian with special training in pain management, such as a Certified Veterinary Pain Practitioner, is also desirable. However, general practitioners can still provide much assistance if a pet owner chooses not to obtain advanced care or if a specialist is not available in the area of the practice.

The application of the Five-Step Strategy for Comprehensive Hospice and Palliative Care, which is discussed elsewhere in this issue, may help guide the veterinary staff through supporting a mobility-impaired pet. When discussing the pet owner's needs, beliefs, and goals for the pet, the veterinarian can develop a personalized plan after the family is educated about the disease and mobility challenge. Developing a personalized plan for the pet and pet owner should take into account the pet and pet owner's needs and ensure that all is being done to maintain quality of life. Next, the pet owner should be shown how to carry out the plan. Technical support staff should review the techniques required to care for the mobility-challenged pet. Emotional support for the owner should begin when the pet enters the palliative care program, because the stress associated with mobility challenges is great.

Box 3
Five common categories of disability
Can stand to support self with minimal lameness, paraparesis, or ataxia
Can stand to support self but frequently stumbles and falls with mild lameness, mild paraparesis, or ataxia
Unable to stand to support self, but when assisted moves limbs yet stumbles and falls frequently with moderate lameness, paraparesis, or ataxia
Unable to support self, has slight movement when supported, with severe lameness or paraparesis
Absence of purposeful movement secondary to disease or near death

Despite the cause of the mobility challenge, there are two main areas of focus when dealing with the mobility-impaired pet. First, preservation of the physical and emotional quality of life is vital. Not tending to mobility challenges can result in pain, urinary tract infections, decubital ulcers, hygromas, decline in range of motion, and pneumonia. Second are the behavioral risks of anxiety and boredom. Through applying basic care tips, such as treating pain in the pet, modifying and enhancing the environment, maintaining hygiene of the pet, offering mobility assistance, and performing simple therapy, many problems associated with mobility impairment can be prevented.

PAIN MANAGEMENT

Pain is often associated with mobility challenges and should be treated immediately or anticipated and prevented. For a pet with hard-to-manage pain, referral to a Certified Veterinary Pain Practitioner may be critical. One remedy for caring for a pet that is experiencing pain is to give pain medications 1 or 2 hours before working with the pet.[1] Signs of pain when performing care include biting, scratching, whimpering, crying out, moaning, wiggling, struggling, reluctance to move, and resisting the care. How to manage pain is discussed elsewhere in this issue.

ENVIRONMENTAL MODIFICATION

When caring for mobility-impaired pets, one should begin with modifying the environment. If the pet is still mobile, having flooring with good traction is imperative to minimize the risks of falls, and can be accomplished by laying down rugs with rubber backing that do not slip and slide. The rubber backing serves a double purpose because it is waterproof and will protect the underlying floor if a pet is urinary incontinent. Rubber floor runners also can be helpful. Commercially available rubberized flooring or garage floor rubber matting can also be used.

Bedding that is soft and easy to clean is recommended to prevent decubital ulcers, hygromas, and irritated calluses. Having at least two sets of bedding is helpful in case one gets soiled. Egg crate foam enclosed in a waterproof mattress cover works well. Covering a bed with plastic makes it slippery and should be avoided. Thermal comfort should be adjusted based on the pet's needs. Some short-coated lean pets prefer warmth, whereas others that are overweight or thick-coated northern breeds prefer cool temperatures. The bedding can be adjusted to accommodate those needs. If a pet is an outdoor animal, care must be given to protect it from temperature extremes and to prevent fly strike in the warmer months and frostbite or freezing when it is cold.

If possible, the pet owner should choose an access to the outside that allows the pet to negotiate the fewest steps. Pet owner assistance or ramps to help the pet navigate any steps would be important to prevent falls. A narrow ramp with a support railing at a low grade of incline works best. Pets with mobility challenges often are too weak to climb steep inclines on ramps. For cats, litter box access should be made easier by moving it close to the cat, lowering the sides of the box, and increasing the size of the box. Some cats can be taught to urinate on hygiene pads sprinkled with a small amount of kitty litter.

Pet owners should block off stairways to prevent falls for pets that are unstable. Some furniture should be moved to prevent a pet from falling into sharp edges or getting stuck between objects. For pets that are allowed on furniture, human beds could be lowered or steps or ramps provided. Mobility-impaired pets often cannot use steps and ramps because the steep inclines make these difficult to navigate.

To minimize the risk of dehydration, all locations where the pet may reside should have access to water so the pet does not have to move to another location to find water. Access to food should also be made easy. Some pets with disabilities may need to be fed with elevated feeders or even hand-fed if their mobility problem interferes with normal eating posture.

HYGIENE ASSISTANCE

A pet's hygiene should be checked a minimum of every 2 hours, and more often for severely debilitated pets. When a pet needs extra care to maintain good hygiene, precautions should be taken to ensure that any lifting or positioning of the pet does not cause pain.

Hygiene aids like absorptive pads, diapers, and incontinence panties may make care easier because they minimize the amount of urine and feces that contacts the pet and contaminates the environment. Also, careful trimming of the hair coat may make hygiene care easier. Care should be taken not to irritate the skin or remove too much hair over pressure points such as the ischium, where the hair may be protective against pressure necrosis. Pet owners and staff should be taught to use baby wipes or mild soap and water to keep the pet clean around the genitals, anus, feet, eyes, and mouth. All of the urine and feces must be cleaned from the hair coat and kept away from the skin. After the fecal material and urine are removed, the area should be cleansed using warm water and mild shampoo. The owner should rinse the area well and then make sure it is dry. A moisture-barrier ointment and cornstarch baby powder should be applied after each cleansing. If a pet is outside, extreme attention must be given to hygiene to protect against heatstroke and fly strike during warm months and freezing during cold months.

ASSISTIVE DEVICES

An assistive device is a type of rehabilitation equipment designed to perform a particular function that makes caring for the mobility-impaired pet easier. It helps a pet live a better quality of life through enhancing its ability to continue to be active in a more comfortable way. Regardless of the type of device, any new piece of equipment must be introduced gradually to avoid complications such as aversion to the device secondary to fear of the novelty of the apparatus. Positive reinforcement and conditioning a pet to accept an assistive device will help ensure that the pet is emotionally comfortable with the new piece of equipment. For pets that are sensitive, hesitant, or fearful, consultation with a pet behaviorist or reputable pet trainer may be helpful.

Gradual introduction also helps ensure proper fit of a device and acceptance of the device by making sure it is comfortable. A device should be removed at designated intervals to allow examination for complications. Close monitoring for evidence that the device may be interfering with respirations is paramount. Examination for pain, abrasions, pressure sores, or pinching of skin should be performed several times per day.[2] Proper padding may be added to the assistive device to help prevent discomfort.

When working with mobility-challenged pets, an inventory of assistive devices of various sizes should be in stock for immediate use. Equipment most commonly used to enhance mobility includes slings, harnesses, splints, and braces. Devices that protect body parts from abrasions secondary to the mobility challenge include boots and other protective garments. Other devices are also available to make caring for these pets less difficult, such as carts and physiorolls for performing simple exercise.

SLINGS AND HARNESSES

Mobility slings and harnesses can be used to move pets more comfortably while minimizing injury to the pet and the pet owners. Slings and harnesses are designed to accommodate forelimbs, hind limbs, or all four legs. When choosing a sling, ease of use should be considered. Observing the pet for pain, discomfort, and respiratory distress is critical. Slings can potentially create pressure on the chest wall, and debilitated pets may experience difficulty breathing if the sling does not fit correctly. This phenomenon can often be remedied by laterally separating the strap away from the body. The sling also should not pinch skin nor cause abrasion or pressure sores. Homemade slings may work well, such as a log carrier for larger dogs, but technical advancements may make commercial products more comfortable for the pet and owner. Some slings, or towels used as slings, may apply added pressure to the bladder and cause the pet to inappropriately urinate. Most commercial slings are designed to prevent this problem.

Orthotic Braces, Prosthetics, and Other Protective Devices

Many different orthotic braces and splints are available to help pets with mobility. Sometimes a pet may have instability of a joint or joints that contributes to a mobility change. A splint or brace provides protection of the affected joints and joint stabilization. Commercially available and customized braces (HandicappedPets.com, Nashua, NH, USA) may help the pet be more comfortable through allowing weight-bearing of the affected limb and preventing further injury. Braces are available for several joints, including the tibial tarsal joint, radial carpal joint, stifle, and elbow. Hinged or dynamic braces support while allowing the joint to bend, which helps prevent muscle atrophy from disuse and strengthen the limb. The dynamic, hinged braces are good for long-term support.[2]

A BIKO Canine Physio Brace (BIKO, Vienna, Austria) is a device to assist dogs that have moderate ataxia and hind limb weakness, and knuckle over but are still able to stand even when requiring effort. The brace helps dogs when walking and turning. The device has elastic straps that run from the dorsal midline harness connection to the tarsal area of the hind feet. The elastic band assists the forward movement of the feet and also protects and prevents the feet from knuckling.

Prosthetic devices restore function after amputation by substituting for the missing limb. Many pets cope well with a missing limb; however, some may benefit from the extra support a prosthetic device can offer. Customized prosthetic devices can be made to attach to the distal site of the missing limb, and have antimigration and rotational stability for comfort and better function.

Protective Wear

Protective devices to prevent and care for abrasions should be considered in the presence of excessive wear on exposed body parts. Splints and braces can also be used for this function, but protective wear made of specialized materials for pressure point protection also can help a mobility-impaired patient. Specialized wear is available for the protection and treatment of areas that are at high risk for irritation and decubital ulcer formation, including the hock, ischium, and greater trochanter in the hind limb and the carpus, elbow, and acromion in the forelimb. Pets with proprioceptive deficits who drag their toes are prone to abrasions to the dorsal surface of the tarsus or carpus. DogLegg Wraps and DogLegg Booties (DogLeggs, Washington, DC, USA) protect pressure points in the legs and feet; they are custom fitted to protect and prevent irritations. In pets with rear limb paralysis, a drag bag (HandicappedPets.com) that covers the pet from abdomen to hind limbs reduces friction and hence abrasions. It is used for pets who have rear limb paralysis but are still able to pull themselves around using their forelimbs when not in their cart.

Mobility Carts

Two- and four-wheeled carts are available for pets that are having difficulty ambulating or are no longer able to ambulate on their own. Carts allow pets to regain their ability to move about, which can improve their quality of life. Previously carts had to be custommade; however, an adjustable cart called Walkin' Wheels (HandicappedPets.com) can be used on a temporary basis to condition pets to a cart and determine whether a cart is the proper choice. This option can also be used long-term when fitted properly. Practices are advised to invest in one adjustable cart so it is immediately available as a mobility choice. The time a pet spends in the cart should be increased slowly and the pet should be monitored closely for side effects. The pet should be removed from the cart at designated intervals to allow examination for complications. As with other assistive devices, pain, discomfort, and respiratory distress should be monitored closely.[2] Carts can potentially create pressure on the chest wall, and debilitated pets may experience difficulty breathing if the cart does not fit correctly. When fitted properly, the pet should not dangle in the cart.

Assistive devices that improve mobility can have an enormous effect on quality of life. No matter what device is used, the pet must be monitored closely for pain and discomfort. The cart should not pinch skin, cause abrasions, or cause pressure sores.

Simulated Mobility

For pets that are not mobile, their emotional well-being may be maintained by allowing them to participate in activities through simulated mobility. Pet owners may choose to hike with their dogs using the Kyjen Backpack Pet Carrier by Outward Hound. Caution should be used to make sure the pet's breathing and comfort are not compromised when in a backpack. Dog bike trailers and bike baskets are available from various online sources so pets can enjoy a bike ride. Wagons and baby (dog) buggies also allow pets to enjoy the outdoors with their owners. Car rides provide another means of emotional stimulation and simulated mobility.

Therapy Techniques

Mobility assistance and simple exercises may preserve remaining strength, improve respiratory function, and prevent decubital ulcers.[2] Appropriate exercise choices for mobility-challenged pets must be performed safely and without pain. Exercise and therapy may be a good substitute for other activities that pet owners can no longer participate in with their pets. Three exercises that require little training but have large benefits are assisted standing, weight-shifting, and range of motion exercises. Massage and positioning also have benefits as therapies. More detailed information on how rehabilitation can help a pet can be found elsewhere in this issue.

Assisted standing helps debilitated pets in several ways. It not only improves mental contentment but also may also improve circulation, respirations, balance, and proprioception.[2] It will relieve the pressure over joints that could result in decubital ulcers. It can be used to maintain strength and slow muscle atrophy.

The amount of effort needed will be determined by the patient's mobility status. This technique is especially useful in pets that have adequate strength to bear some of its own weight but are too weak to bear all. If a pet cannot support at least 75% of its body weight, more assistance will be required. The use of slings and therapy balls called *physiorolls* can make this task more manageable. When the pet is assisted into a standing position through use of a sling, or supported over a therapy ball, the feet should be placed in the normal position and help with support. If placed on a therapy ball with a full bladder, the pet will usually urinate from the pressure applied to the abdomen, which may be a disadvantage for some pet owners. However, this is one way to help manually express the bladder in a pet that cannot void on its own. The duration of assisted standing is determined on a case-by-case basis. Sometimes even 5 minutes may be tiresome for debilitated pets. The technique should be repeated three to six times per day if the pet is comfortable.[2]

Weight-shifting is another method for preventing the side effects of decreased ambulation. With this technique, owners position themselves next to or over the standing pet, place their hands on each side of the pet's hips, and gently sway the pet from side to side. A sway can also be created from front to back and on a right and left diagonal. These motions disrupt the pet's center of gravity and require it to shift its weight through engaging core muscle activity to recenter its balance. This exercise helps maintain and build core strength and balance.

Passive range of motion is used when a pet cannot initiate a voluntary muscle contraction. This type of range of motion is often used with paralysis or immediately postoperatively. Passive range of motion does not increase strength but will help stabilize or improve the movement of joints and increase flexibility and the extensibility of soft tissues. It will also increase blood and lymphatic flow and may increase synovial fluid flow.[1]

Assisted range of motion is used when a pet is able to participate in muscle activity. This type of range of motion may improve strength, and also helps in the reeducation of nerves, proprioceptive training, and gait training. With both passive and assisted active range of motion, the staff and pet owner begin by gently flexing and extending the joints through their comfortable range of motion while stabilizing the limb proximal to the joint to be moved. The lower limb is then gently moved with the hand close to the joint to minimize the force to that joint. This exercise should be performed for all affected joints, including the toes. A bicycling-like motion can also be used to put the joints through their range of motion when time is limited. The frequency may vary from ten to thirty repetitions up to six times daily.[1]

Massage and positioning may also benefit patients with mobility challenges. Pets with mobility challenges will have soreness and weakness associated with the problem, and therefore muscle tension often exists, contributing to discomfort. The pet's position should be changed as frequently as possible, but at least every 2 hours. Massage helps increase blood flow to the massaged area, which helps improve oxygen supply and carry away metabolic wastes. It is also helpful for releasing endorphins and improving lymphatic and venous return.[3] Caution should be used if the pet has bleeding disorders or if the massage causes discomfort. Overzealous massage may cause sensitivity.

Special consideration should be given to nursing the mobility changes of the actively dying pet. If a pet has lost the ability to move on its own, the pet owner must regularly change the position of the pet to prevent decubital ulcers and pneumonia. Ideally, a pet owner should try to move the pet every 30 minutes, but at least every 2 hours. If a pet is actively dying (within hours), a decision must be made whether the treatments create more discomfort than benefit. For example, if moving the pet to perform therapy or maintain hygiene causes pain or distress, that task may be eliminated if the pet is near death.

SUMMARY

Mobility challenges disrupt the relationship between the pet and caretaker. Managing pets with mobility challenges may be one of the most difficult changes for pet owners to deal with, especially when coupled with another serious illness, and even when it occurs in an otherwise healthy patient. Near death, the pet's mobility usually declines to the point of recumbency or becoming moribund, but this varies according to the disease. As the pet's mobility changes, the burden of care will increase. Families enrolled in palliative and hospice care plans will find it easier to care for their pets because they will have supportive resources.

REFERENCES

1. Millis D, Lewelling A, Hamilton S. Range-of-motion and stretching exercises. In: Millis D, Levine D, Taylor R, editors. Canine rehabilitation and physical therapy. Philadelphia: Saunders; 2004. p. 228–43.
2. Hamilton S, Millis D, Taylor R, et al. Therapeutic exercise. In: Millis D, Levine D, Taylor R, editors. Canine rehabilitation and physical therapy. Philadelphia: Saunders; 2004. p. 244–63.
3. Bochstahler B. Massage therapy. In: Bochstahler B, Levine D, Millis D, editors. Essential facts of physiotherapy in dogs and cats. Babenhausen (Germany): BE Vet Verlag; 2004. p. 46.

SUGGESTED READINGS

Millis D, Levine D, Taylor R. Canine rehabilitation and physical therapy. Philadelphia: Saunders; 2004.
Gaynor J, Muir W, editors. Handbook of veterinary pain management. St Louis (MO): Mosby; 2010. p. 588–600.
Shearer T. The essential book for dogs over five. Columbus (OH): Ohio Distinctive Publishing; 2002.
Manning A. Physical rehabilitation for the critically injured veterinary patient. In: Millis D, Levine D, Taylor R, editors. Canine rehabilitation and physical therapy. Philadelphia: Saunders; 2004. p. 404–10.
Taylor R, Millis D, Levine D, et al. Physical rehabilitation for geriatric and arthritic patients. In: Millis D, Levine D, Taylor R, editors. Canine rehabilitation and physical therapy. Philadelphia: Saunders; 2004. p. 411–25.

Comfort, Hygiene, and Safety in Veterinary Palliative Care and Hospice

Robin Downing, DVM, CCRP, CPE[a],*, Valarie Hajek Adams, CVT[b],
Ann P. McClenaghan, BS, CVT[c]

KEYWORDS

• Palliative care • End of life • Safety • Comfort • Hygiene

Palliative care and hospice for animals is a new phenomenon. Palliative care originated in the United Kingdom in the 1960s to address the unmet needs of terminally ill patients and their families. The World Health Organization defines palliative care as "…an approach that improves the quality of life of patients and their families facing the problem associated with life-threatening illness, through the prevention and relief of suffering by means of early identification and impeccable assessment and treatment of pain and other problems, physical, psychosocial and spiritual" (www. who.int/cancer/palliative/definition/en/). Likewise, hospice originated in the United Kingdom with formal facilities for end-of-life patients. Hospice in the United States has developed as a practice involving an interdisciplinary team and a variety of settings. Dr Alice Villalobos, a veterinarian who has practiced oncology since the 1970s, has coined the term pawspice to describe the transfer of principles and practices from human medicine to veterinary medicine. Pets are living longer and better than ever before, and their place in the home is more and more integral to the fabric of the family. Pet owners are understandably expecting and requesting a higher standard of care and a greater variety of options as their beloved animal companions approach the end of their lives. Dr Villalobos is also credited with developing a quality-of-life scale for animal hospice patients (www.veterinarypracticenews. com/images/pdfs/Quality_of_Life.pdf) (see the article by Alice E. Villalobos elsewhere in this issue for further exploration of this topic).

As veterinarians and members of the veterinary health care team expand their practices to include palliative care and hospice for their patients, it is important that they

The authors have nothing to disclose.

[a] The Downing Center for Animal Pain Management, LLC, 415 Main Street, Windsor, CO 80550, USA

[b] Healing Heart Pet Hospice, 4706 New Horizons Boulevard, Appleton, WI 54914, USA

[c] Hearts on the Mend, 1615 North Hills Avenue, Willow Grove, PA 54914, USA

* Corresponding author.

E-mail address: drrobin@downingcenter.com

consider all the diverse aspects of this level and style of care. The reader is directed to other articles in this issue dedicated to pain management, physical therapy, and mobility that address specific techniques to assist the pet in achieving and maintaining acceptable life-quality as death approaches. In addition to the technical strategies and procedures that may be applied to patients, it is equally important for the veterinary health care team to be knowledgeable and forthcoming in addressing the simpler issues surrounding palliative care and hospice: comfort, hygiene, and safety for the patient, for the human family members, and for the members of the veterinary health care team who are overseeing and delivering the palliative care and hospice experience.

Palliative practices should be integrated into the traditional management of disease and not reserved for the final weeks and days of life.[1] It is important to remember that palliative care treats the symptoms of underlying disease within the context of approaching death, but does not involve treatment with the intent to cure. Palliative care and hospice are supportive and encompass aspects of medical care that include and address physical, psychosocial, and spiritual issues. Successful palliative care and hospice for pets engage a collaborative relationship around the pet's human family members, extended family and friends, and the veterinary health care team (which may be an extended group as well). Just as human hospice in the United States has evolved to describe a comprehensive philosophy and approach to care provided by an interdisciplinary team,[2] this is the model veterinary hospice seems to be following as well. In human hospice, four distinct levels of care are defined:

1. Routine home care
2. Continuous home care
3. General inpatient care
4. Respite inpatient care.[2]

These general concepts can easily be adapted to veterinary palliative care and hospice, and their application is dependent on escalating patient symptoms and needs.

In applying palliative care and hospice principles to veterinary patients, it is useful to consider disease-based care tailored to specific issues surrounding the various diseases that may contribute to impending death, such as renal failure, cancer, escalating pain, and liver failure.[2] Regardless of the details of applied palliative care and hospice, it is important to include specific strategies to address the comfort, hygiene, and safety of the hospice patient, the pet's family, and the members of the veterinary health care team involved in delivering palliative and hospice care. This level and style of care needs to be relationship centered, and is best initiated as soon as a terminal diagnosis is in place. Ideally, once the pet owner is educated about the disease process, a plan can be developed that reflects the owner's needs and goals for the pet. Whatever the life-limiting disease, the pet and owner need and deserve to have a personalized plan articulating the palliative care techniques that will be applied to the pet.

COMFORT FOR THE PATIENT

Pain is inevitable; suffering is optional. Buddhist proverb

Maximizing comfort for the veterinary palliative care and hospice patient means tracking a moving target because these patients change with time, and their needs change with time. One of the most important goals of palliative care and hospice is to help patients achieve a good death.[3] In order to accomplish this goal, it is important to prevent and mitigate the suffering associated with whatever disease process the dying pet faces. Suffering takes place if a symptom is out of control or overwhelming,[4] so controlling symptoms forms the foundation of comfort care for patients in palliative care and hospice. Appropriate, aggressive, and comprehensive pain management must be in place and continuously updated as the pet's disease progresses. Controlling nausea is also important to sustaining comfort.

Pain is physiologic, whereas suffering is emotional, and sustaining the emotional comfort of the pet revolves around maintaining the familiar as much as is possible. This means maintaining familiar surroundings, keeping loved ones close, and sustaining familiar routines whenever possible. Continuing the routine of combing, bathing, brushing, and trimming hair and nails for pets used to regular grooming sustains normalcy. The layout of the home is part of the pet's familiarity. For pets losing their mobility, minimize obstacles, do not rearrange furniture, brighten the lights to help with fading vision, and use baby gates to protect from stairs. Maintaining a regular schedule may also be comforting for the pet, so keep to a regular feeding schedule. Increase the frequency of elimination opportunities to accommodate diminished anal and urethral tone.

Mobility issues often emerge in aging pets approaching death as they become weaker and possess less stamina. For detailed information, see the article on mobility and assistive devices by Tamara S. Shearer elsewhere in this issue. Consider the following ideas as a place to start:

Slick floor surfaces need to be covered using nonskid area rugs or runners, or interlocking foam tiles.

Slings designed to assist with walking are more comfortable and ergonomically safe than towels for both the pet and the owner (**Fig. 1**).

Food and water should be moved to the pet when the pet has trouble moving to the feeding area.

Raised food and water dishes protect the pet from having to reach down to the floor (**Fig. 2**).

Consider walkers or wheelchairs to help keep pets active and moving (**Fig. 3**).

Maintaining close contact with the pet is part of maximizing the pet's and the family's comfort during palliative and hospice care. Locate comfortable bedding in the areas where the family congregates to encourage the pet's inclusion. Pets losing their

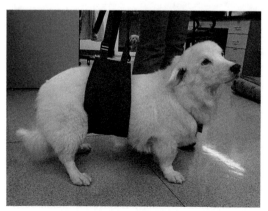

Fig. 1. Slings provide easy support. (*Courtesy of* Robin Downing, DVM, Windsor, CO.)

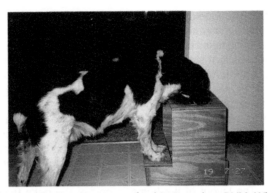

Fig. 2. Homemade raised feeder. (*Courtesy of* Robin Downing, DVM, Windsor, CO.)

hearing can be taught hand signals. Pets with diminished vision and hearing still possess their sense of smell, so outside time gives them sniffing opportunities. (Remember to protect them by using a leash.) Dogs who have enjoyed car rides will appreciate going for the occasional jaunt, even if it is just around the neighborhood. Sitting with and stroking the pet, reading quietly to the pet, and moving the pet's bed near the owner's bed are other strategies for finding comfort in the end-of-life time.

Quality care at the end of life entails knowing the disease trajectory and being able to anticipate physical symptoms.[5] Managing the physical comfort of the pet receiving palliative and hospice care not only benefits the animal but also reinforces the human-animal bond. Thermal comfort must be ensured; not too hot, not too cold. It is important to avoid fly bites and maggots in recumbent pets, and to keep the eyes lubricated and the mouth moist (**Fig. 4**).

For pets that are used to regular exercise, frequent short sessions provide sensory stimulation and also tire them out to enable restful sleep. Although it is technically a matter of hygiene, keeping the genitals, anal area, feet, eyes, nose, and mouth clean contributes significantly to comfort. Once pets become less mobile or completely recumbent, it is critical to prevent ulcerative lesions or pressure sores, which can be

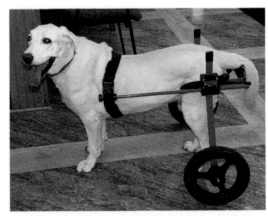

Fig. 3. Carts can restore and maintain mobility. (*Courtesy of* Robin Downing, DVM, Windsor, CO.)

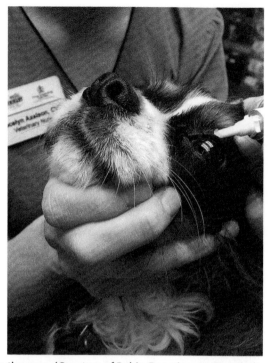

Fig. 4. Lubricating the eyes. (*Courtesy of* Robin Downing, DVM, Windsor, CO.)

a source of pain, anemia, infection, and foul-smelling discharge. These lesions are much easier to prevent than to treat.[6,7] To avoid pressure sores, it is important to keep the skin clean and free of excessive external moisture,[7] and to provide padded surfaces for resting and sleeping (**Fig. 5**).

If the pet is incapable of eating on its own because of oral disease, it may be appropriate to implant a feeding tube (eg, esophagostomy tube). If there is a feeding tube, it is appropriate to teach the client tube management, the feeding protocol, the strategy for managing tube patency, and monitoring the entry site for infection (**Fig. 6**).[6]

Oxygen therapy may be well tolerated by the pet, and, if so, is not a heroic intervention and is easy for the client to manage (**Fig. 7**).

In this same category is the administration of subcutaneous fluids to supplement what the pet drinks. In general, fluids are easy to administer at home and well tolerated by the pet (**Fig. 8**).

From human palliative and hospice care, veterinary medicine can transfer many patient-related considerations that influence the clinician's plan for care to animal patients. Many of these factors are interrelated. These considerations include (but are not limited to)[6]:

- Activities of daily living (ADLs) limitations
- Behavioral/mentation changes
- Chronic illnesses
- Cognitive function
- Disabilities
- Drug considerations
- Environment

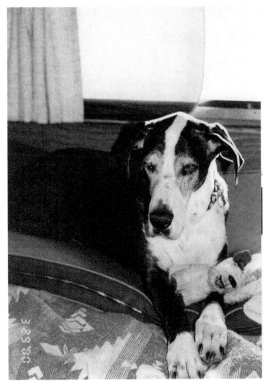

Fig. 5. Orthopedic foam beds provide extra comfort. (*Courtesy of* Robin Downing, DVM, Windsor, CO.)

- Family
- Fatigue
- Functional limitations
- Goals/expected outcomes
- History

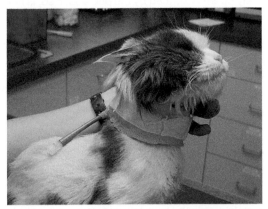

Fig. 6. Esophagostomy tubes are minimally invasive and provide easy delivery of food and medications. (*Courtesy of* Robin Downing, DVM, Windsor, CO.)

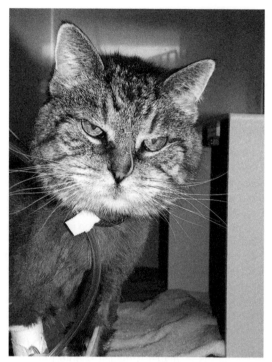

Fig. 7. Nasal oxygen is surprisingly well tolerated. (*Courtesy of* Robin Downing, DVM, Windsor, CO.)

- Home setting
- Medications
- Mobility
- Nutritional status
- Pain
- Pathology
- Physical assessment findings
- Physical setting for care

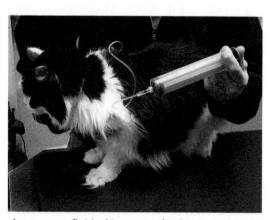

Fig. 8. Delivering subcutaneous fluids. (*Courtesy of* Robin Downing, DVM, Windsor, CO.)

- Polypharmacy
- Rehabilitation needs
- Resources
- Risk factors
- Safety
- Skin integrity
- Swallowing.

COMFORT FOR FAMILY AND PROVIDERS

It is important to remember that the family can be suffering even if the patient is not.[8] So much of helping the veterinary palliative care and hospice family achieve and maintain comfort in the face of palliative care and hospice for the pet involves managing expectations. As was mentioned earlier, this may mean tailoring the palliative care to specific disease-based issues when possible. It also means making plans for the decisions that need to be made at various steps in the journey toward death. In order for advance care planning to be successful, the veterinary health care team must focus on effective communication skills, including active listening.[9] Although it is important to be direct and honest with the client, the veterinary health care team must be careful not to use terms that may be misinterpreted.[9] It is best to make advance care plans before there is a crisis. These discussions must address the issue of resuscitation in the event of a respiratory or cardiac arrest. Something to consider is to refer to an allow-natural-death (AND) policy versus a do-not-resuscitate (DNR) policy (**Fig. 9**).[9]

There are several resources available to assist clients through this most difficult time, and the challenge of planning end-of-life care.[10–15] Because approaching death can feel disempowering, the more active a role the client can play in comfort care for the pet, the more control they have of the overall experience. Teaching simple massage techniques to the pet owner provides a vehicle for mutual comfort and reassurance between pet and human. Activities to reinforce the powerful family-pet bond may also include outdoor activities with the pet, such as car rides, riding in a trailer behind a bicycle, riding in a baby jogger, or being pulled in a child's wagon on a walk. Even pets that are completely immobile can enjoy such activities with the family.

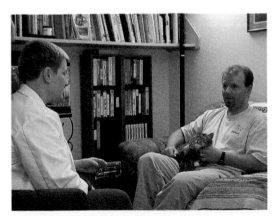

Fig. 9. Comfort Room consultation about end-of-life issues. (*Courtesy of* Robin Downing, DVM, Windsor, CO.)

Comfort for the family members of veterinary patients in palliative and hospice care includes self-support of their personal mental and emotional health. It is important for the veterinary health care team to pay attention and remind the family caregivers to take time for themselves: they need a support system too, whether that involves friends, extended family, clergy, or all of these. As death nears, the family should take care to create respite time for themselves; that is, time away from the pet, allowing the pet to be cared for by a trusted individual. This respite period gives them time to breathe, relax, and refresh. Unrelenting caregiving can be emotionally and physically draining, leading ultimately to an unhealthy day-to-day existence.

COMFORT FOR THE VETERINARY HEALTH CARE TEAM

Many of the strategies for providing comfort to the veterinary health care team members who deliver palliative and hospice care are part of keeping oneself mentally and emotionally safe (discussed later). Overall, comfort care for the professional team is straightforward, and there are resources available for the veterinary team in addition to those listed for the pet hospice family.[16] Team members (including the veterinarian) should get enough sleep, eat well, keep physically active, and engage in ritual or spiritual practices they find comforting (if applicable). Just like the pet's family, the veterinary palliative care and hospice providers need a supportive network. Regular debriefing about individual patients and modifying the care plan can empower the care providers. Acknowledging and working through anticipatory grief as patients approach death also contributes to health care provider comfort and emotional health.

HYGIENE FOR THE PATIENT

As animal patients approach their death, many of them develop fecal and/or urinary incontinence. This incontinence is the most likely hygiene issue pet owners will face during palliative and hospice care. Preventing urine and fecal scald is a priority in these patients. Keep hair trimmed around the genitals and anus, making it easier to clean and dry the skin should it become soiled. In dogs and cats with long hair who do not enjoy or tolerate being groomed, it may be worth considering a whole body trim (eg, a lion cut) to make hair coat management easier. The pet may need a diaper to contain urine and stool. There are several pet diaper options available with replaceable liners. In some pets, human diapers may work. Any time diapers are required for containment, it is important to do regular checks in order to change them when they become soiled (**Figs. 10** and **11**).

If incontinence is intermittent or unpredictable, a diaper may not be necessary. In this case, modifying the environment and the pet's schedule to manage urine and stool may be adequate. Waterproof sheets or mattress covers can be used on pet beds to make cleanup easy. A pet bed can be covered with a trash bag before being inserted into its cover, meaning only the cover need be washed. Carpets can be protected by using waterproof material under drop cloths. Ambulatory issues sometimes make it challenging for a dog to get outside to eliminate. Some dogs easily adapt to using potty pads for elimination in the house, sparing the floor and carpet from soiling (**Fig. 12**).

For cats that develop ambulatory issues as they age and progress through palliative care and hospice, using the litter pan may become a challenge. The litter pan is sometimes on a different floor of the home from where the cat spends most of its time, and stairs have become a problem. Perhaps there is only one litter pan on a particular level of the home, and the cat is less ambulatory. Increasing the number of litter pans and adding locations, including at least one pan on each level of the house, may be enough

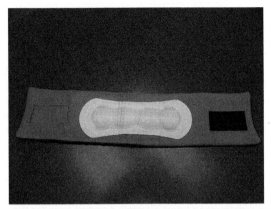

Fig. 10. Sanitary pads can help with urine containment. (*Courtesy of* Robin Downing, DVM, Windsor, CO.)

to solve the problem. Sometimes the cat becomes too weak or uncomfortable to climb over the side and into the litter pan. In this case, a change in litter pan design may be in order. A low-sided, under-the-bed storage box can serve as a litter pan alternative. Likewise, a cardboard box for beverages (also low sided) may be used once it is placed into an appropriately sized trash bag before being filled with litter. The key is low sides. Occasionally, a cat in palliative or hospice care becomes litter pan aversive or litter aversive. It may work simply to choose a different style of litter from what has been previously used. It may be that a completely different substrate is needed (eg, shredded newspaper, sand, sheets of newspaper, shredded or sheets of paper towels). Some cats are happy simply to transfer to using potty pads if the litter pan becomes too much of a challenge.

Some pets may develop devitalized areas over tumors that then secrete serum or develop crusts on the surface. Absorbent fabrics like T-shirts may be used to manage exudates. Waterless shampoo (made for dogs and cats) works well to keep these areas clean. If a particular lesion needs to be bandaged, pet owners can usually be

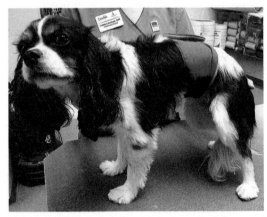

Fig. 11. A belly band with absorbent padding. (*Courtesy of* Robin Downing, DVM, Windsor, CO.)

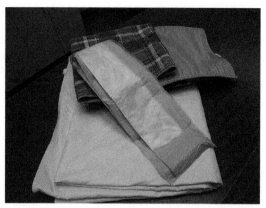

Fig. 12. Various absorptive products. (*Courtesy of* Robin Downing, DVM, Windsor, CO.)

taught how to change dressings. Lemon juice or vinegar in a 1:1 dilution with water may also be used to clean the hair coat. A loofah scrubber may work better than a simple washcloth. Likewise, moist baby wipes may be used for spot cleaning. For animals who become messy eaters, a bib during meals will help contain spills. A tiny bib for a cat or small dog may be fashioned from a coffee filter with the center cut out to slip it over the pet's head.

HYGIENE FOR THE PET OWNER AND VETERINARY HEALTH CARE TEAM

It is important for the veterinary health care team to take the time to educate pet owners and their families in the basics of universal precautions and good hygiene practices as pets enter palliative and hospice care. Universal precautions are infection control guidelines designed to protect people from diseases spread by blood and certain body fluids. It is best to assume that all blood and body fluids are infectious for blood-borne diseases. Universal precautions (second nature to veterinary health care providers) are straightforward and easy to implement. For instance, when cleaning up blood, urine, stool, vomit, or wound secretions, the following steps should be taken:

- Put on disposable gloves
- Wipe up blood or body fluids with absorbent paper towels
- Place contaminated paper towels in a plastic garbage bag
- Clean and rinse area with whatever disinfectant is typically used
- Remove gloves and place into garbage bag
- Secure bag with tie
- Dispose of plastic garbage bag
- Wash hands.

Clients and health care team members should also take precautions to prevent injuries caused by needles if the pet is receiving injectable medication. To prevent needle-stick injuries, needles should not be recapped by hand, purposely bent or broken by hand, removed from disposable syringes, or otherwise manipulated by hand. After they are used, disposable syringes and needles should be placed in puncture-resistant containers for disposal. The puncture-resistant containers should be located as close as is practical to the use area (www.cdc.gov/ncidod/dhqp/bp_universal_precautions.html).

Be ready to offer ordering information for any supplies or products your practice cannot sell to the client. Examination gloves serve as the cornerstone of good hygiene practices for the pet owner. Should clients have any immune-system issues, they should add a surgical mask for protection from dust or aerosolized contaminants. Offer recommendations for cleaning products and odor neutralizers for the home environment. The same guidelines apply to veterinary health care team members as to pet owners for managing hygiene issues.

PATIENT SAFETY

In considering veterinary patient safety during end-of-life care, it is important to emphasize effective communication among the veterinary health care team and the human family members. The best communication is direct communication, so that all parties in the caregiving circle can be confident that they share a common understanding of the plan that is in place for the pet. Providing for the safety of patients in palliative and hospice care means focusing on the big picture of their lives at home and the home environment. Here is a situation in which detailed questioning of the pet owner is critical to success. Likewise, a home visit may provide invaluable insights into the day-to-day life of the pet and its family. In addressing patient safety issues, the owner may need to be guided to protect the pet from access to stairs without supervision. Baby gates at the top and bottom of flights of stairs will prevent a fall. Nonskid floor surfaces are essential; this may mean nonskid area rugs or runners, or interlocking foam tiles, which are easy to install, remove, and clean. Pets that become weaker and more unsteady as they reach their end of life deserve to have secure footing available to them.

If there are other pets in the home, it is important to ensure that the pet receiving palliative or hospice care is not subjected to attack or injury. It is possible for the dynamics among pets to change dramatically when one pet in a household becomes ill; *weak* in the vernacular of the wild world. Perceived weakness can precipitate a power struggle within the family pet hierarchy leading to confrontations, fights, and injury. If there are children in the household, it is important to involve them actively in keeping the affected patient safe. This involvement means protecting the pet from being handled inappropriately or roughly in a way that might cause pain or injury.

Another aspect of palliative and hospice care safety is attention to the details of medication delivery. In human medicine, medical error accounts for an inordinate number of deaths and near deaths in patients. The veterinary health care team has an ethical and medical obligation to the patient and pet owner to assist in appropriate delivery of prescribed medications, food, and supplements. This appropriate delivery may be as simple as providing pill minders (multiday pill holders with a chamber for each day of the week; 1 for morning medications and 1 for afternoon medications, with more if needed). It may help clients to have blank spreadsheets they can customize, fill out, and post in a central location (**Fig. 13**). Memory aids like these serve 2 important purposes: they encourage the delivery of medications to the pet and they help to prevent overdosing.

PET CAREGIVER SAFETY

For pet owners whose animals have entered palliative and hospice care, it is important to help those clients think through the possible consequences of the pet's approaching death so they may stay safe while handling the animal. For instance, they should be supplied with a snap-on fabric muzzle fitted to the pet in case the pet becomes painful

MEDICATION CHECKLIST

Name:_____

Medication

Medication

Medication

Medication

Fig. 13. Medication checklist. (Copyright © The Downing Center for Animal Pain Management, LLC, Windsor, CO. Used with permission.)

but needs to be handled or moved. Four Flags Over Aspen (www.fourflags.com) has an excellent selection of easy-to-use options (**Fig. 14**).

If pets develop either urine or fecal incontinence, pet owners should be clearly directed to use universal precautions (discussed earlier) when cleaning messes either from the pet or from the environment, including disinfecting the soiled areas, using surgical masks when cleaning up messes if the pet owner is sensitive to inhaled irritants, and so forth. It is also important for these pet owners to keep young children

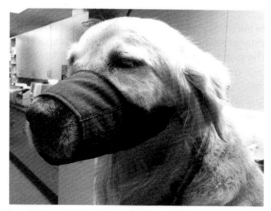

Fig. 14. Soft muzzles can be used when needed for safety. (*Courtesy of* Robin Downing, DVM, Windsor, CO.)

safe from any urine, stool, or vomit contamination. It is important to prevent food contamination in the household. Any humans in the household who are immune compromised (eg, chemotherapy, human immunodeficiency virus/acquired immune deficiency syndrome, rheumatoid arthritis) should be excused from handling the pet's waste if possible. If this is not an option, then these individuals should be especially careful to keep themselves safe by using gloves and a mask during waste disposal and washing carefully afterward. The basics of universal precautions also help pet owners avoid needle sticks as well as preventing infection of any minor wounds they may have. Pet owners need guidance in handling wounds on their pets, whether or not those wounds are infected.

SAFETY FOR THE VETERINARY HEALTH CARE TEAM

Veterinary health care team members who are engaged in palliative and hospice care need to keep themselves safe, both within the veterinary practice and in the field if they are providing services in the home. Universal precautions apply to cleaning up pet waste, preventing needle sticks, handling sharps, and handling wounds or weeping lesions on the patient. Soft, snap-on fabric muzzles in various sizes allow for safe handling of a painful patient.

When providing palliative and hospice care in the home, personal safety must be a priority. The practice should have a written and detailed protocol in place for how this is accomplished. If possible, have two people make these home visits. Here are some details to consider in staying safe[17]:

- Have a full tank of gas
- Carry a blanket, water, and a first aid kit
- Carry a shovel and snow brush
- Be sure the spare tire is in good working order
- Have detailed directions to the home (global positioning system, if possible)
- Call owners to have them watch for the team member
- Carry a cell phone
- Lock car doors while driving and while in the client's home
- Keep maps out of sight; do not look unfamiliar with the area
- Be sure someone else on the team (ideally a supervisor) knows the details and timing of the planned visit
- Be aware of the surroundings and trust your instincts.

Another aspect of veterinary health care team safety is emotional, mental, and physical health, which means getting enough sleep, eating a balanced diet, and engaging in regular exercise. The pet hospice worker needs a support network just as the pet's family does. Regular debriefing about these patients in order to modify the care plan will help with mental health as well.

SUMMARY

Hygiene, comfort, and safety considerations during pet palliative care and hospice are, for the most part, straightforward. All members of the caregiving team deserve to be comfortable and safe as the journey toward the end of life unfolds. It is the obligation of the veterinary health care team to coordinate palliative care and hospice details to ensure that the pet and the family are fully informed and fully engaged in the process. Although end-of-life issues, euthanasia, and death are nearly everyday concerns for most veterinary health care teams, these are typically not everyday concerns for the pet owner. Pet owners and veterinary patients rely on the veterinary health care team to help create the structure within which the pet will die, knowing that each pet's journey is unique. The gift the veterinary team can give the family-pet unit in this circumstance is the gift of structure and multifaceted comfort. The time has come for the veterinary profession to take seriously this unique niche of care.

REFERENCES

1. Kuebler KK, Davis MP, Moore CD, editors. Palliative practices: an interdisciplinary approach. St Louis (MO): Elsevier Mosby; 2005. p. xv.
2. Kinzbrunner BM. Palliative care perspectives. In: Kuebler KK, Davis MP, Moore CD, editors. Palliative practices: an interdisciplinary approach. St Louis (MO): Elsevier Mosby; 2005. p. 5, 9, 19.
3. Vena C, Kuebler K, Schrader SE. The dying process. In: Kuebler KK, Davis MP, Moore CD, editors. Palliative practices: an interdisciplinary approach. St Louis (MO): Elsevier Mosby; 2005. p. 360.
4. Loseth DB, Moore CD, Mulder JA, et al. Cultural and spiritual issues. In: Kuebler KK, Davis MP, Moore CD, editors. Palliative practices: an interdisciplinary approach. St Louis (MO): Elsevier Mosby; 2005. p. 328.
5. Loseth DB. Psychosocial and spiritual care. In: Kuebler KK, Berry PH, Heidrich DE, editors. End of life care. Philadelphia: Saunders Elsevier; 2002. p. 120.
6. Marrelli TM. Hospice and palliative care handbook. St Louis (MO): Elsevier Mosby; 2005. p. 80, 81, 358, 382.
7. Heidrich DE. Ulcerative lesions. In: Kuebler KK, Berry PH, Heidrich DE, editors. End of life care. Philadelphia: Saunders Elsevier; 2002. p. 419, 425.
8. Loseth DB. Psychosocial and spiritual care. In: Kuebler KK, Berry PH, Heidrich DE, editors. End of life care. Philadelphia: Saunders Elsevier; 2002. p. 118.
9. Moore CD. Advance care planning. In: Kuebler KK, Davis MP, Moore CD, editors. Palliative practices: an interdisciplinary approach. St Louis (MO): Elsevier Mosby; 2005. p. 32–4. 38, 39.
10. Downing R. Pets living with cancer. Lakewood (CO): AAHA Press; 2000. p. 81–103.
11. Kaplan L. So easy to love, so hard to lose. Briar Cliff (NY): JanGen Press; 2010.
12. Wolfelt AD. Healing your grieving soul: 100 spiritual practice for mourners. Fort Collins (CO): Companion Press; 2009.
13. Wolfelt AD. When your pet dies: a guide to mourning, remembering, and healing. Fort Collins (CO): Companion Press; 2004.
14. Wolfelt AD, Duvall KJ. Healing your grieving body: 100 physical practices for mourners. Fort Collins (CO): Companion Press; 2009.
15. Yoder G. Companioning the dying. Fort Collins (CO): Companion Press; 2005.
16. Wolfelt AD. Interpersonal skills training: a handbook for funeral home staffs. Florence (KY): Accelerated/Development (Taylor & Francis); 1990.
17. Marrelli TM. Hospice and palliative care handbook. St Louis (MO): Elsevier Mosby; 2005. p. 52–3.

RECOMMENDED READINGS

AAHA/AAFP Pain Management Guidelines Task Force. AAHA/AAFP pain management guidelines for dogs and cats. J Am Anim Hosp Assoc 2007;43:235–48.

Berger AM, Portenoy RK, Weissman DE, editors. Principles & practice of palliative care & supportive oncology. 2nd edition. Philadelphia: Lippincott Williams & Wilkins; 2002.

Downing R. Pets living with cancer. Lakewood (CO): AAHA Press; 2000.

Gaynor JS, Muir WW. Handbook of veterinary pain management. 2nd edition. St Louis (MO): Mosby Elsevier; 2009.

Kaplan L. So easy to love, so hard to lose. Briar Cliff (NY): JanGen Press; 2010.

Kuebler KK, Berry PH, Heidrich DE, editors. End of life care. Philadelphia: Saunders Elsevier; 2002.

Kuebler KK, Davis MP, Moore CD. Palliative practices: an interdisciplinary approach. St Louis (MO): Elsevier Mosby; 2005.

Marrelli TM. Hospice and palliative care handbook. St Louis (MO): Elsevier Mosby; 2005.

Nakaya SF. Kindred spirit, kindred care: making health decisions on behalf of our animal companions. Novato (CA): New World Library; 2005.

Villalobos A, Kaplan L. Canine and feline geriatric oncology: honoring the human-animal bond. Ames (IA): Blackwell Publishing; 2007.

Wolfelt AD. Healing your grieving soul: 100 spiritual practice for mourners. Fort Collins (CO): Companion Press; 2009.

Wolfelt AD. Interpersonal skills training: a handbook for funeral home staffs. Florence (KY): Accelerated/Development (Taylor & Francis); 1990.

Wolfelt AD. When your pet dies: a guide to mourning, remembering, and healing. Fort Collins (CO): Companion Press; 2004.

Wolfelt AD, Duvall KJ. Healing your grieving body: 100 physical practices for mourners. Fort Collins (CO): Companion Press; 2009.

Yoder G. Companioning the dying. Fort Collins (CO): Companion Press; 2005.

A Veterinarian's Role in Helping Pet Owners with Decision Making

Amir Shanan, DVM

KEYWORDS

- End-of-life care • Companion animals • Hospice veterinarians
- Palliative care • Animal quality of life

Hospice veterinarians act as medical experts as well as educators, support persons, guides, and facilitators. In these roles, veterinarians have many opportunities to help owners make end-of-life decisions. The veterinarian makes up the foundation of a palliative and hospice care team. Some veterinarians are gifted in that they possess qualities that are conducive to medically caring for pets and also supporting pet owners emotionally. There are concepts that veterinarians need to be familiar with to be more productive and effective when helping pet owners with end-of-life decisions. The concepts that are unique to the veterinary profession include the relationship between hospice care and the human-animal bond, the nonmedical role that veterinarians play in helping pet owners, and the role euthanasia plays within hospice care.

Communicating with owners of animals approaching the end of their lives is a challenge every veterinarian in small animal practice faces. End-of-life care frequently requires owners and veterinarians to make decisions of monumental consequences while feeling they sorely lack essential information. This feeling can be distressing to both owners and veterinarians and also lead to strains in the relationship between them.

When an attending veterinarian and a terminally ill pet's owner agree that an animal is best served by a hospice approach, they have reached an understanding that

- Preserving QOL takes precedence over measures to prolong life
- The evaluation of QOL is based on the affect-balance model
- Assessment of an animal's affect (feelings and mood) is based on an animal's behavior.

International Association for Animal Hospice and Palliative Care, www.iaahpc.org and Compassionate Veterinary Care, 620 West Webster Avenue, Chicago, IL 60614, USA.
E-mail address: Ashanan1g@gmail.com

Vet Clin Small Anim 41 (2011) 635–646
doi:10.1016/j.cvsm.2011.03.006
0195-5616/11/$ – see front matter © 2011 Elsevier Inc. All rights reserved.

- Evaluating an animal's QOL is primarily the responsibility of the family—especially the family member most attached to the pet and most involved in the pet's care.

Many of the advancements in medical technology of the past half-century have in recent years become available to companion animals. It has become increasingly clear that doing everything medical science can offer to prevent death is not always in an animal's best interest and that prolonging life is not adequate as a sole measure for the success of the health care delivered. The mission of hospice is to ensure that care provided to terminally ill animals remains focused on their interests. To help owners make the best decisions, it is a veterinarian's role to present all options; to provide guidance in assessing QOL; and to respond to owners' emotional bonds with their pets in terms of the way the owners see them, meeting owners at their "model of the world."

This article will help veterinarians improve their palliative and hospice care skills by offering tools necssary to help pet owners make the best end of life decisions for their pets.

ASSOCIATION BETWEEN HOSPICE AND THE HUMAN-ANIMAL BOND

The association between hospice care and the human-animal bond should to be taken into account when assisting pet owners with decision making. The past 3 decades have witnessed an increasing recognition of the depth of emotional connection between humans and their companion animals, termed the *human-animal bond*. In recent studies, a majority of pet owners indicated they consider their pet a family member, that they refer to themselves as their pet's parent, and that their animal is allowed to sleep in bed with them.[1] Extensive literature documents the benefits to humans from having such relationships with animals in their lives[2] and substantiates the loss of such relationships as significant losses associated with grief.[3(p29)] In one study, as many as 30% of pet owners rated their grief over the death of a pet as "severe."[4]

The hospice philosophy originated in England in the 1960s in response to the inadequacy of services for terminally ill patients and to the rising popularity of the Voluntary Euthanasia Society (for humans). Dr Cicely Saunders, founder of the modern hospice movement, commented that both hospice and the Voluntary Euthanasia Society have "a vendetta against pointless pain and impersonal indignity." To sway people away from the idea of voluntary euthanasia, hospice's vision aimed to achieve care of the dying that is "so effective that no-one should reach that desperate place where he could only ask for his life to be taken."[5] For more details on the history of animal hospice, see article by Kathryn D. Marocchino elsewhere in this issue for further exploration of this topic.

Owners of pets with life-limiting conditions are often presented with limited treatment options by their veterinarians. Many owners report feeling abandoned when they perceive the options offered as unacceptable—too aggressive on the one hand or a premature recommendation for euthanasia on the other. Delivering palliative and hospice comfort care may be a veterinarian's best way to serve their needs.

A critical moment in the clinical management of life-limiting medical conditions in companion animals is when an attending veterinarian and/or owner recognize that cure is not an attainable goal. Such a realization is loaded with significance for an attached owner, indicating that a degree of discomfort in the animal's life is inevitable, that caregiving is permanently more complex and demanding, and that the animal's remaining life expectancy is shorter than hoped for. The realization is of great significance to the clinician as well, signaling that it is time to shift priorities from curing the disease to maximizing patient comfort.

The moment of recognizing that cure is unattainable defines the beginning of a hospice stage in an animal's care. When highly attached pet owners recognize that moment, it is normal for them to experience strong emotions, generally termed, *anticipatory grief*. Anticipatory grief is the psyche's way of preparing for impending loss. How a pet owner's anticipatory grief is managed has a strong impact on the grieving process after a loss. The mission of animal hospice is to guide the provision of physical, emotional, social, and spiritual comfort to animal patients and their human families as they approach the end of life.

NONMEDICAL HELPING ROLES OF VETERINARIANS

The nonmedical role that veterinarians play when helping clients with end-of-life decisions is as important to the philosophy of hospice care as is medical expertise. Human hospice organizations use interdisciplinary teams of professionals (physicians, nurses, social workers, and clergy, to name a few) and lay people from a patient's community. Such elaborate organizations are starting to evolve in animal hospice.

Pet owners often trust veterinarians and/or see them as authority figures. During loss, clients may look to a veterinarian to provide strength, guidance, and leadership.[3(p80)] Surveys in human medicine have shown that patients want medical professionals to acknowledge their emotions and listen to their concerns. Effective listening is a significant predictor of patient satisfaction.[6] The manner in which a veterinarian provides care for a client whose pet has died has the potential to alleviate or aggravate grief, influence client and veterinarian satisfaction, and create or destroy long-lasting client-veterinarian relationships. Given clients' expectations and the impact of end-of-life conversations on pet owners and the veterinary team, compassionate communication should be considered both a core clinical skill and an ethical obligation for veterinarians.[7(pp95–7)]

Veterinarians often choose their profession because of a strong internal need to serve people in addition to other reasons. It is not surprising that helping clients has been shown to strongly correlate with job satisfaction among veterinarians and their staffs. Lack of compassionate care, alternatively, may have a negative affect on veterinarians financially, by prompting grieving clients to seek help from other providers.[3(pp80–1)]

Lagoni and colleagues recommend that veterinarians can add 4 specific helping-oriented roles to their role as medical experts: educating (primarily talking), supporting (primarily listening), guiding (primarily suggesting), and facilitating (primarily acting). When a balance between these roles is achieved, helping grieving clients is usually effective.[3(p60)]

Building healthy helping relationships with clients is a skill in which most veterinarians have not been trained. Without training, helping may take the forms of problem solving, advice giving, rationalizing, or rescuing, none of which is appropriate or effective in dealing with other people's emotions. Boundaries between treating animals and treating people must be kept clear. Grieving clients may share with a veterinarian struggles with spiritual and religious beliefs triggered by the loss experience or mention suicidal thoughts or plans. Veterinarians' roles in helping in such matters must be limited to making appropriate referral suggestions or notifying authorities.[3(pp59,60)]

Presenting Options

It is essential that veterinarians offer more than one option when discussing medical care for a terminally ill animal and provide families with sufficient and balanced information to form an opinion on each option.

As a medical expert, a veterinarian is responsible for collecting the information necessary to make a diagnosis and suggesting a plan for an animal's medical and nursing care. Medical expertise addresses primarily patients' physical needs. The degree to which veterinarians address animals' emotional and social needs in making medical decisions is slowly increasing but currently leaves much to be desired. Medical expertise also serves an important need of caregivers, that is, the need to obtain competent medical advice for their animal.

The objective of discussing options is to give families some control over the process leading to the inevitable loss, by helping them find out their view of what constitutes the best way to care for their animal. A sense of control—even if limited—has been shown to correlate with healthy grieving and emotional healing. To achieve this objective, veterinarians should be attentive to clients' reactions when discussing options for end-of-life care, maintain eye contact as much as possible, and acknowledge when they respond.

Euthanasia is frequently one of the options discussed, because most pet owners struggle with it at some point. Euthanasia should never be the only option offered, however.

Veterinary Hospice and Euthanasia

Veterinarians' role in helping clients make decisions about their animals' end of life invariably involves discussing and struggling with the option to intervene and end a patient's suffering and life by euthanasia. Opinions about the relationship between hospice care and euthanasia in veterinary medicine vary widely. Some veterinarians in the field believe that some aspects of hospice care, when not properly managed, may prolong suffering, whereas others see euthanasia as interfering with the process of natural dying.

The original vision of hospice care was developed a half-century ago as a solution for the pointless pain and indignity that the health care system prescribed for dying patients at the time. The capabilities of twenty-first century medical sciences to extend life could hardly be imagined then, when open heart surgery, pacemakers, organ transplants, parenteral nutrition, fiberoptic endoscopy, cancer chemotherapy, and computers were all in their infancy. Since then, life-prolonging technology has rendered the term, *natural death*, progressively meaningless, giving rise to complex ethical struggles with medical futility and who decides when to pull the plug and why.

The line separating medical care and euthanasia is further blurred by the principle of double effect, that is, permitting relief of a terminally ill patient's suffering using medications that may also cause the patient's death. Similarly, the objective of euthanasia is to relieve suffering, and the ending of life is the undesirable outcome when there is no other way to end suffering.[8] Medical science has rendered obsolete centuries of experience, tradition, and language about mortality and created a new difficulty for humankind: how to die.[9]

In veterinary medicine, euthanasia is a legal and widely accepted solution to protecting dying patients from pointless pain and indignity. Veterinary patients cannot communicate their wishes verbally and it cannot definitively be determined whether or not an animal prefers euthanasia at a given point in time. It is the responsibility of an animal's proxy to decide if and when euthanasia is a better option than life for an animal that is suffering despite receiving the best comfort care available.

Ultimately, the answer to the question, "Which is better—euthanasia or 'natural' death?" depends on how death is experienced by a dying animal. At this time, such information is not available and veterinarians and pet owners must humbly accept that, in scientific terms, the subjective experience of dying is a great mystery.

Proxies are free to make decisions based on beliefs as long as a realistic assessment of an animal's QOL remains supreme to any ideology. They must be prepared to change course of action as dictated by a sense of empathy with the patient to truly fulfill their responsibility.

The realities of the twenty-first century have rendered the 1960s' definition of hospice care, as the antithesis to euthanasia, outdated. I propose the following definition: animal hospice is care for nonhumans with life-limiting illness, focused on the patient's and family's needs, on living life as fully as possible until the time of death (with or without intervention), and on the end of life as an opportunity for closure and growth.

QUALITY OF LIFE AND QUALITY OF DEATH

When considering the options for end-of-life care for an animal, an animal's owner or caregiver acting as a proxy is charged with the responsibility of making the decisions a patient would consider the best. The strongest desire of highly attached pet owners facing the loss of a beloved companion is to do what is best for the animal. Attaining this goal depends heavily on humans' ability to define and determine what is best for an animal approaching the end of life. The widespread use of hospice services for terminally ill humans has offered many insights into the experiences, wishes, and goals of humans as they approach the end of life. This knowledge was obtained primarily by recording patients' verbal accounts of their feelings and thoughts. There are, however, human patient populations that do not have the capacity to communicate verbally due to brain lesions, neuromuscular deficits, or simply young age. Medical and other decisions are made for these individuals by family members or by medical and/or social service providers, collectively termed, *proxies*. Studies designed to correlate decision making by proxies to the decisions made by their charges (using charges who can communicate) revealed that even close relatives and highly competent health professionals have only a limited ability to correctly predict a patient's perception of what the patient considers "best for myself."[10(p193)]

The past 50 years have seen the accumulation of knowledge from long-term studies—some decades long—of the behaviors of many species of social animals in their natural environment. These ethological studies have established solid documentation supporting a new paradigm: that humans are not the only creatures with minds capable of solving problems; capable of love, joy, fear, sorrow, and despair; and capable of experiencing happiness and suffering, without quotations marks.[11] Hence, if companion animals are considered capable of feelings and some thinking but incapable of expressing those feelings and thoughts verbally, it is evident that doing what is best for an animal becomes an elusive goal, inescapably subject to a proxy's interpretation.

Owners anguish as they repeatedly ask themselves whether their beloved animal's QOL is acceptable (defined as staying alive is in the patient's overall best interest) or unacceptable (defined as staying alive is against the patient's overall best interest). A veterinarian can help by educating an owner in how to assess an animal's QOL. Assessing an animal's QOL depends on attributing relative weight to specific experiences—like the presence or absence of joy or the presence or absence of pain or frustration. These relative weights are determined by the psychological impact of the experience on the individual animal and are therefore by definition subjective.

Animals can only communicate their QOL nonverbally. Knowledge of animal behavior provides a basis for interpreting the affect expressed by animals' specific actions or reactions or lack thereof. Another form of nonverbal communication is interspecies empathy. Empathy is described as the intellectual and emotional comprehension of someone else's condition or being in someone else's shoes.[3(p99)] This is closely related to the ability of persons most closely bonded with an animal to feel in their gut what the animal is experiencing. Owners who are motivated by the profound desire to do what a pet would have wanted must be encouraged to humbly accept that some components of their animals' experience cannot be fully understood or recognized by any human. They can be supported, however, by reassurance that after processing information provided by a veterinarian and others, they have no better tool for answering the question of whether or not their beloved animal is better off dead or alive than their own interspecies empathy. QOL life has been adopted to serve as a complementary objective for health care decisions, a means of assuring that the perspective of the patient remains the focus of the medical care.[10(p184)]

McMillan[10] uses an affect-balance model to define QOL as follows:

Quality of life is the affective and cognitive (to the degree that the animal can form such a cognitive construct) assessment that an animal makes of its life overall, of how its life is faring, experienced on a continuum of good to bad. This assessment is derived from the balance between the various pleasant and unpleasant affects experienced by the animal at and recently preceding the QOL assessment. In general, the further the affect balance tips toward the pleasant side, the higher the QOL. The contributory weights of the specific affects vary between individuals and are determined by the psychological impact of the affects on that individual.[10(p193)]

The affect-balance model definition of QOL means, in plain English, that QOL is influenced by the balance between levels of happiness and distress. Following is a brief summary of McMillan's analysis of the meaning of these terms as applied to animals.[10]

McMillan defines distress as "the unpleasant affective state, akin to or the same as anguish, resulting from an inability to control or otherwise cope with or adapt to the unpleasant affect generated by altered or threatened homeostasis." For example, a surgical incision constitutes an alteration to tissue homeostasis; pain sensation is the unpleasant affect generated; however, the degree of distress experienced by a patient depends on the ability to control, cope with, or adapt to the physical pain. McMillan makes no distinction between distress and suffering, describing both as "unpleasant affective mental states attributable to an underlying unpleasant affect."[10(p105)]

McMillan distinguishes between the terms, *happy*, which refers to "short term experience of pleasant feelings," and *true happiness* as "the long-term mood state associated with one's evaluative overview of life."[10(p222)] Forming an evaluation of one's life overall as satisfactory or unsatisfactory requires a cognitive capacity to conceptualize the future and the past. If the commonly held view of nonhuman animals as being aware of the present only is accurate, then by definition animals lack the mental faculty needed to form a concept of life as a whole and experience true happiness.

An increasing number of studies and anecdotal observations, however, offer substantial evidence that animals do form life-as-a-whole evaluations. These evaluations are likely not as cognitively complex as those in humans, but they do seem to represent an assessment of an animal's life satisfaction. Readers are referred to the discussion in McMillan for the detailed arguments supporting the existence of true happiness in animals that bears a strong resemblance to that in humans.[10(pp228–31)]

QOL is considered strictly a view from within—how individuals feel about the circumstances and events making up their lives and what they mean to them alone. Applying this QOL to animals dictates that it should be assessed from the perspective of an individual animal. Because the experience of QOL depends on what matters to an individual animal, which varies greatly, and due to obvious communication barriers, it is reasonable to assume that some components of animals' QOL will never be fully understood or even recognized.

QOL is viewed as a continuum, ranging from high to low. Various scales and instruments for measuring animal QOL have been proposed in recent years, for example, as described by Villalobos,[12(pp304–6),13(pp581–6)] and summarized by Wiseman-Orr and colleagues,[6] but no consensus exists on how to measure happiness, QOL, emotional health, or psychological well-being in any animal. There are no clear-cut demarcations or recognizable cutoff points on the QOL continuum. Most significantly, there is no objective point below which QOL is unacceptable.

QOL issues need to be revisited often by veterinarians when helping pet owners with decision making because of changes in patient status. Veterinarians can provide education and guidance to families to assure their competence in carefully monitoring QOL by observing, recording, and interpreting animals' behaviors. The author recommends to owners the following protocol:

- Determine which behaviors are pertinent to an animal's affect balance and compile an inventory list of those behaviors.
- Divide the list into behaviors indicating positive affect (joy, companionship, mental engagement and stimulation, control, and others) versus those indicating negative affect (fear, anxiety, boredom, isolation, depression, pain, hypoxia, hunger, nausea, and others).
- Keep a journal or otherwise document observations of the behaviors listed in the inventory.
- Use the journal to detect trends—changes in the frequency of behaviors and in the intensity of affect they reflect (eg, How happy is the pet this week compared with last week? How much discomfort is the pet in today compared with an average day this week?).

If a terminally ill animal is not experiencing significant observable emotional distress (anxiety or fear, for example) but also is not experiencing any observable joy, considerations other than the animal's QOL can play a role in making end-of-life decisions, such as

1. Owner's concern about and/or desire to avoid further deterioration in the animal's QOL
2. Owner's desire to continue to enjoy the animal's physical presence
3. Owner's perception of euthanasia or natural death as a better way to die
4. Owner's QOL. Although frequently laden with guilt, a decision to euthanize a terminally ill beloved pet to improve the owner's life may be justified when all of the following are true:
   a. The owner has carefully reviewed every possible way to determine what the animal would want, and the results of the review are inconclusive.
   b. The animal's QOL is not expected to improve.
   c. The owner can be assured that ending a pet's life by euthanasia will be peaceful.

Ultimately, veterinarians must fulfill their role as animal advocate, however, and speak to what matters to the animal if an owner's primary motivation seems to be ideas or feelings other than the animal's best interests.[14]

MAKING DECISIONS ABOUT TIMING: TOO EARLY VERSUS TOO LATE—PREPARING FOR GUILT

Guilt and anxiety may seriously complicate grieving, and veterinarians can offer education and support to minimize the negative impact. In some cases, this may be a veterinarian's most significant contribution to an owner's healing. Owners of terminally ill pets frequently experience emotional distress as they struggle with the questions, "How will I know if it is time to euthanize?" and "Which is better (or worse)—making a euthanasia decision too early or making one too late?" Making a euthanasia decision too early may lead to feeling guilt for taking away from an animal (and/or themselves) the possibility of enjoying more time together. It may even lead to guilt about having killed a beloved creature. Letting an animal die naturally or making a euthanasia decision too late may lead to guilt for allowing a beloved companion to suffer more than the animal "should have."

The time most often considered the right time for euthanasia is when an animal's QOL is recognized as having crossed the line from acceptable to unacceptable (as defined previously). Unfortunately, there are no generally accepted standards in society defining the line between acceptable to unacceptable QOL. In the end, owners must carry the burden of drawing it—a lonely, often overwhelming task. Feelings of anxiety and guilt are particularly common when making the decision involves a struggle with uncertainty. These feelings intensify later on, when owners second-guess their own decisions.

Making end-of-life decisions is associated with anxiety—about death, about suffering, about finances, and about the uncertainty of a future without the loved one. To be helpful, it is essential to listen to what is most important to a family under the circumstances—what their concerns are, how they want to spend their time as options become limited, and what kinds of trade-offs they are willing to make—before offering further information and advice.[9]

Guilt is a common experience when coping with actual or anticipated loss. It is commonly associated with decisions to abandon efforts to cure and with decisions to euthanize a beloved companion. Guilt often stems from owners' perceptions (which may or may not be justified) that they have failed in their responsibility to keep their pets safe, healthy, and alive.[3(p397)] Many owners feel some relief when presented with the clear notion that making a decision perceived as too late and making a decision perceived as too early lead to the same outcome: guilt. Seeing the commonality between the two opposite situations helps owners accept the reality that it is not always possible to assure making the perfect decision. Veterinarians can help by encouraging owners to focus on the more attainable goal of making the best possible decision. Knowing they did their best with the information they had, owners have an easier time forgiving themselves when haunted by thoughts that the decision to end their pet's life was made a little too early or a little too late.

ACTIVE DYING AND EUTHANASIA

Final details about the active dying process and euthanasia, including how and where the process should take place and who should be present, should be discussed ahead of time with pet owners. When an animal is actively dying or when a decision has been made that euthanasia is necessary, an owner should be in a position to exercise control over the physical and social environment that surrounds a beloved pet during the last moments of life. Veterinarians can educate owners by providing information about available options and by encouraging owners to formulate a plan in advance. Veterinarians can then facilitate decisions at the time of crisis by reminding owners of the plans they have already made and/or by pointing toward options veterinarians believe most consistent with owners' values.

If an owner's choice is natural death, the owner can be encouraged to take part in making decisions about desirable and acceptable comfort-oriented interventions using medications, touch, massage, and other alternative and spiritual healing modalities. If an owner's choice is euthanasia, the owner can be encouraged to take part in deciding if it is desirable to place an intravenous catheter, if and how to administer sedative before euthanasia, and other technical details.

Many options are available regarding who is present during an animal's last moments (or hours) and immediately after death. Some owners feel they must be alone, but most prefer to be in the company of someone supportive. Options include family members, friends, and trusted individuals from the community. An animal's last moments can be experienced in somber prayer, ritual, or reflection, or they can be experienced as a party celebrating a pet's life and death. The number of people present varies accordingly. Decisions must be made about the presence of a family's other animals and younger children.

Veterinarians can inform owners of the options available and encourage them to choose the location where their beloved pet will die. At a veterinary clinic, options may include a comfort room or an examination room; at a client's home, it could be the kitchen, the living room, and so forth. In either case, it can be on the floor or on a table, sofa, favorite chair, or an animal's own bed. It can be on a soft blanket or on an owner's lap. An animal's last moments can also be outdoors—on a porch, in the backyard, at a favorite park or beach, or in a vehicle. Veterinarians can provide support by encouraging owners to make a choice they feel is most appropriate and facilitate by making the necessary accommodations so owners' desires can be performed.

Last, but not least, veterinarians can help by preparing owners that they may experience unexpected emotions when their pet is actively dying and encourage them to give themselves permission to deviate from their own plans as needed. Veterinarians must be prepared to answer owners' questions and accommodate owners' preferences whenever possible. The extent of conversation and amount of information owners want when in acute grief must be carefully gauged.

Facing the Loss: After Death Care and Coping with Grief

Grief is a term used to describe the emotions that are common and normal when experiencing a significant loss. An understanding of those emotions can help pet owners make better decisions and make the challenging task of coping with grief easier. Veterinarians can help by finding opportunities to provide clients with information about grief before, during, and after the loss. The book, *The Human-Animal Bond and Grief*,[3] provides detailed information veterinarians can use when educating clients about grief.[3(pp29–51)]

A veterinarian's presence at the time a pet dies or immediately afterwards offers a unique opportunity to help a client in a vulnerable emotional state. Pet owners may be overwhelmed or in a state of shock. They may be crying, feeling physically sick, or feeling numb. They may also be surprised, confused, or embarrassed by their own emotions.

While experiencing these intense emotions, pet owners have to make decisions. The most immediate decisions include

1. The length of time until the deceased animal is removed from the room (or owner's home, and so forth)
2. The length of time the owner stays in the room with an animal's body
3. The presence of other people and/or animals after an animal's death
4. When, how, and who covers or wraps the body
5. Appropriately modifying the environment (light, sound, and/or fragrance)
6. Performing a ritual or saying a prayer.

Other decisions that are of a less immediate nature are

1. Where and when will the body be transported? By whom?
2. Will the body be cremated or buried? Where?
3. If cremated, how will the cremains be handled?
4. How will the deceased be memorialized?

It is common for owners in acute grief to struggle even when decisions have been made in advance, because they feel insecure, guilty, or confused. Veterinarians can remind them of the decisions that they have to make or have already made. That can be best accomplished by asking guiding questions in a quiet, patient manner. Closely watching owners' emotional state helps veterinarians choose the most appropriate time to offer such guidance. Veterinarians can also help owners make decisions by answering questions and by encouraging them to trust themselves. Owners' ideas should be supported but any risks involved pointed out.

Veterinarians' role as medical expert after a patient's death is minimal and limited to discussing reasons for a postmortem examination and to requests by a family to review events that preceded the death. Veterinarians' helping roles, alternatively, are of great significance. Support for owners can be offered by validating and normalizing owners' emotions. Nonverbally communicating respect for the body and an owner's feelings is extremely important, often more so than words. It is essential that veterinarians or others not attempt to talk owners out of their feelings, even if they are in great pain. Showing empathy by acknowledging and accepting what owners are feeling can be done in silence or with few words and do more to relieve the pain than trying to distract them or tell them what they should be doing, thinking, or feeling. The book, *The Human-Animal Bond and Grief*, provides a useful guide to effective verbal and nonverbal communication in helping relationships.[3(pp118–65)] Of particular significance to end-of-life communications is to recognize and avoid the clichés of grief.[15–17]

Many owners look for confirmation from a veterinarian that they have made good decisions up to this point. If a veterinarian disagrees with some of the decisions or feels that the owners had made mistakes, this is not the time to educate them. To be helpful, a veterinarian must affirm as many of an owner's decisions as possible without being dishonest.

SUMMARY

Highly attached owners of pets approaching the end of life want to be faithful to what pets would have asked for and to do what is best for the animals as they face many difficult decisions. If companion animals are considered capable of feelings and some thinking but incapable of expressing those feelings and thoughts verbally, doing what is best for an animal is an elusive goal, subject to proxy interpretation.

Assessing animals' QOL can only be based on nonverbal communication. Veterinarians can play a crucial role in pet owners' decision making by educating them about animal behavior and interspecies empathy—their ability to put themselves in an animal's shoes—thus enabling owners to assess their animals' QOL most accurately and consistently.

Veterinarians should offer more than one option when discussing medical care for terminally ill animals and information sufficient for owners to form an opinion on each option. Euthanasia is an option most pet owners struggle with at some point but should never be the only option offered. The objective of discussing options is to help families find the best way to achieve what they want to accomplish. This gives families some control over the process leading to the inevitable loss, which in turn promotes healthy grieving and emotional healing.

Owners feel anxiety and guilt when facing end-of-life decisions, which may complicate grieving. Veterinarians can help minimize those feelings and help owners make better end-of-life decisions by adding specific helping-oriented roles to their role as medical experts. Lagoni and colleagues recommend 4 such roles: educating (primarily talking), supporting (primarily listening), guiding (primarily suggesting) and facilitating (primarily acting).

Pet owners have to make decisions while experiencing the intense emotions of acute grief. Those decisions greatly influence some owners' subsequent grief and healing process. A veterinarian's presence offers a unique opportunity to help owners make those decisions. An important goal is to help owners accept that making a perfect decision is not always possible.

The mission of animal hospice and palliative care is to guide the provision of physical, emotional, social, and spiritual comfort to animal patients and their human families as they approach the end of life. Veterinarians' efforts and skills in helping families make the best possible decisions is paramount to realizing this mission.

ACKNOWLEDGMENTS

Many of the author's ideas have been strongly influenced by the books, *The Human-Animal Bond and Grief*[3] and *Mental Health and Well-being in Animals*,[10] and the author feels deeply indebted to the pioneering scholarship of Laurel Lagoni, MS; Carolyn Butler, MS; Suzanne Hetts, PhD, and Franklin McMillan, DVM, DACVIM.

REFERENCES

1. APPMA. National pet owners survey (NPOS). Washington, DC: American Pet Products Manufacturers Association; 2005–2006.
2. McNicolas J, Gilbey A, Rennie A, et al. Pet ownership and human health: a brief review of evidence and issues. BMJ 2005;231:1252–4.
3. Lagoni L, Butler C, Hetts S. The human-animal bond and grief. Philadelphia: Saunders; 1994.
4. Adams J, Bonnett B, Meek A. Predictors of owner response in companion animal death. J Am Vet Med Assoc 2000;217:1303–9.
5. James N. From vision to system: the maturing of the hospice movement. In: Morgan D, Lee R, editors. Death rites: law and ethicat the end of life. London: Routledge; 1996. p. 102–8.
6. Wanzer M, Booth-Butterfield M, Gruber K. Perceptions of health care providers' communication: Relationships between patient-centered communication and satisfaction. Health Commun 2004;16:363–84.

7. Shaw J, Lagoni L. End of life communication in veterinary medicine. Vet Clin North Am Small Anim Pract 2007;37:95–108.

8. McMillan F. Rethinking euthanasia: death as an unintentional outcome. J Am Vet Med Assoc 2001;219:1204–6.

9. Gawande A. Letting go. NewYorker Magazine; 2010. Available at: www.newyorker.com. Accessed March 4, 2011.

10. McMillan F, editor. Mental health and well-being in animals. Hoboken (NJ): Blackwell; 2005.

11. Goodall J, Bekoff M. The emotional lives of animals. Foreword. Novato (CA): New World Library; 2007.

12. Villalobos A, Kaplan L. Canine and feline geriatric oncology. Hoboken (NJ): Blackwell; 2007.

13. Gaynor J, Muir W. Handbook of veterinary pain management. 2nd edition. Maryland Heights (MO): Mosby/Elsevier; 2009.

14. Rollin B. Euthanasia and quality of life. J Am Vet Med Assoc 2006;228:1014–6.

15. Online Ministries. Avoiding the cliches of grief [Online]. Available at: http://onlineministries.creighton.edu/CollaborativeMinistry/Grief/avoid-cliches.html. Accessed August 20, 2010.

16. Butler C. Pet owner care in a bond-centered practice [Online]. WSAVA World Congress; 2001. Available at: http://www.vin.com/VINDBPub/SearchPB/Proceedings/PR05000/PR00145.htm. Accessed August 10, 2010.

17. M Wiswman-Orr J, Reid A, Nolan E, et al. Quality of life issues [book auth.]. In: Muir W, Gaynor J, editors. Handbook of veterinary pain management. St louis (MO): Mosby Elsevier; 2009. p. 578–87.

Ten Tips for Veterinarians Dealing with Terminally Ill Patients

Azaria Akashi, PhD, MCC

KEYWORDS

• Suicide • Support • Belief • Euthanasia

TIP ONE

Take good care of yourself physically. Get enough to eat. Schedule breaks in your day for genuine rest, relaxation, and, yes, of course, exercise. Get adequate sleep at night, because insufficient sleep has been scientifically linked to disease, increased stress, and poor functioning. Leave enough leisure time for activities that bring you pleasure.

TIP TWO

Take good care of yourself mentally. Rest your brain often and effectively. Seek continuing education on hospice care and on the latest information about illnesses that are typically terminal in pets sufficient to boost your confidence in dealing with patients. Arrange your schedule to give enough time to each patient. Doctors of humans have largely lost this prerogative, but it is not too late for veterinarians to insist on it.

TIP THREE

Take good care of yourself spiritually. Become clear with yourself about what you really believe about the life and death of pets. Be clear with yourself about how much control you truly have so that when it is time to offer options to extend life or to end life, you are comfortable with what you recommend. Reserve in your treatment facility a space that is yours alone, to which patients or staff never come, to which you can retreat for renewal or eat your lunch.

TIP FOUR

Explore your beliefs about your role in a pet's dying process. Do you see yourself as "the answer" to an owner's situation? An owner has a dilemma and you know the

The author has nothing to disclose.
6885 Alloway Street West, Worthington, OH 43085, USA
E-mail address: aakashi@columbus.rr.com

answer and expect the owner to follow it. Or, do you see yourself as a conveyor of information? An owner has a dilemma and you provide several options among which the owner chooses. You may offer options that an owner is unaware of, like pain protocols. Or, do you see yourself as part of an owner's support system, a facilitator? An owner has a dilemma, you offer options, and you support the owner in choosing among them. Or, do you see yourself as detached from an owner's process? An owner has a dilemma, which you expect the owner to have resolved before coming to you to carry out what has been decided. These different ways of relating to pets and owners are all within the acceptable range of the profession, and you need to know where you stand on this continuum.

TIP FIVE

Explore your beliefs about your role in relation to both pet and owner. Do you see yourself as an advocate for the pet to the owner? Or, are you principally responsible to the owner? Which is your primary relationship, to the pet or owner? Or, do you attempt to take a more holistic and flexible view, dealing with the pet family system? It is helpful to articulate your role to yourself so that when called on, you can share it with those consulting you.

TIP SIX

If you regard yourself as a facilitator in primary relationship to owners, you need to carefully consider who are the "pet's people." What are their resources, strengths, and struggles? Is the owner a single mom with three children and limited financial resources who needs to be taken off the hook of expensive treatment? Are the owners a wealthy couple whose resources are best spent lavishly keeping alive and then memorializing their pet for their own peace of mind? Is the family conflicted about the pet and its treatment, faced with a decision whether to treat or to euthanize and with differing opinions? If you take a role in their negotiations, you need to gain the skill of giving up outcome so that you may extricate yourself from making the decision and still do your job in carrying out the decision.

TIP SEVEN

Study the ethics of end-of-life treatment of pets so that you are clear about where you stand, particularly in a situation in which a pet develops severe behavioral problems near the end of life. A family with a newly decorated house and a suddenly incontinent pet has difficult decisions to make and you should know what you would recommend if asked. When you give your opinion, you can then step back and leave moral decisions to the owners. Your moral obligation is to state what you regard as ethical. It is not your moral obligation to see that an owner carries it out. An attitude of nonjudgment at that point is both self-protective and lucrative. If a family makes a decision that is not consistent with your ethics, you can refer to another veterinarian to assist the family in carrying out their wishes.

TIP EIGHT

Learn when to refer an owner to psychotherapy. You may be asking another highly trained professional to deal with situations for which you have no training. An owner who regards a pet as part of the family may be at as great a risk of depression or desperation when the pet dies as when a child does. An owner who identifies with a pet may wish to die when the pet does and be at risk of suicide. An owner who regards the human-animal bond as deeper than a person-to-person bond may seek to die before the pet dies, another suicide risk. An owner who has used the veterinary office and staff as both a location for and source of emotional support may be vulnerable when losing the occasion to come there after a pet dies. Having an obituary board for pets and allowing owners to post pet obituaries may allow for another level of closure. Some signs to watch for are owners reporting not having eaten regular meals, grief consuming their time, extreme levels of anxiety and/or anger, having difficulty sleeping, or sleeping all the time. In these cases, you want to ask if they want a referral to someone who can help them explore the impact of their pet's death on their life.

TIP NINE

Take good care of your staff. Recognize that staff may create bonds with some terminal pets, causing grief and longing when the death occurs. Give staff members an opportunity to discuss their feelings, if not with you, then with someone who can help them. Sending sympathy cards signed by all staff members is a way for a practice to acknowledge a death and also to get closure. If you learn that a staff member has been greatly helpful to an owner, pass that information along with expressions of your gratitude. Be sure your staff members have the option of a mental health day as needed.

TIP TEN

If possible, give yourself, the staff, and owners room and time to change your minds.

Euthanasia, Moral Stress, and Chronic Illness in Veterinary Medicine

Bernard E. Rollin, PhD

KEYWORDS

• Euthanasia • Moral stress • Chronic illness

A recent study published in England confirms what has been widely believed on the basis of anecdotal evidence over a long period of time, namely that suicide among veterinarians is higher than in any other profession. In the 1980s, I identified a problem that is pervasive among humane society and animal shelter workers, laboratory animal personnel, and veterinarians, and called it "moral stress."[1] Moral stress is a unique and insidious form of stress that cannot be alleviated by normal approaches to stress management. It arises among the people identified previously, whose life work is aimed at promoting the well-being of animals. There is little doubt that people who volunteer or work in animal shelters are there out of concern for animals. Yet in far too many cases, their major activity turns out to be killing unwanted dogs and cats. Many research technicians too go into the field of animal research to help the animals, yet their day-to-day work ends up being the killing of animals or being complicit in creating pain, distress, disease, and other noxious states demanded by the research enterprise. Equally certain is the fact that most veterinarians enter the field to treat disease, alleviate pain and suffering, and provide high-quality of life for the animals to whom they minister. Yet historically, veterinarians, like humane society workers, have been called upon to kill unwanted animals for appalling reasons, what has been called convenience euthanasia.

This state of affairs creates moral stress in the groups identified previously. This kind of stress grows out of the radical conflict between one's reasons for entering the field of animal work, and what one in fact ends up doing. Furthermore, normal avenues for alleviating stress are not available in this area. If one is stressed by normal stressors, standard stress management vehicles are quite helpful, for example relaxation techniques or talking it out with peers and family; these modalities are not available for moral stress, however. As one woman who worked in a shelter told me, "I tried to

Department of Philosophy, Colorado State University, 240 Eddy Hall, Fort Collins, CO 80523-1781, USA
E-mail address: Bernard.Rollin@colostate.edu

Vet Clin Small Anim 41 (2011) 651–659
doi:10.1016/j.cvsm.2011.03.005
0195-5616/11/$ – see front matter © 2011 Elsevier Inc. All rights reserved.

explain to my husband at dinner that I had killed the nicest dog earlier in the day. He responded by clapping his hands over his ears and telling me he did not want to hear about it." The eventual effect of such long-term, unalleviated stress is likely to be deterioration of physical and mental health and well-being, substance abuse, divorce, and even, as I encountered on a number of occasions, suicide.

I did not realize the full impact of moral stress on companion animal practitioners until the early 1980s, when I was part of a group that held a symposium on client grief sponsored jointly by the Animal Medical Center and the Columbia University College of Physicians and Surgeons. During the first question period a veterinarian stood up and commented that "if I did not know how to deal with client grief, I could not have stayed in business. What I really need to know, is how I deal with my own grief when I am constantly confronted with demands to kill healthy animals."

Convenience euthanasia was, for a long time, perhaps the major ethical issue confronting companion animal practitioners. Imagine the psychological impact of constant demands to kill healthy animals for appalling reasons: "the dog is too old to run with me anymore; we have redecorated, and the dog no longer matches the color scheme; it is cheaper to get another dog when I return from vacation than to pay the fees for a boarding kennel," and, most perniciously, "I do not wish to spend the money on the procedure you recommend to treat the animal," or "it is cheaper to get another dog." Small wonder that veterinarians' mental well-being and job satisfaction can be eroded. In Western democracies, who one is, one's personal identity, is inextricably bound up with what one does, with one's job. Most veterinarians, particularly companion animal veterinarians, but also veterinarians in other fields, see their raison d'être as being improving the health, well-being, and happiness of animals in their societal roles. When companion animal veterinarians face regular requests for convenience euthanasia, sometimes for animals that they have labored mightily to save in the past, it is no wonder that they face moral stress and loss of joy in their work.

Somewhat compensatory for the moral stress attendant upon a steady stream of requests for convenience euthanasia, is what has been called the gift of euthanasia. Whereas human physicians are not empowered to help horribly suffering patients end their pain by providing access to euthanasia, veterinarians are fortunately blessed to be able to end suffering by providing a peaceful and painless death.

As the vast and international movement in favor of assisted suicide attests—laws in Belgium, the Netherlands, and Oregon, the work of Dr Kevorkian, pleas for death with dignity—it has become clear that many if not most human patients fear pain, and the suffering and degradation that extreme pain inflicts on patients and families, more than they fear death.

It was the recognition of this point that led to the organization of a unique conference on euthanasia in 1980 in New York sponsored jointly by the Columbia University College of Physicians and Surgeons and the Animal Medical Center, a major veterinary hospital. The ideas of the planners (myself included) were that the power of euthanasia as an ultimate modality for alleviation of suffering was well-recognized in veterinary medicine, but insufficiently so in human medicine. This was well-illustrated by the conundrum that a person who fails to euthanize a suffering animal is societally perceived as morally blameworthy, while a person who helps a suffering grandmother, begging to die, end her life is also seen as blameworthy. The organizers felt that as companion animals become increasingly perceived as members of the family and less like livestock, the moral imperative to end suffering might transfer to human medicine.

With the wisdom of hindsight, it is now clear that the hopes of the organizers were bound to be dashed. The social willingness to use euthanasia for animals stemmed not so much from their assuming a new and higher moral status in society as from the view of animals as replaceable. The proliferation of veterinary specialty practices and social willingness to spend vast amounts of money for animal treatment was not yet present in a widespread way. And in human medicine, quality-of-life considerations were not yet dominant values.

The assimilation of medicine to science in the early 20th century following the publication of the Flexner report was not without costs. As medicine became applied biology or biomedical science, certain key aspects of traditional medicine were suppressed. For example, as rational treatments for diseases like cancer emerged, physicians marked their success by measurably empirically indisputable parameters. Notable among these measures was additional life garnered by way of the treatments. Such a scoring system, however, entailed a studied neglect of quality-of-life considerations. While chemotherapy or radiation did indeed prolong life in many instances, medicine failed to ask "at what cost?" Qualitative considerations, such as patient subjective experience, became invisible to scientific medicine in the face of the assumption that more life was always better, a victory against the disease.

Social, cultural, idiosyncratic, and moral dimensions of a person—features essential to being a person—came to be seen as irrelevant to the task of medicine, or as mystical or metaphysical and therefore outside of the physician's purview. Thus physicians too often treated illnesses as bodily malfunctions and saw no need to be more than polite and competent applied scientists. A great deal has, of course, been written about the tendency of physicians to forget that patients are persons and to designate patients by such locutions as "the kidney in room 422," "the osteosarcoma," "the gomer." The repeatable, universal features of bodies are interesting to medicine, not the individuality of persons. Hospitals and hospital garb suppress even external manifestations of individual uniqueness.

Palliative care was forgotten in the zeal to preserve life. Two examples will make this manifest. In 1972, psychiatrists Marks and Sacher were called into the Sloan-Kettering Cancer Center to consult on an outbreak of insanity characterized by patients engaging in extreme and emotional behavior.[2] The psychiatrists soon realized that the issue was not madness, but rather patient response to extreme and untreated cancer pain. As recently as 1991, it was reported that although 90% of cancer pain was manageable with available modalities, 80% was not controlled.[3] In the same vein, hospice was a concept developed almost wholly by nurses, not scientific physicians, to help preserve patient quality of life. As one nursing dean stated, "Physicians worry about cure; nurses worry about care." If pain was ignored as scientifically unreal, what hope was there for other negative sequelae to treatment, such as loss of dignity?

In a major ironic twist of fate, rather than human medicine learning the wisdom of euthanasia for suffering animals from veterinary medicine, in the ensuing 30 years veterinary medicine assimilated some of the more pernicious aspects of human medicine. In particular, as animals became increasingly viewed as members of the family, the reluctance to euthanize began to enter veterinary medicine.

Various surveys have been conducted on the percentage of pet owners who view their animals as members of the family. The lowest number attributes such a view to 88% of the pet owning population; the highest ascribes it to some 98%. While one may quibble about the accuracy of such polls, it is indubitable that so viewing one's companion animals is a dominant mode of societal thought. Every veterinary school and major clinic has provisions for grief counseling for owners who have lost an animal. More and more people will respond to the question "do you have children?" by saying "no, we have dogs."

Thus companion animals, in today's world, provide people with love and someone to love, and do so unfailingly, with loyalty, grace, and boundless devotion. In a book that should be required reading for all who work with animals, author Jon Katz has chronicled what he calls "the new work of dogs,"[4] all based on his personal experiences in a New Jersey suburban community. Here one reads of the dog whom a woman credits with shepherding her through a losing battle with cancer, as her emotional bed rock. Katz tells of the "Divorced Women's Dog Club," a group of divorced women united only by divorce and reliance on their dogs. He tells the tale of a dog who provides an outlet for a ghetto youth's insecurity and rage, and who is beaten daily. He relates the story of a successful executive with a family and friends, who in the end deals with stress in his life only by long walks with his Labrador, totaling many hours in a day. While raising the question of whether we are entitled to expect this of our animals, Katz explains that we do, and that they perform heroically.

Our pets have become sources of friendship and company for the old and the lonely, vehicles for penetrating the frightful shell surrounding a disturbed child, beings that provide the comfort of touch even to the most asocial person, and inexhaustible sources of pure, unqualified love.

The rise of deep love-based relationships with animals as a regular and increasingly accepted social phenomenon came from a variety of converging and mutually reinforcing social conditions.[5] In the first place, probably beginning with the widespread use of the automobile, extended nuclear families with multiple generations living in one location or under one roof began to vanish. At the beginning of the 20th century, when roughly half of the public produced food for themselves and the other half of the public, significant numbers of large extended families lived together manning farms. The safety net for older people was their family, rather than society as a whole. The concept of easy mobility made preserving the nuclear family less of a necessity, as did the rise of the new idea that society as a whole rather than the family was responsible for assuring retirement, medical attention, and facilities for elderly people.

With the concentration of agriculture in fewer and fewer hands, the rise of industrialization, and as the Depression, Dust Bowl and World War II introduced migration to cities, the nuclear family notion was further eroded. The tendency of urban life to erode community, to create what the Germans called "Gesellsohaft" rather than "Gemeinschaft," mixtures rather than compounds, as it were, further created solitude and loneliness as widespread modes of being. Correlatively, as selfishness and self-actualization were established as positive values beginning in the highly individualistic 1960s, the divorce rate began to climb, and the traditional stigma attached to divorce was erased. As biomedicine prolonged human life spans, more and more people significantly outlived their spouses, and were thrown into a loneliness mode of existence, with the loss of the extended family removing a possible remedy.

In effect, there are now lonely old people, lonely divorced people, and most tragically, lonely children whose single parent often works. With the best jobs being urban or quasi-urban, many people live in cities or peripherally urban developments such as condominiums. In New York City, for example, one can be lonelier than in rural Wyoming. The cowboy craving camaraderie can find a neighbor from whom he is separated only by physical distance; the urban person may know no one, and have no one in striking distance who cares. Shorn of physical space, people create psychic distances between themselves and others. People may (and usually do) for years live 6 inches away from neighbors in apartment buildings and never exchange a sentence. Watch New Yorkers on an elevator; the rule is stand as far away from others as one can, and study the ceiling. Making eye contact on a street can be taken as a challenge, or a sexual invitation, so people do not. One minds one's own business; one steps over and around drunks on the street. "Don't get involved" is a mantra for survival.

Yet people need love, companionship, emotional support, and to be needed. In such a world, a companion animal can be one's psychic and spiritual salvation. An animal is someone to hug and hug one back; someone to play with, to laugh with; to exercise with; to walk with; to share beautiful days; to cry with. For a child, the dog is a playmate, a friend, someone to talk to.

For many old people, the dog (or cat) is a reason to get up in the morning, to go out, to bundle up and go to the park ("Fluffy misses her friends, you know!") to shop, to fuss, to feel responsible for a life, and needed. Thus companion animals then, in today's world, provide people with love and someone to love, and do so unfailingly, with loyalty, grace, and boundless devotion.

But a dog is more than that. In New York, and other big, cold, tough cities, it is a social lubricant. One does not talk to strangers in cities, unless he or she—or preferably both of you—are walking a dog. Then the barriers crumble. Among the most extraordinary social phenomena I have ever participated in were the dog people in the Upper West Side of Manhattan. These were people who walked their dogs at roughly the same time—morning and evening—in Riverside Park. United by a common and legitimate purpose, having dogs in common and thereby being above suspicion, conversations would begin spontaneously. To be sure, one usually did not know people's names—they were "Red's owner," "Helga's person," "Fluffy's mistress." But names did not matter. What mattered was that people began to care for each other through the magic of sharing a bond with an animal and the animals not knowing New York etiquette and playing with one another.

Whether as a cause or an effect or both of the rise in status of companion animals, the last 40 or so years have witnessed an enormous and proliferative explosion in the number of specialty veterinary practitioners treating companion animals. Veterinary hospitals now deploy many of the most sophisticated diagnostic and treatment modalities found in human medicine to treat companion animals. These include radiation treatment, transplant surgeries, open heart surgeries, computed tomography scans and magnetic resonance imaging diagnoses, particle accelerators, stem cells, immunotherapy, dialysis, and a vast panoply of other expensive approaches to animal disease. The financial barriers to widespread use of such treatments seem to be crumbling, or at least irrelevant to much of the companion animal owning population.

As laudable as the societal change regarding companion animals may be, it creates a new source of moral stress for veterinarians. Whereas, as seen previously, veterinarians were faced with stressors growing out of client demand for convenience euthanasia, this issue remains and is compounded by an opposite source of stress, clients being unwilling to euthanize suffering animals and instead holding on and continuing treatments regardless of the cost to the animal's quality of life. Thus, it is quite possible that a veterinarian may find himself or herself advocating for a healthy animal in the face of client demand for convenience euthanasia, and then later, that very day, advocating to end suffering in a different, chronically ill animal by euthanasia with a client unwilling to give up on treatment. Counterintuitively, the augmented moral status of the companion animal compounds veterinarians' job-created moral stress. Given that the legal status of animals decrees that they are the property of owners, whether the situation be that the client demands euthanasia in morally unjustifiable circumstances, or refuses to terminate the suffering of a sick animal, the veterinarian is in a highly untenable position of knowing the right thing to do, yet being unable to implement his or her expertise. Adding to the problem is the fact that trying everything is what veterinary specialists do, and that the specialist probably does not have the sort of relationship with the clients where he or she can straightforwardly advise that it is time to let go. A good general practitioner staying involved even after referral can help serve as a check against well-intentioned but excessive zeal by the specialist.

Furthermore, today's society is one in which medical paternalism is a dirty word, and patient or client autonomy is a trendy slogan. (I personally believe that paternalism is not always bad, given public appalling ignorance of science and medicine; autonomy requires knowledge.) Nonetheless, a powerful element of paternalism is alive and thriving and can be deployed to good effect by veterinarians.

I am referring here to a veterinarian's Aesculapian authority, the singular authority possessed by physicians and veterinarians in virtue of being medical professionals.[6] It is Aesculapian authority that allowed Hitler's physician to scold him for his diet, when anyone else doing so would be summarily shot. To deploy such authority on behalf of the animal to end suffering is, in my view, not only permissible but also obligatory. When clients ask "what would you do if it were your dog, Doctor?" they are appealing to Aesculapian authority. I thus categorically reject the dictum, sometimes pronounced in veterinary circles, that a practitioner should never suggest or advocate euthanasia, lest the client later blame the veterinarian for killing his or her beloved animal. Part of a veterinarian's job, as an animal advocate, is to forthrightly respond to such a cry for exoneration under difficult circumstances.

Inextricably bound up with successful deployment of such authority regarding the need for euthanasia to alleviate suffering is the issue of explaining to clients some fundamental differences between human and animal mental life that have major and radically distinct implications for quality of life in people versus companion animals.[7,8] Human thought is irreducibly tied to language, which allows us ingression into modes of thought closed to animals. Humans can think in very abstract terms (eg, mathematics and logic); in negative terms ("there are no dragons in the library"); in conditional terms ("if it does rain, we will hold graduation indoors"); in future terms ("I wish to retire in Iceland someday"); in universal terms ("all triangles have three sides"); in fictional terms (writing novels); in counterfactual terms ("if Darwin had not discovered natural selection, someone else would have"). These are all made possible by being able to structure thought linguistically, which in turn allows linguistic syntax to transcend thought rooted in immediate experience.

As one who did much to restore the credibility of talking about animal pain, distress, and emotion, I certainly do not deny the richness and moral relevance of animal mental life. There is, however, a striking dissimilarity between people and animals facing life-threatening illnesses, even as the tools of medicine dealing with such crises converge in the two areas. Human cognition is such that it can value long-term future goals and endure short-run negative experiences for the sake of achieving them. Examples are plentiful. Many people undergo voluntary food restriction, and the unpleasant experience attendant in its wake, for the sake of lowering blood pressure, or looking good in a bikini as summer approaches. People memorize volumes of boring material for the sake of gaining admission to veterinary or medical school. People endure the excruciating pain of cosmetic surgery to look better. And people similarly endure chemotherapy, radiation, dialysis, physical therapy, and transplants to achieve longer life and a better quality of life than they would have without it, or, in some cases, merely to prolong the length of life to see their children graduate, or to complete an opus, or fulfill some other goal.

In the case of animals, however, there is no evidence, either empirical or conceptual, that they have the capability to weigh future benefits or possibilities against current misery. To entertain the belief that "my current pain and distress, resulting from the nausea of chemotherapy, or some highly invasive surgery will be offset by the possibility of indefinite amount of future time," is taken to be axiomatic of human thinking. But reflection reveals that such thinking requires some complex cognitive machinery. For example, one needs both temporal and abstract concepts, such as "possible future times" and the ability to compare them; a concept of death, eloquently defined by Heidegger as grasping "the possibility of the impossibility of your being;" the ability to articulate possible suffering, and so on. This, in turn requires the possibility to think in an if–then hypothetical and counterfactual mode (ie, "if I do not do X, then Y will occur"). This mode of thinking in turn seems to necessitate or require the ability to possess symbols and combine them according to rules of syntax.

To treat companion animals morally and with respect, one needs to keep in mind their mentational limits. Paramount in importance is the extreme unlikelihood that they can understand the concepts of life and death in themselves, rather than the pains and pleasure associated with life or death. To the animal mind, in a real sense there is only quality of life (ie, whether its experiential content is pleasant or unpleasant in all of the modes it is capable of—bored or occupied, fearful or not fearful, lonely or enjoying companionship, painful or not, hungry or not, thirsty or not). There is no reason to believe that an animal can grasp the notion of extended life, let alone choose to trade current suffering for it.

This in turn entails that one realistically assesses as far as possible what animals are experiencing. An animal cannot weigh being treated for cancer against the suffering that entails. An animal cannot affirm or even conceive of a desire to endure current suffering for the sake of future life, cannot choose to lose a leg to preclude metastasis. One must remember that an animal is its pain, for it is incapable of anticipating or even hoping for cessation of that pain. Thus when one is confronted with life-threatening illnesses that afflict animals, it is not axiomatic that they be treated at whatever qualitative, experiential cost that may entail. The owner may consider the suffering a treatment modality entails a small price for extra life, but the animal neither values nor comprehends extra life, let alone the trade-off this entails. (Treatment for minor illnesses or injuries can be justified by the virtual certainty of a long pleasant life thereafter.) The owner, in turn, may ignore the difference between human and animal mind and choose the possibility of life prolongation at any qualitative cost. It is at this point that the morally responsible veterinarian is thrust into his or her role as animal advocate, speaking for what matters to the animal.

I am not, of course, denying that animals can have short-term futural expectations and projections. This is evidenced by the cat waiting outside the mouse hole, anticipating the mouse's appearance, or the dog waiting at the door for a walk. These limited futural anticipations can be explained by associative learning. What I am denying is that animals can conceptualize accepting current major suffering in exchange for the possibility of an extended lifespan. There is no reason to believe that an animal can grasp the notion of extended life, let alone choose to trade current suffering for it.

Quality-of-life considerations should be introduced at the beginning of a veterinarian–client relationship, not suddenly sprung on a client when treatment is over. In particular, it is useful to recall Plato's dictum that, when dealing with ethics and adults, it far better to remind than to teach. For this reason, the client, who after all knows the animal better than the veterinarian, should be encouraged from the beginning to help define quality of life for that animal.

From the outset, then, I would recommend that the veterinarian obtain from the client, a list, as long as possible, of what makes the animal happy or unhappy, and how he or she knows. This list, written down as part of the medical record, can serve to remind the owners of their own criteria for quality of life at the point when treatment is failing, when wishful thinking and essentially selfish desires may replace objectivity. I used this method with a friend of mine who asked me how to judge when it was time for euthanasia and how to avoid compromising his animal's quality of life by overly prolonging treatment. He later thanked me and told me that, were it not for his own encoded notes defining the animal's quality of life while it was still well, he would have rationalized trying a variety of modalities that would have greatly impaired the animal's quality of life. Unquestionably, he said, denial would have distorted his perception, but for his own reflective, codified deliberations on that animal's quality of life which, even in extremis, were impossible to ignore. In the end, such dialogue, while awkward, difficult, and emotional, can nevertheless benefit the animal, the owner, and the veterinarian's own peace of mind.

An additional ethical issue regarding end-of-life for companion animals has been created by the advent of "pawspice," hospice for animals. In many ways, this is a good thing. Many owners do not have either the time or the ability to provide the regular treatments that tending to a chronically or terminally ill animal entails. An animal hospice can be extremely valuable in performing such services. However, given that the hospice profits for as long as the animal requires hospice care, there may well arise a pernicious tendency on the part of those running hospice to keep the animal alive as long as possible, thereby failing to reckon quality-of-life issues arising under such circumstances. I have heard anecdotally of some hospice veterinarians catering to owner reluctance to euthanize by their willingness to pursue all sorts of unproven and untested, evidentially baseless alternative modalities to save the animal's life. This can go as far as going to Mexico to acquire such cancer drugs as Laetrile, declared worthless in the United States, to pander to owner false hopes and thereby prolong the revenue stream.

Unfortunately, this is not only a hospice issue, but it may well arise in all practices when clients are unwilling to give up and the veterinarian is reluctant to fight for euthanasia as control of pain and suffering. One should recall that in a deep sense there is no alternative medicine; there is medicine that has sound scientific evidence in its favor, and various modalities that have no evidence, or indeed can only be true if modern chemistry is false, such as homeopathy. To the question "what harm can an ineffective alternative do?" I would answer a client in a very straightforward fashion. It can cater to owner wishful thinking while prolonging unnecessarily the animal's suffering. The longer one pursues useless remedies, the longer the animal experiences negative quality of life, and the longer the veterinarian can suffer moral stress.

In sum, euthanasia is a double-edged sword in veterinary medicine. It is a powerful and ultimately the most powerful tool for ending the pain and suffering that may well be an animal's entire life. Demand for its use for client convenience is morally reprehensible and creates major moral stress for ethically conscious practitioners, and goes against the very essence of a veterinarian's goal to alleviate pain and maximize animal health and quality of life. But equally reprehensible and stressful to veterinarians is the failure to use it when an animal faces only misery, pain, distress, and suffering. Finding the correct path through this minefield may well be the most important ethical task facing the conscientious veterinarian.

REFERENCES

1. Rollin BE. Euthanasia and moral stress. Loss, Grief and Care 1987;1(1):115–26.
2. Marks RM, Sachar EJ. Undertreatment of medical inpatients with narcotic analgesics. Ann Intern Med 1973;78(2):173–81.

3. Ferrell BR, Rhiner M. High-tech comfort: ethical issues in cancer pain management for the 1990s. J Clin Ethics 1991;2:108–15.
4. Katz J. The new work of dogs: tending to life, love and family. New York: Villard; 2003.
5. Rollin B, Rollin M. Dogmatisms and catechisms: ethics and companion animals. Anthrozoos 2001;14(1):4–11.
6. Rollin BE. The use and abuse of Aesculapian authority in veterinary medicine. J Am Vet Assoc 2002;220(11):1.
7. Rollin BE. Euthanasia and quality of life. J Am Vet Med Assoc 2006;228(7):1014–6.
8. Rollin BE. Preserving quality of life in oncology. In: Dobson JM, Lascelles BDX, editors. BSAVA manual of canine and feline oncology. 3rd edition. Gloucester (UK); British Small Animal Veterinary Association; 2011. p. 40–4.

Legal Concerns with Providing Hospice and Palliative Care

Amir Shanan, DVM[a], Vandhana Balasubramanian, JD[b]

KEYWORDS

• Hospice • Palliative care • Companion animals
• Legal responsibility

Palliative and hospice care for companion animals is a rapidly growing field in veterinary medicine. Most veterinary hospice services are provided in locations other than veterinary facilities; most commonly, in the pet owner's home. Recognized standards of care have not yet been established in this emerging field, although several organizations are in the process of developing such standards.[1,2] The combination of offering services off-site, lack of recognized standards, and absence of legal precedents pertaining to practicing veterinary hospice is a source of apprehension to current and potential providers in this field.

This article explores the legal implications surrounding the provision of veterinary hospice care in the United States[1]; and provides veterinarians with the legal information necessary to determine whether and how to prepare for offering palliative and hospice care services. The authors' opinion is that the legal issues that may arise in the context of veterinary hospice are largely duplicative of those that arise in the course of other types of small animal veterinary practice.

THE VETERINARY HOSPICE RELATIONSHIP

A veterinarian offering hospice care services is engaging in a distinct veterinarian-client-patient relationship characterized by the pursuit of 2 parallel goals: to ensure the best possible quality of life for animals who are suffering from life-limiting illness, and to provide their human caregivers with the emotional support and guidance

[a] International Association for Animal Hospice and Palliative Care, www.iaahpc.org and Compassionate Veterinary Care, 620 West Webster Avenue, Chicago, IL 60614, USA
[b] 1517 West Addison Street, Suite 2, Chicago, IL 60613, USA
E-mail address: ashanan1g@gmail.com

[1] This article is intended as a general legal overview for veterinarians on the main issues that are likely to arise in the veterinary hospice setting, rather than as a comprehensive case law analysis for lawyers. Because each state's laws may differ on several of these issues, veterinarians are strongly encouraged to consult with a legal professional to determine the specific rules of laws in the state in which they are practicing.

Vet Clin Small Anim 41 (2011) 661–675
doi:10.1016/j.cvsm.2011.03.007
0195-5616/11/$ – see front matter © 2011 Elsevier Inc. All rights reserved.

vetsmall.theclinics.com

needed to cope with a significant loss and to make difficult end-of-life decisions. To accomplish this challenging undertaking, a relationship must be developed in which veterinarians assume helping roles in addition to their recognized roles as a medical experts (see article by Shanan elsewhere in this issue for the further exploration of this topic). The veterinarian-client-patient hospice relationship develops in 3 distinct phases: (1) identifying a hospice patient (pet), (2) formulating a hospice plan for the patient and the caregiver (owner), and (3) implementing the hospice plan. Frequent, open, and honest communication between the veterinarian and the client is crucial during all phases for the successful provision of hospice care.

Identifying a Hospice Patient

Before undertaking hospice care, veterinarians should conduct an intake interview to determine whether hospice care is the most appropriate course of action for a particular patient. During the intake interview, the veterinarian obtains the relevant medical and behavioral history of the animal and identifies the concerns and expectations of the client/caregiver, which may include concerns about pain and suffering, uncertainty regarding decision making, spiritual or religious views about death and dying, and the financial impact of veterinary services.[3(p590)]

Formulating a Hospice Plan

The hospice plan must take into consideration the patient's diagnosis, prognosis, and available treatment options; as well as the family's values, beliefs, goals, concerns, and available resources. Clients should be advised of all treatment options, including the risks and costs associated with each. With input from both the veterinarian and the family, priorities can be established that will best serve both the patient and the family.

Implementing the Hospice Plan

Implementation of the agreed hospice plan involves veterinarians, their staff, pet owners and their family members, and others in the community. The respective roles of the clinical staff, the owner, and others should be clearly delineated, preferably in writing.

When the patient is receiving hospice care at home, the veterinarian largely depends on the owner's objective and subjective observations of the patient's symptoms and behaviors in assessing the success or failure of a given course of treatment. Clearly communicating all parties' specific responsibilities is essential to ensure that the animal receives the care and treatment prescribed in the hospice plan.

As the patient's condition changes, so may the client's perceptions and priorities. Frequent reappraisal of the diagnostic and prognostic information and of the various treatment options is often necessary to accomplish the goals of hospice care.

LEGAL ANALYSIS: RELEVANT LEGAL PRINCIPLES

Most veterinarians are already familiar with the legal issues that could arise in their private practices. This article does not address those issues in detail; it uses those issues as a starting point for analysis of what, if any, additional legal risks a veterinarian may face in providing veterinary hospice services. The main legal principles that are likely to be implicated in the veterinary hospice process are explored. This analysis is not intended as an exhaustive resource for attorneys, but aims to provide veterinarians with a basic understanding of the most common issues that are likely to arise.

Legally Responsible Party

The first step, before undertaking any treatment, is to identify the individual who is legally and financially responsible for the care of the animal.[2] In the eyes of the law, animals continue to be viewed as items of personal property, and not as legal entities of their own.[3] The right to make decisions regarding the care and treatment of a companion animal rests exclusively with its owner, who is considered the legally responsible party.[4] During the hospice intake interview, the legally responsible party should be identified in writing as the person who has ultimate decision-making authority and who will be held financially responsible for the treatment and care rendered to the animal. Treatment decisions made pursuant to the direction of persons other than the legally responsible party could result in the veterinarian's inability to collect payment for those services, and, although unlikely, could potentially result in lawsuits alleging unauthorized treatment.[5]

Informed/Owner Consent

The single most useful tool in minimizing legal risk to the veterinarian in providing hospice care is the informed/owner consent form. This form, prepared by the veterinarian and signed by the client, is a comprehensive document that apprises the client of all of the risks, responsibilities, and other considerations in the hospice relationship. It should include detailed information on the following topics: the legally responsible party; the diagnosis and prognosis of the patient; the various treatment options discussed with the client and the risks, benefits, and costs of each; the agreed treatment plan; the specific details on how care is to be rendered; relevant risks to the patient, the caregiver, and any other pets; and payment agreements.

The purpose of the informed consent form is twofold: first, the more information that is conveyed to the client, the better suited the client is to making the difficult and often painful decisions that hospice care involves. Second, it serves as an acknowledgment that the client was made aware of, and fully understood, all of the relevant risks before deciding on a particular course of treatment.[6] Claims that a veterinarian failed to warn the client of risks to either the client or the animal from a prescribed course of treatment are common types of professional negligence claims. Informed consent forms are extremely useful in promptly resolving, or precluding altogether, such litigation.

---

[2] Because this principle applies to all aspects of veterinary care, veterinarians in private practice should already be in the habit of identifying and dealing with the legally responsible party.

[3] See, for example, New Mexico Stat. Ann. § 77-1-1 (1978) ("dogs, cats and domesticated fowls and birds shall be deemed and considered as personal property"); Jones v. Collins, No. 3:09CV-394-H, 2010 WL 2572811, at *3 (W.D. Ky. June 23, 2010) (Under Kentucky law, "[i]t remains … that a dog is property"); Kaufman v. Langhofer, 222 P.3d 272 (Ariz. Ct. App. 2009) ("Arizona law is consistent with the majority position classifying animals as personal property"); Phillips v. Baus, No. DBDCV054003065S, 2007 WL 1976219, at *4 n. 7 (Conn. Super. Ct. May 24, 2007) (Connecticut law classifies dogs as personal property).

[4] See, for example, Grabowicz -Kretunski v. ASPCA, 867 N.Y.S.2d 374 (N.Y. Sup. Ct. 2008); McAdams v. Faulk, No. CA 01-1350, 2002 WL 700956 (Ark. Ct. App. Apr. 24, 2002).

[5] See, for example, Loman v. Freeman, 890 N.E.2d 446 (Ill. 2008) (horse owner sued veterinarian for negligence based on allegations of unauthorized treatment of horse).

[6] Except in certain limited situations, a veterinarian must receive the approval of the client before undertaking any treatment. Lawrence v. Big Creek Veterinary Hosp., L.L.C., No. 2006-G-2737, 2007 WL 2579436, at *3 (Ohio Ct. App. Sept. 7, 2007) (Under Ohio law, a veterinarian has a duty to obtain the client's informed consent before undertaking veterinary treatment).

They foreclose the possibility that the client can claim that the veterinarian did not provide sufficient information or proper warnings, or undertook a course of treatment that was not authorized. Throughout this article, relevant topics for inclusion in an informed consent form are individually identified. Appendix 1 contains a sample informed consent form that can be used as a basic model, subject to the appropriate modifications of state law.

Professional Negligence (Veterinary Malpractice)

The primary legal risk to veterinarians in providing hospice care is exposure to claims of veterinary malpractice (ie, misdiagnosis or mistreatment of an animal's illness).[7] However, in the authors' opinion, the risk of professional malpractice exposure is no greater in the hospice context than when providing routine care; a claim of professional malpractice is less likely to be successful in the hospice context than in routine practice because of certain evidentiary problems that hospice litigants face.

In most states, claims of veterinary malpractice are subject to the same evidentiary standards as claims of medical malpractice.[8] That is, they are adjudicated under principals of professional negligence. In this context, a litigant must offer sufficient evidence of 4 specific elements:

1. the veterinarian owed a specialized duty of care to the client
2. the veterinarian breached that duty by failing to meet the recognized standard of professional care
3. the veterinarian's acts or omissions caused the injury to the animal, and
4. that injury resulted in identifiable damages to the client.[9] Litigants commonly face hurdles in establishing breaches of the duty of care and legal causation. In the hospice context, these 2 elements provide even greater obstacles to a litigant's success.

Expert Testimony

To prevail in a veterinary malpractice claim, a claimant must introduce evidence that (1) the veterinarian owed a duty of care to the claimant, and (2) the veterinarian's actions or omissions failed to meet that generally recognized standard of care.[10] In

---

[7] Sherman v. Kissinger, 195 P.3d 539 (Wash. App. Div. 1, 2008) (medical malpractice act did not apply to veterinary claims, and owner could bring claims of breach of fiduciary duty, negligent misrepresentation, conversion and trespass to chattels, and breach of bailment contract against veterinarian); McAdams v. Faulk, No. CA 01-1350, 2002 WL 700956 (Ark. Ct. App. Ct. Apr. 24, 2002) (under Arkansas law, client could advance a claim of breach of fiduciary duty against a veterinarian). In addition to veterinary malpractice claims, which are based on negligence principles, litigants have advanced other types of claims against veterinarians, including breach of contract, breach of fiduciary duty, conversion, trespass to chattels, and breach of bailment contract. These types of claims are less likely to arise in the hospice context than in nonhospice care.

[8] See, for example, Lauderbaugh v. Gellasch, 2008 WL 5182915, at *1 (Ohio Ct. App. Dec. 11, 2008) ("A veterinary malpractice claim has similar elements to a medical malpractice claim").

[9] See, for example, Berres v. Anderson, 561 N.W.2d 919, 924 (Minn. Ct. App. 1997) (Under Minnesota law, a veterinarian "has a duty to exercise the ordinary care, skill, and diligence as established by the standards of veterinary care in his community"); Lauderbaugh v. Gellasch, 2008 WL 5182915, at *1 (Ohio Ct. App. Dec. 11, 2008).

[10] See, for example, Austin v. State of Illinois, No. 98-CC-0388, 2002 WL 32705296 (Ill. Ct. Cl. Feb. 4, 2002) (veterinary malpractice claim was dismissed because litigant could not produce any evidence that veterinarian's treatment of animal was below the standard of care).

most states, evidence of these 2 elements must be presented through the testimony of an expert witness.[11] Some states require the affidavit of an expert witness alleging some negligence on the part of the defendant as a precursor to even filing suit.[12]

An expert witness is an individual who has training and experience in the same area of practice as the veterinarian.[13] Hiring an expert witness to testify at trial can cost litigants a considerable amount of money. Given the limitations on recoverable damages in any veterinary malpractice suit, such expenditures can be cost-prohibitive enough to discourage the filing of some claims.

Moreover, because veterinary hospice work is still new, the ability of a litigant to find an expert witness for a hospice case is likely to be more limited than in non–hospice-related claims of veterinary malpractice. In many instances, litigants would be required to hire expert witnesses residing in another state. Litigants may try to overcome this hurdle by seeking to use a nonhospice veterinarian in a hospice case.[14] However, consistent with the legal principals in medical malpractice cases, the veterinarian could object to the use of a nonhospice veterinarian's testimony in a veterinary hospice case.

Legal Causation

Proof of legal causation is likely to be the more insurmountable burden in claims of veterinary malpractice relating to hospice care. A successful litigant must introduce evidence, again through the testimony of an expert witness, that the clinician's negligent actions or omissions caused the animal to suffer an injury. In hospice situations, this requirement poses unique problems to potential litigants.

The provision of hospice and palliative care presumes that the animal in question suffers from a terminal or incurable illness.[15] It is end-of-life care. Because the animal in question was suffering from a terminal or incurable illness, litigants will be virtually unable to prove that any hospice care provided by a clinician caused the animal to

---

[11] See, for example, Zepecki v. Arkansas Veterinary Medical Examining Bd., No. CA09-266, 2010 WL 645847 (Ark. App. Ct. 2010) (veterinary standard of care must be presented through expert testimony); Diakakis v. W. Res. Veterinary Hosp., No. 2004-T-0151, 2006 WL 156732 (Ohio App. Ct. Feb. 24, 2006) (case dismissed for claimant's failure to produce expert testimony that veterinarian breached the standard of care); Sumner v. Bridge, No. 04 LM 1489, 2005 WL 2414718, at *3 (Kan. Dist. Ct. May 10, 2005) ("Kansas law recognizes a requirement of expert veterinary testimony involving animal diseases."); Hight v. Dublin Veterinary Clinic, 22 S.W.3d 614 (Tex. Ct. App. 2000) (dismissing veterinary malpractice claim because expert testimony presented by claimant was insufficient); Williamson v. Prida, 75 Cal. App. 4th 1417, 1424 (Cal. Ct. App. 1999) (Standard of care "is a matter peculiarly within the knowledge of experts; it presents the basic issue in a malpractice action and can only be proved by their testimony").

[12] See for example, Collins v. Newman, 517 S.E.2d 100 (Ga. Ct. App. 1999) (Under Georgia law, if an expert affidavit is not filed along with the complaint, a claim of veterinary malpractice will be dismissed).

[13] Hendrick v. Ashburn,No. 09-92-260 CV, 1993 WL 389197, at *4 (Tex. Ct. App. Sept. 30, 1993) ("A doctor of the same school of practice as the defendant must testify that the defendant's diagnosis or treatment was negligent and proximately caused the injury").

[14] This issue has yet to be put the courts, and, at the time of publication, the authors are unaware of any published decisions regarding expert testimony in veterinary hospice cases.

[15] The informed consent form should include a statement that the animal in question already suffers from a terminal illness, and therefore the goal of hospice care is to provide palliative end-of-life care aimed at ensuring quality of life rather than longevity.

suffer legally compensable injuries.[16] Absent any such proof, a claim for veterinary malpractice will not be successful.[17]

Damages

Most states limit the types of damages that are recoverable in a veterinary malpractice action, unlike cases involving medical malpractice. Because animals are considered items of personal property, damages in veterinary malpractice claims are generally not recoverable for pain and suffering, wrongful death, and emotional distress.[18]

Courts will award successful litigants the loss of the fair market value of the animal (ie, the difference between the value of the animal before and immediately after the claimed injury or death).[19] In some instances, the replacement value of the animal may be awarded, again by determining the value of the animal immediately preceding the claimed injury. In the hospice context, the market value of the animal immediately before the hospice care is nominal, because hospice patients are critically and terminally ill.[20] In some instances, courts have also awarded successful litigants their costs of veterinary treatment, both past and anticipated future, burial/cremation expenses, and the costs, including lost income, incurred by the owner in caring for the animal as a result of the claimed injury.[21] However, damage

---

[16] See, for example, McAdams v. Curnayn, 239 S.W. 3d 17 (Ark. Ct. App. 2006) (expert testimony that dog's organ failure resulted from a preexisting spinal infection and not the defendant veterinarian's conduct resulted in dismissal of veterinary malpractice claim); Mathew v. Jerome L. Klinger, D.V.M., P.C., 686 N.Y.S.2d 549 (N.Y. Sup. Ct. 1998) (dog's owner was not entitled to fair market value of dog in a successful veterinary malpractice action because the dog was not healthy, but was in a life-threatening situation when it was brought to the defendant veterinarian).

[17] See, for example, Peltier v. McCartan, No. 17-05-14, 2005 WL 1798543 (Ohio Ct. App. Aug. 1, 2005) (although veterinarian misread ultrasounds and incorrectly informed owner that her pet was pregnant, there was no evidence presented that the veterinarian's actions caused the owner to suffer damages, and the claim was therefore dismissed).

[18] See, for example, Jones v. Collins, No. 3:09CV-394-H, 2010 WL 2572811, at *3 (W.D. Ky. June 23, 2010) (Under Kentucky law, "[t]he loss of love and affection resulting from the loss or destruction of personal property is not compensable"); Kaufman v. Langhofer, 222 P.3d 272 (Ariz. Ct. App. 2009) (under Arizona law, damages for emotional distress cannot be recovered in an action for veterinary malpractice); McMahon v. Craig, 176 Cal. App. 4th 1502 (Cal. Ct. App. 2009) (discussion of reasons why emotional distress damages to owner are not available in veterinary malpractice cases under California law); Carbasho v. Musulin, 618 S.E.2d 368 (W.Va. 2005); Oberschlake v. Veterinary Assoc. Animal Hosp., 785 N.E.2d 811 (Ohio Ct. App. 2003); Zeid v. Pearce, 953 S.W.2d 368 (Tex. Ct. App. 1997) (Under Texas law, one may not recover damages for pain and suffering or mental anguish for the loss of a pet); Jason v. Parks, 638 N.Y.S.2d 170 (N.Y. App. Div. 1996) ("It is well established that a pet owner in New York cannot recover damages for emotional distress").

[19] See, for example, Fleischer v. Henvy, No. CV960324902, 2000 WL 1889703 (Conn. Super. Ct. Dec. 7, 2000).

[20] See, for example, Sherman v. Kissinger, 195 P.3d 539 (Wash. Ct. App. 2008) (a toy poodle with a rare clotting disorder did not have a fair market value because it was not suitable for sale; as such, the owner was entitled, under Washington law, to provide evidence as to the intrinsic value of the dog); Vazquez v. Cragg, No. 09-94-240CV, 1996 WL 87222 (Tex. Ct. App. Feb. 29, 1996) (it was a defense to a claim of veterinary malpractice that the client's pet had a terminal condition before the veterinarian undertook any treatment).

[21] See, for example, Saratte v. Schroeder, No. 08-BE-18, 2009 WL 685272 (Ohio Ct. App. March 10, 2009) (damages for veterinary expenses of injured dog awarded in dog bite case); Brooks v. Goettl, No. A-05-CA-642-LY, 2006 WL 3691000 (W.D. Tex. Dec. 12, 2006) (claim for lost wages of owner was allowed to stand against veterinarian for owner's time spent caring for herd of sick horses).

awards are generally extremely nominal, if at all, in cases of veterinary hospice malpractice.[22]

In contrast, because a significant portion of hospice care is provided in-home, the caregiver may sustain personal injuries in the course of providing care to the animal. In such cases, the scope of recoverable damages would be much greater, and could include damages for pain and suffering, emotional distress, lost income, medical expenses, and wrongful death. In this context, legal principles such as informed consent, assumption of risk, and contributory negligence can serve to minimize or altogether bar liability of the veterinarian for injuries to the caregiver.

Ordinary Negligence

A veterinarian also faces liability exposure under principles of ordinary negligence.[23] Unlike professional negligence, which holds veterinarians to a higher standard of care based on their education, training, and experience, a claim of ordinary negligence is assessed under the level of care that the average person would exercise in a given situation. The most helpful way to illustrate the difference between claims of professional versus ordinary negligence is by example. A professional negligence claim may allege, for example, that a veterinarian misdiagnosed a patient, or prescribed an improper course of treatment. Ordinary negligence claims would arise in situations in which an animal escapes from the clinic because of a failure to properly secure the animal, or the wrong animal is operated on. That is, it has little to do with the practice of veterinary medicine, but, rather, of exercising ordinary care in common, everyday situations. The testimony of expert witnesses is not required in ordinary negligence claims.

Assumption of Risk/Contributory Negligence

As discussed earlier, the existence of an informed consent form signed by the client may serve to bar claims of malpractice against hospice veterinarians. The informed consent form should identify potential risks, not only to the animal, but to the caregiver, that may arise during the course of treatment. The legal doctrine of assumption of risk bars recovery in claims for injuries in which the evidence shows that the caregiver was fully apprised of the relevant risks but nonetheless voluntarily chose to engage in a particular conduct.[24] This defense is of great value in cases in which the client sustains injuries during the rendition of hospice care to the companion animal. However, to be invoked, the client must have been fully apprised of the potential risks of injury.

---

[22] Oberschlake v. Veterinary Assoc. Animal Hosp., 785 N.E.2d 811, 813 (Ohio Ct. App. 2003) ("damages will seldom be awarded for the loss of a family pet, since pets have little or no market value").

[23] See, for example, McGee v. Smith, 107 S.W.3d 725 (Tex. Ct. App. 2003) (discussing difference between professional and ordinary negligence); McAdams v. Faulk, No. CA 01-1350, 2002 WL 700956 (Ark. Ct. App. Apr. 24, 2002) (claim that someone in veterinarian's office choked owner's dog to stop its barking was a claim for ordinary negligence and not veterinary malpractice).

[24] See, for example, Bailly v. Thompson, No. 06-4925, 2008 WL 2229022, at * 4 (D. Minn. May 27, 2008) ("Primary assumption of risk bars recovery in a negligence action if the plaintiff: (1) has knowledge of the risk, (2) appreciates the risk, and (3) has a choice to avoid the risk but voluntarily chooses to accept the risk"); Priebe v. Nelson, 140 P.3d 848 (Cal. 2006); Brady v. White, No. 04C-09-262-FSS, 2006 WL 2790914, at *2 (Del. Super. Ct. Sept. 27, 2006) ("If the plaintiff knows of the existence of risk, appreciates the danger of it and nevertheless does not avoid it, [s]he will be held to have assumed the risk and may not recover").

Another bar to claims of professional malpractice is the concept of contributory negligence (ie, the failure of the caregiver to exercise due care). In the context of veterinary hospice, this issue is likely to present itself in 2 ways. First, the client may have chosen to forgo appropriate diagnostics.[25] If this is the case, the client will be precluded from later accusing the clinician of failing to properly diagnose the animal, because of insufficient diagnostics.[26] As previously stated, documentation of each decision made during the treatment process will be extremely advantageous in defending against malpractice claims.[27] The second way in which a client's contributory negligence may affect litigation is the client's failure to properly execute treatment. Any injuries to the animal or to the caregiver resulting from the client's inaction or mistakes generally will serve to reduce, or, in some cases, completely bar, recovery from the veterinarian.[28]

LEGAL ANALYSIS: TYPES OF CLAIMS
The Caregiver's Inability or Failure to Render the Necessary Care

The hospice plan will most likely involve the caregiving family administering various treatments at home. If a particular treatment is difficult or potentially hazardous, a demonstration should be provided by the veterinarian's staff to ensure that the caregiver becomes comfortable with the proper way to administer treatment. In the case of potentially hazardous treatments, such as those involving needles or harmful chemicals, specific warnings should be given regarding not only the need for caution but as to the potential injuries to the caregiver. If possible, such warnings should be given in writing and specifically acknowledged by the client.

The veterinarian runs the risk that the caregiver may be unable to provide the necessary treatment, or will fail to do so. Veterinarians have indicated that, in their experience, caregivers are typically forthcoming about any difficulties they are

---

[25] The inability or refusal by a client to conduct the necessary diagnostics should be documented on the informed consent form.

[26] See, for example, Kyu Son Yi v. State Bd. of Veterinary Medicine, 960 A.2d 864 (Pa. Commw. Ct. 2008) (veterinarian did not commit malpractice in improperly treating a dog's broken leg because the client refused to authorize a radiograph of dog's leg, which was the necessary diagnostic tool to determine the appropriate course of treatment); Downing v. Gully, 915 S.W.2d 181 (Tex. Ct. App. 1996) (claim of veterinary malpractice arising out of the death of a dog immediately after a neuter surgery was dismissed because the veterinarian did not deviate from the standard of care during anesthesia protocol, where client refused preanesthetic blood work).

[27] Although major treatment decisions are best incorporated into the informed consent form, the veterinarian's progress notes should also provide a sufficient evidentiary basis of the agreed course of treatment. See, for example, Austin v. State of Illinois, No. 98-CC-0388, 2002 WL 32705296, at *2 (Ill. Ct. Cl. Feb. 4, 2002) ("This Court recognizes that a veterinarian cannot remember everything that was said and done in regard to a specific patient. Therefore, great weight is given to the veterinary records."); Restrepo v. State, 550 N.Y.S.2d 536 (N.Y. Ct. Cl. 1989) (veterinary medical records and radiographs were admissible as evidence as business records).

[28] See, for example, Smith v. Hugo, 714 So.2d 467 (Fla. Dist. Ct. App. 1998) (issue of owner's contributory negligence was properly considered by the jury where owner was bitten by his cat during vaccination by the veterinarian); see also Mazella v. Fairfield Equine Associates, P.C., No. 02 CV 7391, 2005 WL 2452908 (S.D.N.Y. Oct. 3, 2005) (issue of plaintiff's contributory negligence in veterinary malpractice was allowed to go to the jury); Workman v. B. H. Grim, No. 83-S-143, 1986 WL 20569 (Pa. Com. Pl. Sept. 30, 1986) (jury award in veterinary malpractice case was reduced by the amount of the plaintiff's comparative fault).

experiencing in rendering treatment. A caregiver who goes to the trouble of procuring hospice care for a companion animal is unlikely to neglect the animal's treatment. Caregivers should also be advised that, if they are uncomfortable with administering treatments at home, alternatives exist, such as home visits by the veterinarian's staff, or hospitalization.

Likely injuries to the caregiver from the rendition of in-home care include needle wounds, improper disposal of sharp objects, or being scratched or bitten by the animal while administering medications. Once a treatment plan is formulated, the informed consent form signed by the caregiver should specifically describe the treatment that the caregiver has agreed to administer at home, should identify the possible risks to the caregiver, and should state that the caregiver has agreed to voluntarily assume those risks and therefore holds the veterinarian harmless if an injury is sustained. Because contributory negligence and assumption of risk are important legal defenses to claims involving injuries to the caregiver from in-home treatment, a detailed informed consent form is the best mechanism to prevent against needless litigation.

The risk of injuries to a caregiver from in-home treatment does not arise solely in the hospice context. In their private practices, veterinarians routinely prescribe medications and treatments that must be rendered by the caregiver. Although hospice care requires in-home treatments more often than in the traditional clinical setting, the range of potential claims against veterinarians in the hospice setting is virtually identical to the range that they already face in their daily practices.

Liability for Transmission of Zoonotic Diseases

A veterinarian may face litigation for injuries to clients from transmission of zoonotic diseases. Courts considering this subject have concluded that veterinarians do have an affirmative duty to warn the caregiver of the risks of contracting those illnesses.[29] In cases in which an animal has been diagnosed with a zoonotic disease, the veterinarian should warn the caregiver of the potential for contracting that illness and advise that alternative options, such as hospitalization, exist. Specific warnings should be given by veterinarians based on their knowledge of the particular circumstances of the caregiver, such as pregnancy or small children in the family. If in-home care is the agreed course of action, the informed consent form should explicitly advise of the risk of transmission of zoonotic diseases, and should include a statement that the caregiver was notified of such risks and has assumed those risks voluntarily.

Liability for Transmission of Diseases to Other Animals

Although veterinarians are generally not ascribed with a legal duty for human care, they do have a duty to protect the companion animals they routinely treat.[30] If

---

[29] See, for example, Langley v. Shannon, 628 S.E.2d 608 (Ga. Ct. App. 2006) (veterinarian had duty to warn client of possible risk of contracting rabies); Sloan v. Canadian Valley Animal Clinic, Inc., 719 P.2d 474 (Okla. Ct. App. 1985) (volunteer at clinic could advance claim against veterinarian for injuries from contracting brucellosis); McNew v. Decatur Veterinary Hospital, 68 S.E.2d 221 (Ga. Ct. App. 1951) (veterinarian had duty to warn owner of risk of contracting rabies).

[30] Berres v. Anderson, 561 N.W.2d 919 (Minn. Ct. App. 1997) (there was a genuine issue of fact whether a veterinarian had a duty to warn the owner of a herd of cattle of the risk of spreading Johne disease to other cattle); Fitch v. Prather, 502 So.2d 573 (La. 1987) (there was a genuine issue of fact whether a veterinarian had a duty to warn an individual, who owned horses the veterinarian had treated in the past, that the individual's neighbor's horse had tested positive for equine infectious anemia).

a caregiver has other animals at home, those animals are likely also patients of the veterinarian. As such, veterinarians may owe those other animals a duty if they are aware that they are at risk of contracting an illness from the animal under hospice care. As in the case of transmission of zoonotic diseases, the informed consent form should contain the appropriate statements regarding the veterinarian's communication of those risks and the caregiver's voluntary assumption thereof.

Misuse/Abuse of Controlled Substances

Veterinarians are often called on to dispense controlled substances in their routine practices; thus, the liability risks in doing so should already be familiar to them. In the hospice setting, the only major difference is the frequency with which controlled substances are prescribed to companion animals, because pain management is a primary focus in hospice and palliative care. Clinicians should adhere to the standards they already have in place regarding their dispensation of narcotics and other controlled substances, and should advise the client to use due care based on the regulated nature of the substances in question. Ideally, such risks should be documented in the informed consent form. Accidental overmedication or overdose by a well-meaning caregiver could form the basis of a failure-to-warn claim against a clinician. Likewise, the painful effects of certain medications on the companion animal could result in injuries to the caregiver. Proper warnings and instructions by the clinician should accompany the dispensation of all drugs, but particularly controlled prescription drugs.

Risks to Veterinary Staff in Providing Home Care

Veterinarians and their staff members are often required to provide in-home care for companion animals. This practice is likely to be a departure from the range of services currently provided by veterinarians in their private practices. Thus, certain legal risks can arise in this context above and beyond the veterinarian's current exposure.

Traveling to and from the client's home by clinic staff carries the risk of automobile accidents en route, resulting in injuries or property damage to either the staff or third parties. Clinic staff may suffer injuries at the client's home; for example, slipping and falling on icy steps. In most states, workers compensation laws are the exclusive remedy against an employer for injuries sustained by an employee during the course of employment.[31] That is, an injured employee can only seek recovery against the employer through workers' compensation, and is prohibited from bringing additional lawsuits against the employer.[32] Veterinarians undertaking expansion of their current practices are advised to consult with their workers' compensation insurance carriers regarding the nature and scope of their coverage.

Injuries to third parties carry a risk of litigation if the accident occurred during the ordinary course of the veterinarian's business. For example, accidental damage could occur in the caregiver's home during the provision of hospice care, giving rise to claims of property damage by the caregiver. The veterinarian may carry liability insurance, which would cover those costs. As a general rule, it is preferable that a member of the caregiving family be present in the home while veterinary staff members are

---

[31] Town and Country Animal Hosp. v. Deardorff, No. 0047-08-4, 2008 WL 2338602 (Va. Ct. App. June 10, 2008) (workers compensation act applied to veterinary clinic employee's claim for injuries when she was crossing busy street to retrieve a dog, because she was injured during the course of her employment).

[32] See, for example, Kolacki v. Verink, 893 N.E.2d 717 (Ill. App. Ct. 2008).

present. However, this is not always possible. The informed consent form should reflect that veterinary staff members have permission to enter the home in the caregiver's absence to provide treatment to the animal, and, if possible, should include a hold harmless provision regarding any accidents that may occur in the home.

In-home care will often be performed by clinic staff who take on the role of independent contractors to the owner; that is, they contract directly with the caregiver to perform certain services, and they are compensated for their work by the caregiver and not the veterinarian. In such instances, staff members are acting independently of the veterinarian, and, as such, any accidents or injuries to staff would not be attributable to the veterinarian. If the veterinarian is aware that such a situation exists, the informed consent form should include a disclaimer that work performed by independent contractors falls outside the scope of services that are being provided by the veterinarian, and for which the veterinarian cannot be held liable.

Providing 24-hour Accommodations Within the Clinic

Some veterinarians may choose to provide 24-hour accommodations in the clinic for caregivers whose companion animals are hospitalized. In such cases, legal exposure to the veterinarian would arise in the premises liability context. The veterinarian's liability insurance should be adjusted to reflect such an expansion of services. In many cases, an insurance settlement to an injured client eliminates the possibility of a lawsuit against the veterinarian. However, regardless of the availability of insurance, a client who is injured during an after-hours stay at the clinic may opt to bring a lawsuit against the veterinarian.

Premises liability law is fairly involved, and is not explored in this article. Logistically, veterinarians are advised to locate overnight rooms away from the main portion of the clinic, and provide an entrance/exit that does not require the client to walk through the clinic to reach the room. The less contact the client has with the main clinic, the less likely injuries, and potential lawsuits, are to occur.

Many defenses are available to veterinarians defending premises liability claims. The concepts of assumption of risk and contributory negligence, discussed earlier, would most likely come into play.[33] The informed consent form should include acknowledgment of the risks inherent in staying in the clinic after hours, and a statement that the client assumes those risks and holds the veterinarian harmless for any injuries that may be sustained.

As a practical matter, the veterinarian would be required to provide 24-hour staffing if after-hours accommodations are offered. The presence of a staff member should minimize the possible injuries a client could sustain. Any injuries to staff or property damage to the clinic that may occur during after-hours care would be within the scope of state workers' compensation laws and the veterinarian's liability insurance.

Responsibility for Body Care

Most municipalities have regulations governing the proper way to dispose of the body of a deceased companion animal, setting out the procedures for both burial and cremation. It is unlikely that a veterinarian would face any legal risk stemming from a client's improper disposal of a companion animal's remains. However, because the nature of hospice care contemplates the imminent death of the companion animal,

---

[33] Senkus v. Moore, 535 S.E.2d 724 (W.Va. 2000) (claim against veterinarian was dismissed based on contributory negligence, where owner tripped on veterinary scale on exiting an examination room and sustained injuries).

courts could find that a veterinarian has an affirmative obligation to advise the patient of the proper way to dispose of the animal's body.

Veterinarians can, and most already do, encourage the use of private crematory or burial services. If clients chooses not to employ such a service, veterinarians should take the following steps to ensure that they are not under any obligation to ensure that the client's disposal of the animal's body comports with local law. First, the veterinarian should advise the client of any local ordinances governing proper disposal of companion animal remains. Most local animal shelters or government animal control agencies are able to provide this information. Second, they should include a statement in the informed consent form, whereby the client acknowledges the existence of the local ordinance(s) and agrees to be solely responsible for disposal of the body in a legally permissible manner.

RECOMMENDATIONS

From a medical standpoint, the existence of frequent, detailed, open, and honest communication between the veterinarian and the client is crucial to the successful provision of hospice care to companion animals. From a legal standpoint, that same communication is the best tool to minimize the likelihood of successful litigation against the veterinarian.

Patients are less likely to sue practitioners with better communication skills.[4] It is estimated that 35% to 70% of medicolegal actions result from poor delivery of information, failure to understand patient and family perspectives, failure to incorporate patients' values into the plan of care, and perceptions of desertion.[5]

The veterinarian's ability to show a written record of all communications with a client significantly strengthens a veterinarian's defense when facing potential or actual litigation. In addition to a detailed medical record, an informed consent form signed by the client and the veterinarian can be an effective deterrent against litigation. The sample informed consent form in Appendix 1 presents a comprehensive list of the specific items for inclusion in an informed consent form that are referenced throughout the various sections of this article. This sample form is intended to serve only as a starting point for veterinarians in preparing their own informed consent forms, and is not meant to be used without modification. Veterinarians should customize the form for their practice and, ideally, for each patient. It is critical that each provision accurately reflect the laws of the particular state in which the veterinarian practices. The authors suggest that veterinarians consult with an attorney and/or the insurance carrier to ensure that their informed consent form comports with all applicable provisions of state law.

Although it may appear daunting, an informed consent form is nothing more than written documentation of what has already been discussed by the veterinarian and the client. Once a standard template has been prepared for use by the veterinarian, modification of the template for an individual client should not be a difficult task. Much needless litigation can be avoided by the existence of a detailed informed consent form, and veterinarians are well advised to prepare such a form, which is certain to inure to their benefit in the long run.

SUMMARY

The legal risks faced by a veterinarian in providing hospice and palliative care arise in 2 main contexts: (1) veterinary malpractice claims arising out of diagnosing and formulating a treatment plan for the companion animal; and (2) execution of that treatment plan by the veterinarian, by the veterinarian's staff, and/or by the caregiver. Because the practice of hospice and palliative care involves animals who are critically and/or terminally ill, litigants can face several potentially insurmountable challenges in bringing a successful veterinary malpractice claim in this context. The more likely type of claim arises from injuries to the caregiver, to technical staff, or to third parties during the execution stage of hospice care.

The legal issues that may arise in the context of veterinary hospice described in this article are largely duplicative of those that arise in the course of other types of small animal veterinary practice. Provided they take the steps recommended by the authors to reduce the risks of legal liability, such risks should not deter current and potential providers from offering palliative and hospice care services.

APPENDIX 1: SAMPLE INFORMED CONSENT FORM
Section 1: Authorization for Treatment

The following informed consent form has been executed by [owner's name], of [owner's address] for the veterinary hospice care and treatment of [patient's name], a [description of patient: age, breed, sex]. [Owner] represents that she/he is the legal owner of [patient], and is authorized to make all treatment decisions pertaining to [patient]. [Owner] accepts sole responsibility for the payment of veterinary costs and expenses relating to [patient]'s treatment. Pursuant to the terms set forth below, and as may be added from time to time with the express consent of [owner], [owner] authorizes Dr [name], of [clinic name, if applicable], along with members of Dr [name]'s staff, whether named or unnamed in this document, to provide veterinary care and treatment of [patient] as follows:

Section 2: Diagnosis and Prognosis

[Patient] has been diagnosed with [list diagnoses]. Include statements as to whether the diagnosis was made by the hospice veterinarian or by another veterinarian, and, where applicable, whether the diagnosis was based on objective tests such as radiographs, ultrasounds, and blood tests.

[Owner] has been advised by Dr [name] that the prognosis for [patient] is [provide any relevant information].

Section 3: Treatment Options

Dr [name] has advised [owner] of the various options for treatment of [patient], as follows:[Identify the various treatment options that were discussed with the owner, including curative options, additional diagnostics, hospice and palliative care, and euthanasia, as applicable. List the risks associated with any of these options that were discussed with the owner.]

[Owner] acknowledges that the approximate costs, as well as the risks and benefits of each of the treatment options identified above, have been discussed by him/her and Dr [name], and that [owner] has been fully advised of the various options available to him/her before consenting to the particular course of treatment set forth below.

Section 4: Treatment Plan

Having been fully advised by Dr [name] of the various treatment options for [patient], and the risks associated with each option, [owner] has agreed to the following treatment plan for [patient].

- Identify treatment plan. Include:
- How often the veterinarian/staff will examine patient, and whether the examinations will be in-home or in the clinic
- What tasks the owner must perform, how, and how often

- Include a statement, if applicable, that the owner received a demonstration on how to perform a particular treatment, and that the owner agrees to perform the treatment in the manner prescribed by the veterinarian
- State risks to owner, if any, from performing each task, and any risk of transmission of a zoonotic disease.

Owner has been advised of these risks by Dr [name], understands these risks, and, by agreeing to this particular course of treatment, has hereby agreed to assume those risks and hold Dr [name] harmless for any injuries to [owner] or family resulting from [owner's] rendering of veterinary care and treatment to [patient];

[Identify risks to patient, if any, from owner's performing each task.] Owner has been advised of these risks by [veterinarian], understands these risks, and, by agreeing to this particular course of treatment, has hereby agreed to assume those risks and hold [veterinarian] harmless for any injuries to [patient] resulting from [owner's] rendering of veterinary care and treatment to [patient];

[Identify, where applicable, risks to other pets within owner's household.] Owner has been advised of these risks by Dr [name], understands these risks, and, by agreeing to this particular course of treatment, has hereby agreed to assume those risks and hold Dr [name] harmless for any injuries to [other household pets] resulting from [owner's] rendering of veterinary care and treatment to [patient];

Whether treatment includes dispensation of controlled substances, and acknowledgment by owner that medication is a controlled substance, and will be dispensed in strict accordance with the veterinarian's instructions;

[Owner] understands that, because the care of [patient] will be rendered at home, Dr [name] will be limited in [his/her] ability to observe [patient's] symptoms, progress, and reactions. [Owner] understands that Dr [name] is relying on [owner's] prompt and accurate reporting of [patient's] condition, and agrees to promptly and thoroughly report to Dr [name] any reactions, problems, symptoms, or conditions of [patient] on a frequent and regular basis. [Owner] agrees to hold Dr [name] harmless for any injuries arising from or relating to [owner's] reporting, or failure thereof, of [patient's] symptoms, conditions, or difficulties rendering the agreed treatment.

Owner acknowledges that Dr [name] has provided information to [owner] regarding professional pet crematory and/or burial services. If, on [patient's] death, [owner] does not wish to use the recommendations provided by Dr [name] regarding disposal of the body, [owner] assumes full and sole responsibility for disposal of the body in accordance with any and all state and local laws, rules, and regulations. Owner agrees further to indemnify and hold harmless Dr [name] for any liability arising out of improper disposal of [patient's] body.

If Dr [name] and staff are to provide in-home care to [patient], [owner] authorizes the following individuals to provide such treatment at [owner's] home: [list individuals]. [Owner] agrees to indemnify and hold harmless Dr [name] for any physical injury to [owner] and family or damages to [owner's] property that may arise in the course of such in-home treatment except where occasioned by the sole negligence of Dr [name] or staff.

[24-hour clinic accommodations]

[Owner] acknowledges that the following procedures and treatments were recommended by Dr [name] but declined by [owner] after being satisfactorily informed of their potential benefits, costs and risks. [List recommended procedures and treatments the owner has elected not to pursue.]

[Owner] acknowledges and understands that [patient] has a terminal illness. Any care rendered by Dr [name] as identified above, is not intended to cure [patient's] condition, but is aimed at managing [patient's] pain and maintaining [patient's] quality of life for his/her remaining days.

[Owner] agrees to pay for the costs of all treatment and services rendered by Dr [name] and staff at the rates set by Dr [name], as discussed with [owner].

Any future modifications to the treatment plan for [patient] shall be made in writing and executed by [owner], and shall be deemed incorporated herein. Such future modifications shall have the full force and effect of the provisions set forth herein.

Signed and dated by owner and veterinarian.

REFERENCES

1. AVMA. AVMA guidelines for veterinary hospice care (March 2007). Schaumburg (IL): AVMA; 2007.
2. AAHA. AAHA senior care guidelines for dogs and cats. J Am Anim Hosp Assoc 2005;41:81–91.
3. Shearer T, Muir W, Gaynor J. Hospice and palliative care. Handbook of veterinary pain management [book auth.]. St Louis (MO): Mosby Elsevier; 2009. p. 588–600.
4. Hickson G, Wright Clayton E, Githens P, et al. Factors that prompted families to file medical malpractice claims following perinatal injuries. JAMA 1992;267:1359–63.
5. Levetown M. Communicating with children and families: from everyday interactions to skill in conveying distressing information. Pediatrics 2008;121:e1441–60.

A Case Report: Veterinary Palliative Care and Hospice for a West Highland Terrier with Transitional Cell Carcinoma

Robin Downing, DVM, CCRP, CPE

KEYWORDS

• Palliative care • End of life • Hospice • Metronomic
• Multimodal

Palliative care and hospice principles are now being applied to companion animals as practitioners recognize and realize that there is usually a space between identifying a terminal diagnosis and the time for death, whether natural or as a result of humane euthanasia. There are many excellent resources from human medicine that can give the veterinary practitioner ideas about how to structure and choreograph the end-of-life experience for both the pet and the pet owner (resources and recommended reading are listed at the end of this article). Villalobos and Kaplan[1] devote an entire chapter to end-of-life care for pets. Dr Villalobos has coined the term pawspice to describe this adaptation of human medical principles and practices to companion animals. In any event, as our cultural investment in the human-animal bond continues to grow, veterinarians recognize the need to squire their animal patients and their clients through the end-of-life process.

Palliative care and hospice are not places where the end of life arrives for the pet, but rather reflect a philosophy of care that focuses on comfort and support rather than on the cure of a disease process. One could make the case that any disease that is managed rather than cured requires palliative care (eg, congestive heart failure, chronic renal disease, or diabetes mellitus). However, in the truest sense, the term palliative care is most often reserved to describe the overall support and symptom management offered to an animal who no longer has curative options available or

The author has nothing to disclose.
The Downing Center for Animal Pain Management, LLC, 415 Main Street, Windsor, CO 80550, USA
E-mail address: drrobin@downingcenter.com

for whom care with the intention to cure has been withdrawn. It may be most useful to think of palliative care and hospice as care beyond a cure.

Traditional palliative care typically targets patients who have cancer and often involves a modification of conventional cancer therapies to slow progression or relieve cancer-related symptoms. This type of patient management may involve surgery to debulk a tumor mass, chemotherapy to shrink a tumor, radiation therapy at lower doses than considered curative, or some combination of these. At the heart of palliative care, whether for the patient who has cancer or the pet without cancer, is the commitment to balance the effects of the treatments provided with the outcomes faced by the patient. Always the target is to keep the patient in palliative care and hospice at the center of the care-giving circle, and to keep that pet as comfortable as possible as death approaches. Our practice regularly choreographs end-of-life care for both dogs and cats, and it is rewarding to be able to offer pet owners the opportunity for additional quality time with their beloved animal companions.

BUDDY'S STORY

Buddy was 9 years old when he was diagnosed with transitional cell carcinoma (TCC) originating in his prostatic urethra. He was a neutered male West Highland white terrier who had, until the time of his cancer diagnosis, enjoyed an uneventful health history beyond the occasional upset stomach from dietary indiscretion. Because the tumor originated in the prostatic urethra, the mass was surgically unresectable. In a case like this, the patient enters directly into palliative care because there is no realistic curative treatment option available. All treatment activities are directed at suppressing tumor activity and delaying progression versus treating with intended cure (**Fig. 1**).

Urinary bladder cancer accounts for approximately 2% of all reported malignancies in the dog,[2] with TCC being the most common among these. At the time of his diagnosis and staging, Buddy showed no evidence of metastatic disease, only local invasion. With no treatment at all, rapid tumor growth would be expected, ultimately preventing urination and resulting in euthanasia within a few weeks. With chemotherapeutic management, including ongoing piroxicam as a COX-2 inhibitor, survival may

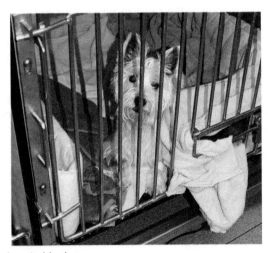

Fig. 1. Buddy in a hospital bedroom.

stretch to 150 days or longer.[2] After much discussion with Buddy's human family members, we embarked on a plan to manage his tumor disease as well as possible without resorting to more invasive options such as surgery or radiation therapy.

Buddy's first round of palliative care involved intravenous (IV) infusions of doxorubicin at 30 mg/m[2] every 3 weeks for a total of 5 treatments. For all of our oncology patients, our commitment is to minimize the adverse effects of these powerful drugs. Buddy enjoyed little interruption of his lifestyle and routine during the course of his chemotherapy: no nausea, no vomiting, no diarrhea, and no loss of appetite. Because chemotherapy in this setting is palliative in nature, and because we needed to confirm its positive effect on Buddy's tumor, we performed an abdominal ultrasound after his third dose of doxorubicin to mark progress. The ultrasound confirmed that the tumor had regressed, which encouraged us to finish his 5-dose protocol. Part of his palliation included daily piroxicam at a dose of 0.3 mg/kg by mouth. This medication was compounded by a local pharmacy.

Once Buddy's doxorubicin protocol was complete, he continued on medication within a metronomic context. Metronomic therapy uses low doses of chemotherapeutic or other tumor-inhibiting agents delivered more frequently than conventional chemotherapy regimens (eg, daily). The principle of metronomic therapy is to target micrometastasis, preventing microscopic islands of tumor cells from taking hold and growing into tumors.[3] In Buddy's case, he took daily doses of piroxicam as well as doxycycline (which inhibits angiogenesis) and was scheduled for regular reassessment of his mass via ultrasound. In the meantime, however, at 9.5 years of age, Buddy developed chronic back pain localized to the thoracolumbar (T/L) area, the lateral lumbar muscles, and the iliopsoas muscles that interfered with his comfort, mobility, stamina, and quality of life. There were no radiographic changes noted in the spine, decreasing our index of suspicion of metastasis to the spine and/or pelvis. Instead, we presumed early osteoarthritis changes to the facet joints of the spine.

This turn of events illustrates the commonly encountered scenario faced by veterinary palliative care and hospice patients who develop and deal with comorbidities in addition to their primary disease entity. In Buddy's case, he experienced pain independent of his urinary tract cancer that needed to be managed appropriately. Because he was taking piroxicam to help manage his TCC, he could not take additional nonsteroidal anti-inflammatory drugs for his back pain. The multimodal pain management strategy we developed for him included the following elements:

1. Dry-needle acupuncture delivered twice weekly for 4 weeks, then weekly for 4 weeks, then once monthly for maintenance
2. Therapeutic laser treatments (class IV, 6W, 980 nm) to the T/L, lateral lumbar, and iliopsoas muscles at 20 J/cm[2] delivered at the surface. Therapeutic laser treatments occurred on the same schedule as the acupuncture treatments
3. Gabapentin at 200 mg (17.5 mg/kg) by mouth twice a day to address the maladaptive nature of his pain.

Within 10 days of initiating this multimodal pain management regimen, Buddy's back pain score was reduced from Visual Analog Scale (VAS) 5/10 to VAS 1/10. With occasional escalations of his gabapentin dose, he maintained that comfort level until the time of his euthanasia.

More than 1 year after completing his doxorubicin protocol, it was determined that Buddy's TCC was again progressing in spite of his ongoing doses of doxycycline and piroxicam. On the advice of a medical oncologist at the Animal Cancer Center at the Colorado State University College of Veterinary Medicine, we proceeded through a course of 4 IV doses of carboplatin at 300 mg/m^2 delivered once every 4 weeks. Abdominal ultrasound assessments confirmed that tumor progression was slowed. Throughout this second course of palliative chemotherapy, Buddy's quality of life remained excellent. We continued management of his chronic maladaptive back pain as well. Once he completed his carboplatin regimen, Buddy's owners decided that they would not pursue any aggressive palliative options, focusing instead on Buddy's day-to-day quality of life. The Villalobos Quality of Life scale[1] provided them with an instrument by which they could attempt an objective measurement of a subjective experience.

More than 2.5 years passed between Buddy's diagnosis of terminal, or life-limiting, TCC with ensuing palliative care, and the time chosen for humane euthanasia. Buddy's human family opted for humane euthanasia based on a rapid decline in his interest in them, in his interest in his surroundings, and in his interest in eating (food motivation remained exceptionally high throughout his palliative care). His quality-of-life score had decreased precipitously to less than 30/70. We were able to provide Buddy and his human family with the ultimate gift of release from his suffering.

SUMMARY

Buddy's case illustrates a straightforward approach to providing palliative care and hospice in a veterinary outpatient primary care setting. It illustrates the importance of managing all aspects of the patient's needs (in this case chronic maladaptive back pain) as well as the primary disease process. This sort of case could easily be managed in the same comprehensive fashion shown here in any number of primary care practices. It is important to understand that veterinary palliative care and hospice do not require a special degree or board certification. They only require compassion for the terminally ill patient and the human family members, a commitment to keeping patients united with their families for as long as they are comfortable, and a willingness to keep a comprehensive perspective on the patient's changing needs as death nears. The rewards are many.

REFERENCES

1. Villalobos A, Kaplan L. Canine and feline geriatric oncology: honoring the human-animal bond. Ames (IA): Blackwell Publishing; 2007. p. 304.
2. Knapp DW. Tumors of the urinary system. In: Withrow SJ, Vail DM, editors. Withrow and MacEwen's small animal clinical oncology. 4th edition. St Louis (MO): Elsevier Saunders; 2007. p. 649, 653.
3. Chun R, Garrett LD, Vail DM. Cancer chemotherapy. In: Withrow SJ, Vail DM, editors. Withrow & MacEwen's small animal clinical oncology. 4th edition. St Louis (MO): Elsevier Saunders; 2007. p. 170–1.

RECOMMENDED READINGS

AAHA/AAFP Pain Management Guidelines Task Force. AAHA/AAFP pain management guidelines for dogs and cats. J Am Anim Hosp Assoc 2007;43:235–48.
Berger AM, Portenoy RK, Weissman DE, editors. Principles & practice of palliative care & supportive oncology. 2nd edition. Philadelphia: Lippincott Williams & Wilkins; 2002.
Downing R. Pets living with cancer. Lakewood (CO): AAHA Press; 2000.
Gaynor JS, Muir WW. Handbook of veterinary pain management. 2nd edition. St Louis (MO): Elsevier Mosby; 2009.
Kaplan L. So easy to love, so hard to lose. Briarcliff (NY): JanGen Press; 2010.

Kuebler KK, Berry PH, Heidrich DE, editors. End of life care. Philadelphia: Elsevier Saunders; 2002.

Kuebler KK, Davis MP, Moore CD. Palliative practices: an interdisciplinary approach. St Louis: Elsevier Mosby; 2005.

Marrelli TM. Hospice and palliative care handbook. St Louis: Elsevier Mosby; 2005.

Nakaya SF. Kindred spirit, kindred care: making health decisions on behalf of our animal companions. Novato (CA): New World Library; 2005.

Villalobos A, Kaplan L. Canine and feline geriatric oncology: honoring the human-animal bond. Ames (IA): Blackwell Publishing; 2007.

Wolfelt AD. Healing your grieving soul: 100 spiritual practice for mourners. Fort Collins (CO): Companion Press; 2009.

Wolfelt AD. Interpersonal skills training: a handbook for funeral home staffs. Florence (KY): Accelerated/Development (Taylor & Francis Group); 1990.

Wolfelt AD. When your pet dies: a guide to mourning, remembering, and healing. Fort Collins (CO): Companion Press; 2004.

Wolfelt AD, Duvall KJ. Healing your grieving body: 100 physical practices for mourners. Fort Collins (CO): Companion Press; 2009.

Yoder G. Companioning the dying. Fort Collins (CO): Companion Press; 2005.

A Case Report: Pawspice for a Visla with Splenic Lymphoma

Alice E. Villalobos, DVM, DPNAP[a,b,c,*]

KEYWORDS

- Splenic lymphoma • Pawspice • Cancer cachexia
- Comorbid conditions

This author's 40 plus years of experience in oncology proposes Pawspice. It is a new concept that offers early supportive care for pets with life-limiting disease, embracing both palliative care and standard care. Pawspice offers compassionate and comprehensive symptom relief at diagnosis while addressing cancer and other life-limiting diseases. The concept of Pawspice is to enthusiastically maintain quality of life with effective palliative care that improves the patient's concurrent debilitating conditions by 30% to 50% while simultaneously administering standard care via gentle chemotherapy modified for low toxicity. The purpose of Pawspice is to elevate quality of life, which reliably extends quantity of life.[1] Pawspice is truly reaching out to help terminal pets at diagnosis with kinder more gentle protocols than those used in definitive therapy. This combination makes Pawspice different than palliative care (pain and symptom relief) or hospice (intense comfort care that precedes imminent death), which prevail in most conventional thinking. Pawspice is a viable third option that should be inserted between the either–or models often pushed upon pet owners at emergency facilities and conventional general and referral practices that inadvertently pressure pet owners to unwillingly elect early euthanasia. The Pawspice philosophy guided Murphy Johnson's 20-month quality survival with splenic lymphoma.

CASE REPORT: MURPHY JOHNSON'S COMORBIDITIES

Murphy Johnson, a frail, nervous 22.7 kg, 12-year-old, female spayed Visla, presented on Oct. 28, 2008, with a history of bilateral hip and stifle degenerative joint disease, hypothyroidism, urinary tract infections (UTIs), multiple dermal nodules, eyelid

[a] Pawspice at VCA Coast Animal Hospital, Hermosa Beach, CA 90254, USA
[b] Pawspice at Beachside Animal Referral Center, Capistrano Beach, CA 92627, USA
[c] Animal Oncology Consultation Service at Animal Emergency and Care Center, Woodland Hills, CA 91364, USA
* Pawspice at VCA Coast Animal Hospital, Hermosa Beach, CA 90254.
E-mail address: pawspice@msn.com

Vet Clin Small Anim 41 (2011) 683–688
doi:10.1016/j.cvsm.2011.03.015   **vetsmall.theclinics.com**
0195-5616/11/$ – see front matter © 2011 Elsevier Inc. All rights reserved.

melanocytomas, dental staining with erosions, and typical aging changes such as energy decline, muscle atrophy, and facial graying. Her previous prescription history included Deramax, Dasequin, 3-V caps, and soloxine 0.5 mg twice daily from her local veterinarian. Murphy was slowing down and had developed several skin tumors that concerned her family. She was referred by a friend for cryotherapy of her skin and eyelid tumors, tumor watch, and longevity counseling. The author placed Murphy on multimodal pain management for her arthritis with metacam, gabapentin, and tramadol and started immunonutrition.

MURPHY DIAGNOSED WITH SPLENIC LYMPHOMA

On Feb. 17, 2009, Murphy presented with weight loss depression, anorexia, severe lameness, and inability to rise. On physical examination, Murphy was 8% to 10% dehydrated, thin, and nearly moribund. Her oral mucus membranes were hyperemic and bleeding from numerous petechiae. Murphy had extreme halitosis with only mild tartar and gingivitis. On abdominal palpation, she was painful with organomegaly. Intravenous fluids were started, and blood and radiographs were taken. Her complete blood cell (CBC) count and chemistry panel were within normal range. Radiographs revealed splenomegaly. On abdominal ultrasonography, the enlarged spleen contained several hypoechoic nodules. The liver was evenly hypoechoic with a dilated gall bladder and calcification of the common bile duct. Fine needle aspiration (FNA) cytology of the splenic nodules revealed sheets of lymphoblasts, which confirmed the diagnosis of splenic lymphoma. Liver cytology was unremarkable but cholangiohepatitis was a suspected complication. The prognosis for Murphy's survival without treatment was grave. Dogs with nodular splenic lymphoma can survive 6 to 8 months with treatment. The family declined immunophenotyping, which can distinguish between T-cell versus B-cell lymphoma due to immediate financial concerns.

PAWSPICE USING WISCONSIN PROTOCOL CUSTOMIZED FOR MURPHY

At diagnosis, Murphy was entered into the author's Pawspice program and given supportive care with intravenous fluid therapy, ursodiol at 300 mg once daily, Clavamox, famotidine, Cerenia, and palliative chemotherapy. She responded very well to induction chemotherapy with a customized version of the modified Wisconsin protocol using vincristine and L-asparaginase and steroids. Evidence of remission was observed on follow-up ultrasound as regression of the splenic nodules, but her body condition score dropped to 3. The known cardio toxicity and gastrointestinal (GI) toxicity of doxorubicin were minimized for Murphy's frailty by using this author's split-dose protocol, which delivers 20 mg/M^2 for 2 consecutive weeks. This technique increases the area under the curve (AUC) dose over a longer period of time but does not put older, frail patients at risk for adverse events (toxicity). If 30 mg/M^2, the standard maximum tolerated dose (MTD) of doxorubicin, were used, it would have been too harsh for old Murphy. The Pawspice rationale with suggestions to reduce toxicity from other chemotherapy drugs for geriatric and frail patients is described in greater detail in this author's textbook, *Canine and Feline Geriatric Oncology: Honoring the Human–Animal Bond*.[2,3]

RELAPSE WITH HYPERCALCEMIA

On April 7, 2009, only 7 weeks later, Murphy relapsed with the previously reported severe symptoms along with azotemia, kidney disease, and cachexia. This first relapse followed the second cycle of doxorubricin (doxorubicin) chemotherapy.

Murphy's relapse was confirmed by identifying splenic nodules on ultrasound and ultrasound-guided FNA of these nodules. Cytology revealed sheets of lymphoblasts once again. It was important to inform Murphy's family that recurrent lymphoma would be more difficult to treat. The family elected to attempt a second remission, because they wanted Murphy to be at their wedding.

Murphy most likely had T-cell lymphoma, which was probably resistant to doxorubicin. Therefore, it was decided to use a COP based protocol (cyclophosphamide, oncovin [vincristine], and prednisone) enhanced with Cytosar and L-asparaginase, which was given twice during the first week as reinduction therapy. Murphy developed azotemia and early kidney disease that required daily subcutaneous (SQ) fluids for optimal maintenance. Murphy's "grandmother" took her to their local veterinarian for SQ fluids, and Pawspice nurses visited the family home to administer SQ fluids and treatments when needed. Reinduction was successful for Murphy. She recovered her happy personality and attended the family wedding. Murphy's second remission lasted almost 6 months, much longer than expected.

IMMUNONUTRITION FOR CANCER CACHEXIA, UTIs, CHRONIC KIDNEY DISEASE, COMORBIDITIES

Cancer cachexia haunted Murphy with body scores as low as 3 during the beginning and end of her Pawspice despite having a fair appetite most of the time. When she lost weight, she was given mirtazapine to increase her appetite and periodic injections of nandrolone at 0.15 mL intramuscularly, Depo-Provera at 30 mg intramuscularly, Glutimmune (glutathione) powder, and ImmunoPro (purified whey) powder and Hill's anorexia diet (Topeka, KS, USA). It also seemed reasonable to lower her soloxine dose from 0.5 mg twice daily to 0.3 mg twice daily. Murphy's original immunonutrition protocol was composed of the following supplements: Agaricus Bio 600 mg twice daily, IP-6, Canine Platinum Performance Plus and Ortho-Chon (a pain control formula by Platinum Performance), and Standard Process (SP) Musculo-Skeletal Support to address her comorbid osteoarthritis and muscular weakness. After being diagnosed with life-limiting splenic lymphoma, the author added Rx Vitamin's Onco Support and Hepato Support (New York, NY, USA), and Auburn Lab's APF Drops (Auburn, CA, USA), which contain Siberian ginseng. Later she was given SP Canine Renal Support then Azodyl, Epikatin and Ultra EFA oil (OM-3 fatty acids) to support renal function and Bio Sponge to control occasional bouts of loose stools.

Murphy thrived on her maintenance chemotherapy and immunonutrition protocols. She regained her weight and reached a stunning 59.8 pounds. Family members reported that Murphy's quality of life was improved over previous years. This was due mainly to the high-quality nutraceuticals and supplements used for supportive care of her immune system and comorbidities. One recheck led to the next, and the summer passed with great happiness knowing that Murphy's Pawspice was successful and that the author were giving her the opportunity to give her family an extended farewell.

RELAPSE IN LIVER AND SPLEEN

On Nov. 3, 2009, at 7.5 months following diagnosis, Murphy lost 5 pounds in 2 weeks. She became azotemic again with a rising alkaline phosphatase (ALP) despite maintaining a normal energy level. The Nov. 17, 2009, blood work revealed that Murphy's serum Ca^{++} was rising to high normal, and her ALP was 2240 U/L (N = 20–150). Another ultrasound indicated the liver and spleen were grainy and hypoechoic. Ultrasound-guided FNA cytology revealed lymphoblasts in both Murphy's liver and spleen along with many atypical lymphocytes. Murphy was in the midst of a smoldering second recurrence of lymphoma and presumptive cholangiohepatitis, and she had already reached the historical prognosis for further survival.

The author counseled the family, explaining that Murphy's chances for a third remission would be reduced and the duration of a third remission is generally half of the second remission. These are very sad consultations and yet, with compassion and regret, the author offer the prognosis based on evidence-based medicine so that the family knows what to expect. Of course, one always remains hopeful.

Prioritizing the principles and philosophy of Pawspice care was first and foremost. The author did not want to cause harm to Murphy's already compromised frail body. The goal was to gain control of the lymphoma, which would increase her quality of life.

Rescue protocols for resistant lymphoma are well known to cause an increased risk of adverse events ranging from grade 1 (mild) through grade 4 (severe). Chemotherapy toxicities generally involve the GI tract and the hematopoietic system. Grade 4 toxicities are life threatening and require costly hospitalization for supportive care. The last thing the author would want for Murphy's end-of-life Pawspice care would be hospitalization, because she was a nervous dog. Being away from home would have a negative impact on her quality of life.

There are several chemotherapy rescue protocols for lymphoma such as mustargen, oncovin, procarbazine, prednisone (MOPP), dexamethazone-melphalan, actinomycin D, cytosine arabinoside (D-MAC), adriamycin-dacarbazine (A-DTIC), and mitoxantrone, cyclophosphamide, actinomycin-D, prednisone (MiCAP). There was a lack of evidence-based data to support which rescue protocol was more effective or which protocol would be less toxic for Murphy. It was likely that the recurrent splenic lymphoma cells had developed multiple drug resistance (MDR) to previously used chemotherapy.

Personal communication from Veterinary Cancer Society meetings recently informed the author that doxorubicin was unhelpful against presumptive T-cell lymphoma and that single-agent mitoxantrone given intravenously at 5 to 6 mg/M^2 every 21 days yielded a 47% overall response rate for dogs with resistant lymphoma. Since mitoxantrone is kinder than its analog, doxorubicin, the author discussed this option with the family. The family elected to go with mitoxantrone reinduction along with injectable dexamethazone every 3 days for Murphy. Surprisingly, Murphy achieved and maintained a prolonged third remission. To temper the high cost of mitoxantrone, 10 mg lomustine was given on day 21–24 to increase the interval between visits. During this time, Murphy's kidney disease was controlled with SQ fluids, Azodyl, and Epikatin. Severe lipemia occasionally obfuscated her serum CA^{++} readings and other serum chemistry values.

At the March 30, 2010, visit, Murphy's serum CA^{++} elevated to 14.4 mg/dL (N = 8.6–11.8). Serum Ca^{++} levels can be used as a tumor marker for recurrence of hypercalcemic lymphomas. When serum Ca^{++} is elevated, the attending doctor can presume that the patient is in relapse. This spared the Johnson's from the cost of repeat ultrasounds and splenic FNAs. Murphy's chemotherapy intervals were adjusted to maintain as low a serum Ca^{++} as possible. The family was quite' satisfied with Murphy's prolonged stable partial remission.

Cancer cachexia plagued Murphy's entire 20-month Pawspice. Her dramatic weight losses and gains coincided with her relapses and remissions. She began losing weight again in May 2009. She was able to gain back a few pounds, but she exhibited a steady weight loss down to 18.7 kg by the end of September 2010. She developed another UTI, which yielded *Escherichia coli* on culture that was responsive to antibiotic therapy. Murphy's body condition score was back down to

3/9 when she began to exhibit signs of physical and mental stress during her clinic visits.

On August 31, 2010, the author applied for a compassionate use permit from AB Science in Paris, France for the tyrosine kinase inhibitor, masitinib, hoping to gain a fourth remission for Murphy. The masitinib dose for Murphy was 150 mg by mouth mornings and 100 mg by mouth evenings. Pretreatment with metoclopramide 30 to 60 minutes before masitinib avoided emesis. Murphy tolerated masitinib very well.

MURPHY'S PAWSPICE TRANSITIONS TO HOSPICE

Murphy's Pawspice began February 17, 2009, on the day that she was presented in a nearly moribund condition. The diagnosis of canine splenic lymphoma precludes long-term survival and justifies entering the patient into Pawspice. The author counseled the Johnsons to stay in touch with reality regarding the prognosis and encouraged them to celebrate Murphy's wonderful days of wellness and to value her good times. The Johnsons knew that each day brought Murphy closer to that bumpy road at the very end of life.[2,4,5]

On Sept. 14, 2010, Murphy presented in a weak and very thin body condition from cancer cachexia. She was being hand feed at home and was very cooperative. During her stay, she was her nervous happy and attentive self, but she exhibited profound muscle quivering. At 2:15 PM, Murphy exhibited neurologic signs and a mild seizure as we held her in the author's arms. Following a 20 mg injection of diazepam, she recovered within minutes and remained very relaxed. During a consultation with the family, it was decided that Murphy's Pawspice would transition to the hospice phase and that she would need house calls and home care from the author's nursing staff. The author dispensed injectable diazepam for intranasal use to control any further seizures.

It was easy to be in touch with the Johnsons via text messaging and phone calls during Murphy's month-long hospice. The family reported that Murphy was in a good mood, still played with her ball, would still walk up and down the stairs, sleep on the couch and that she seemed happy despite continued weight loss with a body score of 2/9 from cancer cachexia. We discussed the HHHHHMM (Hurt, Hunger, Hydration, Hygiene, Happiness, Mobility, More good days than bad days) Quality of Life Scale criterion and her daily score. The Johnsons were in agreement to provide Murphy with the gift of euthanasia when she needed it. This part of the hospice vigil is the most difficult time, because patients are very much alive showing spirited pleasure responses from being petted and talked to despite their physical deterioration and weakness.[5] Murphy's Pawspice nurses, Lena and Melissa, made regular home visits to monitor her vital signs, examine her for distress, administer SQ fluids with vitamins, collect blood samples for evaluation, and monitor her decline. During her 1-month hospice, Murphy's serum urea nitrogen (BUN) went from 80 up to 117, creatinine from 1.8 to 2, alanine aminotransferase (ALT) from 429 down to 181, and ALP from off range down to 2400 as per the VETSCAN readings. Her serum Ca^{++} went from 13.5 to 13 using Miacalcin (calcitonin–salmon) at 48 mg given SQ SID to control malignant hypercalcemia. Everyone involved was satisfied with Murphy's last days under the circumstances.

Preneed discussions regarding euthanasia and after life care were about being prepared to accept plan A, B or C. Plan A would be for me to go to the house, along with one of Murphy's caring Pawspice nurses, and help Murphy peacefully change worlds. Plan B would be for a house call doctor to come to their home. Plan C would be to heavily sedate Murphy with SQ nalbuphine (an injectable pain medication) and diazepam (previously sent for seizure control) and bring her to the hospital for euthanasia. All 3 plans included private cremation and return of her cremains for safe keeping.[6]

How did the final moments go for Murphy? Was plan ABC successful? The Johnsons made their final call early Sunday morning on October 10, 2010. Since I was out of the state at a meeting, I called my colleague, Dr Ben Rosnik, and he was at the Johnson home within the hour and kindly assisted Murphy with a peaceful and painless passing.

REFERENCES

1. Temel JS. Early palliative care for patients with metastatic nonsmall cell lung cancer. N Engl J Med 2010;363:733–42.
2. Villalobos A, Kaplan L. Canine and feline geriatric oncology: honoring the human–animal bond. Ames (IA): Blackwell Publishing; 2007.
3. Villalobos A. Oncology outlook, sensible supplements. Irvine (CA): VPN; 2004.
4. Kaplan L. Help your dog fight cancer. Briarcliff (NY): Jangen Press; 2008.
5. Kaplan L. So easy to love, so hard to lose. Briarcliff (NY): Jangen Press; 2010.
6. Villalobos A. The bond and beyond, cremains create moments of emotion. Irvine (CA): VPN; 2008.

A Case Report: Caring for a Golden Retriever with Nasal Cancer

Tamara S. Shearer, DVM, CCRP[a,b,*]

KEYWORDS

• Cancer • Surgery • Chinese medicine • Protocols • Euthanasia
• Quality of life

When working with hospice and palliative care patients, I always follow the 5-step strategy for comprehensive palliative and hospice care protocol.[1] I developed it years ago to help me organize my examinations, consultations, and conversations with my clients. I found that the protocol is flexible and allows for care on a case-by-case basis.

Dolly was a happy, 14-year-old, spayed golden retriever when she was referred to us for palliative and hospice care. She had been diagnosed with a nasal tumor, and the biopsy performed by her referring veterinarian showed squamous cell carcinoma. As with many nasal tumors, it was unknown when the growth actually started. The surgery performed to retrieve the biopsy over the rostrum of her nose and frontal sinus developed into a nonhealing wound. Her owner was having trouble caring for the wound before seeking our help.

During the visits we proceeded to discuss end-of-life planning by applying the 5-step strategy for comprehensive palliative and hospice care. The initial visit began with step 1 of the care protocol: evaluating Dolly's owner's needs and beliefs. By using the psychosocial concerns assessment table, the following information was gathered (see Box 3 in Pet Hospice and Palliative Care Protocols by Tamara S. Shearer elsewhere in this issue). Dolly had been relatively healthy all of her life, and luckily there were not many physical or emotional barriers that would interfere with her. Dolly's owner wanted to do as much as possible to preserve Dolly's quality of life. She did not want Dolly to suffer. It was okay to track any illness with testing for an increased chance of improving quality of life. Dolly was prone to being a little nervous, especially when away from her owner, so spending time hospitalized was not an option. This would also have been stressful for Dolly's owner. There was interest in palliative care services but not in seeing a medical specialist, such as an oncologist. The owner

The author has nothing to disclose.

[a] Shearer Pet Health Hospital, 1054 Haywood Road, Sylva, NC 28779, USA
[b] Pet Hospice and Education Center, 16111 State Route, 37 Sunbury, OH 43074, USA
* 1054 Haywood Road, Sylva, NC 28779.
E-mail address: tshearer5@frontier.com

was open to alternative medicine options if they helped improve Dolly's quality of life. Dolly's owner's mother was available to help care for Dolly and bring her to appointments when her owner was working. There were no financial barriers to Dolly's health care choices. Her owner's belief regarding death included euthanasia as a last resort if quality of life could not be maintained. Like a lot of pet owners, she had worries about Dolly's quality of life and how to recognize if she was suffering. Her hope was that Dolly would die at home in her sleep before any suffering could manifest itself or that she be present if Dolly had to be euthanized due to a lack of response to the comfort care. She would choose cremation as a means to care for her remains.

At the initial visit, additional support through the aid of a social worker or clergy member was not suggested because Dolly's owner was using her family, personal and professional friends, and our support staff to cope with the changes in her life. She seemed to be coping well with Dolly's disease.

At my office, we try to keep our consultation rooms as comfortable as possible to minimize stress, so the examination rooms look more like comfort rooms. The office follows the feng shui design concept and we also use dog appeasing pheromone diffusers and music to minimize stress. In addition, we provided Dolly with a soft blanket so she could lie comfortably on the floor.

Dolly was happy and had a good appetite. She still enjoyed participating in her regular activities. She was bright and alert but a little nervous during her visits. Dolly's physical examination showed only normal aging changes, such as bilateral lenticular sclerosis. She had a body condition score of 3+ out of 5, it was measured by palpating over her ribs and observing her waste. Her primary problem was a nonhealing incision from the biopsy site that was infected and necrotic. The wound had a putrid odor and was draining a mucopurulent discharge. The site was deformed. The area of the lesion was quite painful to the touch, especially in the most ventral area of the wound. Dolly would jerk her head away when attempts at cleaning the wound were necessary. Even minimal restraint to steady Dolly heightened her anxiety. Her pain score was 2 to 3, using the simple descriptive scale, when the more rostral area of the wound was touched; otherwise, Dolly seemed comfortable.[2]

Step 2 in the palliative and hospice care protocol is education about the disease process. Before discussing details about squamous cell carcinoma, we discussed details on how to assess quality of life (see the article by Robin Downing elsewhere in this issue on how to recognize pain). When I teach pet owners about quality of life, I use several methods, including how to recognize pain. I also use Dr Villalobos' HHHHHMM quality-of-life evaluation, and I discuss in detail each parameter of the scale, putting emphasis on happiness (see the article by Alice E. Villalobos elsewhere in this issue for further exploration of this topic). We discussed what options were available to palliate Dolly's cancer because the prognosis of her cancer was guarded with most interventions. These details included palliative radiation therapy, chemotherapy, immunonutrition, and traditional Chinese medicine. I also shared how to manage the bad side effects of the disease, which included pain, bleeding from the tumor site, and other side effects associated with the close proximity to the affected area.

Next, I began step 3 of the strategy for comprehensive palliative and hospice care, which included designing a personalized plan for Dolly and her owner, taking into account her psychosocial concerns in step 1. Dolly was taking firocoxib when she presented to our office. We added gabapentin and tramadol to her protocol. We talked about changing to a stronger opioid, oxycodone, in the future if needed for pain. Her owner was open to seeking alternative forms of care, so a consultation was submitted to Dr Xie's staff at Jing-tang Herbal, Reddick, Florida. She was placed on

Wei Qi Booster and Stasis Breaker (Dr Xie's Jing-tang). Yunnan Bai Yao was also prescribed for future bleeding events.[3] We also used a therapy laser over the incision to help manage pain and promote healing. We delivered to the area 4 J/cm^2 using a 660 wavelength. Masitinib, a protein kinase inhibitor, was also prescribed for compassionate use in hopes of slowing the progression of the tumor.

In step 4, I gave Dolly's owner written instructions about how to administer and monitor the medications and showed her how we cleaned the wound. Despite her owner medicating Dolly 1 to 2 hours before wound hygiene with gabapentin, tramadol, and firocoxib, Dolly still resisted the cleaning. Even our attempts of trying to manage the wound with the addition of a lidocaine splash were futile. Ultimately, it was determined that an intervention through palliative surgery to debulk and débride the wound would make it easier to care for the wound. This would also reduce some of the pressure from the discharge that was accumulating under the skin's surface. The surgical goal was to make wound care easier and improve quality of life for Dolly and her owner. Surgery was not meant to slow the progression of disease; however, we were hopeful that maybe some of the Chinese herbs and the masitinib might contribute in slowing the growth of the tumor.

Using a surgical laser, the area of the lesion was debulked. Hemostasis during this intervention was good. Large amounts of tumor, necrotic tissue, and foul-smelling discharge were removed from the wound. There was excess tension across the incision and the tissue was not healthy so we did a creative closure using a nonabsorbable suture that was threaded in shoestring-like style through 6 small plastic washers, which were sutured next to the incision so the wound could be easily reopened, débrided, and cleaned. (Dolly's owner thought the lacing system was "really cool.") At the top of the incision, we placed a soaker catheter for the administration of local anesthesia in hopes that future interventions could be done with local anesthesia only. Unfortunately, our soaker catheter worked its way out so we had the owner to administer a lidocaine splash over the incision area and inject lidocaine into the opening left behind by the catheter.

The first surgical intervention improved Dolly's quality of life and made it easier for her owner to care for her. We saw Dolly twice a week for rechecks and cleaned the wound using our modified system by unlacing the suture, wiping out debris, then relacing the site. After 10 days we removed the plastic washers that secured the suture and allowed the incision to granulate in.

Approximately 1 month later, a second anesthesia to facilitate a thorough cleaning of the wound and a touch-up debulking resulted in massive hemorrhage. The bleeding was managed by applying pressure with a gauze sponge and QuikClot (www.z-medica.com, Wallingford, CT, USA) in her incision. The wound was closed and packed with 0.5-inch gauze. The gauze would be removed during the next cleaning scheduled a few days later. Dolly's pain had increased to a 3 to 4, using the canine simple descriptive pain scale, so we changed her to oxycodone (2.5 mg 2 to 3 times daily). We also represcribed Yunnan Bai Yao for bleeding.

Two weeks later, a final wound hygiene session was conducted because of a decline in Dolly's comfort and changes in her activities of daily living. She now had a pain score of 4. Dolly was in pain and was placed on a morphine, lidocaine, and ketamine continuous rate infusion drip before, during, and after her hygiene procedure for the day. We could tell the cancer was increasing in its spread. Dolly was to return 2 days later for a recheck.

We were unable to manage the side effects of Dolly's cancer comfortably. She had a decrease in her appetite and activities to the point that it was an indicator that Dolly was not happy. Physically, there was also a decline because her mentation had changed and she walked slowly because of profound weakness. Her cancer site had also become larger in the past days. Her owner recognized the dramatic decline in quality of life and made an educated decision, based on a review of Dolly's condition and symptoms, that she needed to choose the option that we saved for the last resort: euthanasia. Dolly was euthanized 2 days after her last visit with us at our office. She was accompanied by her owner and support system of friends. I shared with Dolly's owner and friends what they might see during her dying process. Dolly was premedicated with an anesthetic dose of dexmedetomidine, then with a 23-gauge butterfly catheter the euthanasia solution was administered intravenously. She passed peacefully.

In Step 5, as part of the bereavement process, we sent a sympathy card. We were able to check in with Dolly's owner on a regular basis when she adopted a new puppy, named Gus. Dolly's owner misses her greatly but describes Dolly's last months as being more comfortable because of entering into a hospice care plan.

REFERENCES

1. Shearer T. Hospice and palliative care. In: Gaynor J, Muir W, editors. Handbook of veterinary pain management. St Louis (MO): Mosby; 2010. p. 588–600.
2. Mich P, Hellyer P. Objective, categoric methods for assessing pain and analgesia. In: Gaynor J, Muir W, editors. Handbook of veterinary pain management. St Louis (MO): Mosby; 2010. p. 87.
3. Wynn S, Marsen S. Manual of natural veterinary medicine. St Louis (MO): Mosby; 2003. p. 286.

Index

Note: Page numbers of article titles are in **boldface** type.

Vet Clin Small Anim 41 (2011) 693–702
doi:10.1016/S0195-5616(11)00077-5
0195-5616/11/$ – see front matter © 2011 Elsevier Inc. All rights reserved.

vetsmall.theclinics.com

Printed and bound by CPI Group (UK) Ltd, Croydon, CR0 4YY

03/10/2024

01040443-0004